PENICILLIN and OTHER ANTIBIOTIC AGENTS

By

WALLACE E. HERRELL, M.D., M.S., F.A.C.P.

Assistant Professor of Medicine, the Mayo Foundation,
University of Minnesota; Consultant in Medicine, Mayo Clinic,
Rochester, Minnesota

ILLUSTRATED

W. B. SAUNDERS COMPANY

PHILADELPHIA AND LONDON

1945

MADE IN U.S.A.

PRESS OF
W. B. SAUNDERS COMPANY
PHILADELPHIA

TO

DR. DAVID MAYO BERKMAN

*a physician who has retained the enthusiasm of youth
while acquiring the wisdom of experience*

PREFACE

Nearly four years have elapsed since the first report on the clinical use of penicillin was made by the Oxford investigators. Also, nearly four years have passed since my colleagues and I progressed from studies on gramicidin to studies on penicillin. Accordingly, at the request of others, I have tried to bring together in a monograph the fundamental experimental and clinical studies which have been carried out on penicillin and other antibiotic agents. On the subjects of chemistry and production methods of penicillin, this book contains only information which previously has appeared in print. In general, when writing in my own person, I have attempted to make the formal bacteriologic terms which I have used conform with those of "Bergey's Manual of Determinative Bacteriology." On the other hand, many of the original investigators to whose work reference is made in the book did not use these terms and usually, in such instances, I have retained the terms which the investigators employed. It is hoped that this small book will serve as an easily accessible starting point for students of chemotherapy who are interested in the further development and the possible clinical uses of these agents. Obviously, much experimental and clinical investigation on the use of antibiotic substances remains to be done.

It is unnecessary to point out that the modern medical investigator and author is not a lone worker. Many, whose interests were wider than mine, contributed to my efforts. For instance, after it became necessary for government agencies to assume control of the distribution of penicillin, part of the penicillin used at the Mayo Clinic was provided by the Office of Scientific Research and Development, from supplies assigned by the Committee on Medical Research for experimental investigations recommended by the Committee on Chemotherapeutic and Other Agents, of the National Research Council. In the course of the early clinical work with penicillin, the scientific and production staffs of the Abbott Laboratories and of the Winthrop Chemical Company gave invaluable help. The same is true, with reference to the early clinical work with gramicidin, of the staff of Sharp and Dohme, Incorporated.

Moreover, my own work which is recorded in this volume could not have been accomplished without the invaluable assistance of my colleagues. I wish here, therefore, to acknowledge my debt to Dr. Dorothy Heilman, whose collaboration made possible the early studies on antibiotic substances. To Dr. F. R. Heilman I am also profoundly indebted

v

for his help and scientific advice. The members of the clinical section of which I am a member, namely, Drs. D. M. Berkman, D. M. Masson and D. R. Nichols, cheerfully bore part of my practitioner's burden so that I might have time for investigation and for preparation of this book. These colleagues and others also referred to me the patients who formed the basis of my clinical investigations of the years just past. To all of these associates I am sincerely grateful.

With reference to particular portions of this text, I acknowledge with great appreciation the help I received from Lieutenant Colonel Philip S. Hench, Major Edward W. Boland and Colonel Walter Bauer, who were so good as to read critically the section on gonorrheal arthritis. To Dr. Paul A. O'Leary I am indebted for his helpful suggestions with reference to the chapter on syphilis and other spirochetal infections. Dr. F. R. Heilman, whom I have mentioned before, gave particular attention to that part of the text which deals with the activity of penicillin in vitro and in vivo. To Dr. Dorothy Heilman, also referred to earlier, I am indebted for help in connection with the chapter which deals with tyrothricin.

To the members of the Photographic Department, especially Mrs. Daisy G. Shadduck and Messrs. S. J. McComb, H. H. Skoug and L. A. Coffey, I wish to express my thanks for preparation of the photographs which are used as illustrations in this volume. For invaluable assistance I am also indebted to Miss Alice Anderson of the Art Studio and to the personnel of the Laboratory of Chemistry, particularly Miss Elizabeth Waldron. I wish to acknowledge also the help of members of the staff of the Library, especially Miss Violet Vihstadt.

Those of the Division of Publications whom I would like to mention individually are Mrs. Margaret Riley, who did the work of final preparation of the manuscript for the publisher; the Misses Elizabeth Skafte, Margaret Clark and Florence Schmidt, who read the proof, and Dr. Richard M. Hewitt, head of the division, who gave of his experience in the mechanics of preliminary, detailed outlining of the book and who edited the manuscript. If the reader finds the book orderly, much credit for this I accord my colleague and friend, Doctor Hewitt. Finally, it is most difficult for me to express my profound appreciation for the almost incalculable help and the untiring efforts of my secretary, Miss Charlotte Palen, who has given unselfishly of her time and effort in preparation of this volume.

WALLACE E. HERRELL

ROCHESTER, MINNESOTA
April, 1945

CONTENTS

PART I

HISTORY, PREPARATION, PHYSICAL AND CHEMICAL PROPERTIES, ANTIBACTERIAL ACTIVITY, ABSORPTION AND DISTRIBUTION, EXCRETION AND METHODS OF TESTING PENICILLIN

CHAPTER I

CHAPTER II

CHAPTER III

CHAPTER IV

CHAPTER V

CHAPTER VI

CHAPTER VII

PART II

CLINICAL USE OF PENICILLIN: PREPARATIONS, SYNERGISM, ADMINISTRATION AND EFFECTIVENESS AGAINST DISEASES OF CERTAIN SYSTEMS

CHAPTER VIII

CHAPTER IX

CHAPTER X

CHAPTER XI

CHAPTER XII

PART III

CLINICAL USE OF PENICILLIN (Continued): EFFECTIVENESS AGAINST VARIOUS DISEASES AND CONSIDERATIONS OF TOXICITY

PART I

HISTORY, PREPARATION, PHYSICAL AND CHEMICAL PROPERTIES, ANTIBACTERIAL ACTIVITY, ABSORPTION AND DISTRIBUTION, EXCRETION AND METHODS OF TESTING PENICILLIN

CHAPTER I

THE HISTORICAL ASPECTS OF THE DEVELOPMENT OF PENICILLIN

EVENTS PRECEDING FLEMING'S DISCOVERY

As long ago as 1877, Pasteur and Joubert[1] were aware that certain airborne organisms inhibited the growth of the anthrax bacillus and they even suggested that this phenomenon of antibiosis might be of use in the treatment of certain infections. This observation was based on the fact that the growth of certain bacteria could be stopped or prevented by the concomitant growth of another; at least this was true in the test tube. It is now evident that this inhibition of growth produced by certain micro-organisms is due to the elaboration by the antagonistic microbe of certain products which have definite chemical and biologic properties. Here, therefore, is the origin of what have recently been named "antibiotics." It was pointed out by Florey[2] that, while Pasteur recognized the phenomenon and the fact that this phenomenon might be of use therapeutically, the first serious attempt to apply an antibiotic for the purpose of treatment was made by Emmerich and Loew[3] in 1899. These observers suggested that the products of Bacillus pyocyaneus (Pseudomonas aeruginosa) could be used for treating anthrax and diphtheria; however, pyocyanase, which later was found to be a mixture of more than one substance elaborated by the organism named, never has proved of important clinical value. It seems proper, however, to point out that Pasteur and his colleagues rightfully must be considered the parents of modern chemotherapy.

Alexander Fleming[4] of St. Mary's Hospital, London, in describing the discovery of penicillin, emphasized the fact that as a pupil of Almroth Wright he had been deeply interested during his whole career in the

1

destruction of bacteria by leukocytes. During the war of 1914–1918, Fleming spent much time investigating problems in connection with septic wounds. He was impressed with the antibacterial power of leukocytes contained in pus from these wounds. Fleming's interest continued along these lines and he pointed out that if the antileukocytic action of an antiseptic agent was greater than its antibacterial action, such an agent was unlikely to be of value in the treatment of infected lesions. In 1922, Fleming[5] described lysozyme, a rather potent antibacterial ferment which engaged the attention of many investigators for a time following the appearance of his report. These and other investigations were, therefore, the forerunners of intensive studies to follow and these studies resulted in the discovery not only of penicillin but of other antibiotics. The discoveries were consistent with the theory of bacterial antagonism, which had been known since the early days of bacteriology. In 1924, Gratia and Dath[6] described the production of another antibacterial substance, actinomycetin, which appeared to be elaborated by certain strains of Actinomyces. Four years later (September, 1928) Fleming was working on the variation of staphylococcal colonies when probably the world's most remarkable contamination of a bacterial culture occurred.

FLEMING'S DISCOVERY

It is now well known by students of chemotherapy that Fleming reported the discovery of penicillin in 1929,[7] although the actual observation was made in 1928. Fifteen years after the famous contamination occurred, Fleming was asked how he came to discover penicillin. He stated, "It is very difficult to say just what processes of thought were involved." However, according to the report which appeared in the "British Journal of Experimental Pathology," the observation was essentially as follows: Fleming stated that while he was working with staphylococcal variants, a number of culture plates had been set aside on the laboratory bench and had been examined from time to time. In examination of these plates, Fleming naturally had to lift the lids from time to time. This resulted in exposure to air and, therefore, in contamination of the plates by various micro-organisms. All of the foregoing acts and occurrences are common in routine bacteriologic work. The important thing is that Fleming made the acute observation that around a large colony of a contaminating mold the staphylococcal colonies had become transparent and were undergoing lysis. A photograph of this plate is shown in figure 1. This observation having been made, Fleming then preserved the mold and cultivated it in flasks in liquid broth. Here, then, began the steps to obtain the most remarkable therapeutic agent yet known for the treatment of certain types of bacterial infections. Fleming's first act in preserving the mold had been to transfer with a platinum wire some spores from the colony of mold to a culture tube of Sabouraud's medium. It is well known that practically all the penicillin for clinical use prepared in England and in America through 1943 was derived from subcultures of this original tube.

Fleming was aware that the mold belonged to the genus Penicillium and he, therefore, named the derived antibacterial substance "penicillin." Fleming was of the opinion that the mold resembled Penicillium rubrum; however, some time later the mold was identified as Penicillium notatum, a species which, according to Fleming, had been found by Westling in decaying hyssop in Norway. The identification of this mold is accredited

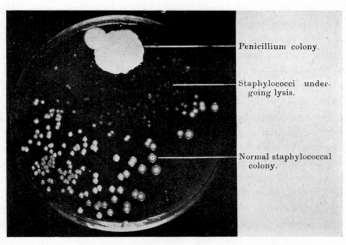

Penicillium colony.

Staphylococci under-
going lysis.

Normal staphylococcal
colony.

Fig. 1.—A culture-plate showing the dissolution of staphylococcal colonies in the neighborhood of a colony of penicillium. (From article by Fleming, British Journal of Experimental Pathology, June, 1929.)

to Charles Thom, the principal mycologist in the U. S. Department of Agriculture. On the request of Clutterbuck and his colleagues of the University of London, Thom carried out studies to identify the mold and reported that it was not Penicillium rubrum but probably Penicillium notatum Westling in the P. chrysogenum Thom series. Thom's report, published by Clutterbuck and others,[8] is of some historical interest: "I have cultivated Fleming's organism under several different conditions and cannot agree with the nomenclature as P. rubrum either in the sense of my 1910 paper or in the sense of Biourge's monograph. In fact, I believe this culture, although showing some divergencies in culture reactions, to be closer to P. notatum of p. 264 in my book than to the groups discovered on pp. 249–50 as indicated by the nomenclature used."

It was evident from Fleming's work with the broth filtrate that penicillin possessed rather remarkable selective antibacterial properties. It produced inhibition of growth of a variety of gram-positive pathogens but was relatively ineffective against certain gram-negative organisms, including Escherichia coli and Bacillus influenzae (Haemophilus influenzae). Fleming made use of this observation to eliminate from cultures of Bacillus influenzae the contaminating gram-positive organisms such as staphylococci. During the years that followed, penicillin (broth filtrates, not purified penicillin) was employed by Fleming in his laboratory in connection with differential culture work. Fleming further made important observations on penicillin to show that it was relatively nontoxic for animals or cellular elements, including leukocytes. He also irrigated human conjunctiva and large infected surfaces and reported that there was no evidence of irritation or toxicity following use of the broth filtrate in this fashion. While Fleming's studies were not clinical, the prize of priority for the use of the material on human subjects must be awarded to him.

Clutterbuck, Lovell, and Raistrick,[8] in 1932, found that the mold could be grown on synthetic media although they were unsuccessful in extracting the penicillin from the liquid in a stable form. Most of the penicillin activity was lost during the process of evaporating the ether into which the penicillin had passed during their attempts at extraction.

In 1935, an American investigator, Reid,[9] and in 1940, another American investigator, Bornstein,[10] published reports on the antibacterial activity of broth filtrates containing penicillin. That is where the matter of penicillin and its possible usefulness rested until the discovery of its chemotherapeutic properties by the able group of investigators[11] under the leadership of Howard W. Florey, at the Sir William Dunn School of Pathology, Oxford, England in 1940.

THE OXFORD INVESTIGATORS' CONTRIBUTION TO THE DEVELOPMENT OF PENICILLIN

According to Florey,[2] he and his colleagues had been interested in antibiotics since 1929 when they began studies on lysozyme which, as I have already mentioned, was discovered by Fleming in 1922. This work on lysozyme continued at Oxford but was not pursued after it became evident that the substance behaved like an enzyme (see Part IV on other antibiotic agents, p. 327) and since the substance was not very effective against micro-organisms which produce disease. In 1938, Chain and Florey decided to make an intensive survey of naturally produced antibacterial substances from a chemical and biologic standpoint. Among the first antibiotics to be examined by Chain and Florey were the products of Pseudomonas aeruginosa and then by good fortune, in 1939, they decided to examine penicillin in spite of the fact that it was said to be very unstable. In the meantime some work by Dubos[12] (1939), which will be described in its proper place, stimulated renewed interest in the study of antibacterial agents of biologic origin. According to Florey, the observations of Fleming and of Clutterbuck and others, that the substance could be maintained in the original medium for some weeks, led the Oxford investigators to believe that penicillin would not be too unstable to work with.

In August, 1940, the results of the co-operative study on penicillin by the investigators at the Sir William Dunn School of Pathology at Oxford were reported in "Lancet."[11] This work has been extended through the close collaboration of a large number of scientists. In addition to Florey and Chain, there were E. P. Abraham, A. D. Gardner, N. G. Heatley, M. A. Jennings, J. Orr-Ewing, A. G. Sanders, C. M. Fletcher and Mary Florey, along with a number of surgeons and physicians. Florey also has acknowledged the work of technical assistants including J. Kent, D. Callow, G. Glister and, as Florey puts it, his "penicillin girls." The 1940 report by the Oxford investigators included details of their methods of purification of penicillin, their studies on the bacteriostatic properties of penicillin in vitro and also its chemotherapeutic action in animals. The fairly purified penicillin used by these investigators was the sodium salt. The magnitude of the investigation undertaken and accomplished by the Oxford investigators becomes increasingly striking when it is realized that their work was accomplished under the stringencies imposed by the war in which the British were involved at that time. One of the great difficulties encountered during the early days of their work, in addition to the rather labile nature of the substance with which they worked, was the problem of producing enough of the material. For example, nearly 100 liters of the mold brew were required to obtain enough penicillin with which to treat one patient for one day. The mold was first grown in flasks and later, as Florey pointed out, when more material was required, it was grown in large vessels. Because of the inactivation of penicillin by heavy metals, the investigators actually employed bed pans in which to grow cultures of Penicillium notatum.

One year later, in 1941, this same group[13] of investigators reported on the preparation of a fairly purified product of penicillin and included the first reports on the possible clinical value of the material. After they had completed their experiments in vitro and on animals, which enabled them to predict that the material could be used for treatment of man, and after months of labor, they obtained enough of the material to give a small injection to a human being. Florey stated that much to their consternation the patient started shivering and the temperature rose. Fortunately, this reaction was then found to be due not to penicillin but to certain impurities which produce pyrogenic reactions and which could be removed by chemical methods. The precious penicillin was recovered from the urine of one of these early patients in a fairly purified state. In other words, passage through the human filter turned out to be part of the early process of purification. Case 1 in the 1941 report from Oxford was that of a policeman who was suffering with a severe pyogenic infection due to Staphylococcus aureus and Streptococcus pyogenes. He was treated with penicillin, some of which had been recovered from urine. The story is told that one of the professors at Oxford University was heard to tell his students, "My fellows, you should learn about this penicillin, a remarkable substance. It is grown in bed pans and purified by passage through the Oxford police force."

FLOREY'S VISIT TO THE UNITED STATES

I have already mentioned the extreme difficulties under which the work at Oxford was done. It is obvious that the intensive bombing of England, together with the limited personnel, made almost impossible an attempt at large-scale production of penicillin in England. Florey's bed pans would hardly satisfy the requirements for wholesale production of penicillin. In the summer of 1941, through the sponsorship of the Rockefeller Foundation, Florey visited the United States. With him came one of his associates, N. G. Heatley, whose work on methods of assay of penicillin had proved invaluable in connection with the studies on antibacterial products under way at Oxford. Florey arrived in this country in July, 1941. He was anxious not only to stimulate interest in penicillin but also to secure help in the problems involved in its production on a large scale.

Florey and his colleague were soon referred to those individuals most interested in mycology. It is natural that they turned to Charles Thom, principal mycologist in the United States Department of Agriculture at Washington, D. C., whose work in connection with the identification of Penicillium notatum I have already mentioned. Florey also consulted with the Committee on Medical Research of the Office of Scientific Research and Development. He and his colleague were referred by Thom to the Northern Regional Research Laboratory, Department of Agriculture, in Peoria, Illinois. There, under the direction of Robert D. Coghill, was a group of microbiologists in the Fermentation Division who had had much experience with molds. There also was A. J. Moyer who was later to find that by adding corn steep liquor to the medium in which cultures of Penicillium grew, the yield of penicillin could be greatly increased. Heatley remained at Peoria for several months and contributed greatly to the early studies carried out there. Of especial importance was his help in connection with the method of assay for penicillin which he had devised at Oxford University.

Dubos, of the Rockefeller Institute, had informed Florey shortly after his arrival in America of our interest at the Mayo Clinic in studies on antibiotic agents, including our preliminary studies on penicillin. I was glad to receive word from Dubos saying that Florey was coming to visit our laboratories after his stay at Peoria. Dorothy Heilman and I had been working with penicillin since the early part of 1941. Florey expressed satisfaction with the studies we had under way. He also had Heatley supply us with approximately 100 mg. of penicillin. Half of this material had been prepared in the laboratories at Oxford and was called at that time Batch NH2 and contained 42 units of penicillin per milligram; the other half was from that small supply which had been recovered from the urine of one of the patients treated at Oxford and was called Batch NHU6 and contained 20 units per milligram. Heilman and I profoundly appreciate the interest and helpful suggestions given us by Florey in connection with our work on penicillin. I often think of his entirely respectful but humorous reference to the brilliant group at Peoria as the "mold merchants."

I had the pleasure of introducing Prof. Florey to the members of the staff of the Mayo Clinic at its weekly meeting on August 20, 1941. My colleagues and I were much impressed with his report, which was based on the material contained in his article which appeared in "Lancet" for August 16, 1941.[13] Florey described, in addition to the experimental studies, the clinical results obtained in ten cases at Oxford. These cases represented the first attempts to use penicillin systemically for treatment of man.

Florey then returned to Washington for further consultation with those connected with government agencies such as the United States Department of Agriculture and the Committee on Medical Research of the Office of Scientific Research and Development, which is a division of the Office for Emergency Management. Under the chairmanship of Dr. A. N. Richards of this committee, it appears that arrangements had been made for consultation with commercial houses interested in development of penicillin. Merck and Company, Inc., E. R. Squibb and Sons, Charles Pfizer and Company, Inc., Abbott Laboratories and Winthrop Chemical Company were pioneers in this country in the development of penicillin suitable for clinical use, and their accomplishments are a great tribute to that part of American industry which is engaged in the manufacture of pharmaceutical and biologic preparations. By this time, Florey had created remarkable enthusiasm among all of the investigators with whom he had communicated and now the studies on penicillin seemed certain to receive the intensive interest not only of independent investigators but also of government agencies and commercial producers of penicillin.

In the autumn, Florey returned to England to continue his studies with his colleagues at Oxford. He later carried the experiences of his group to the battle fronts in North Africa and Sicily and, later still, to our allies in Russia. Thereafter, together with Prof. Fleming, he was knighted by his Majesty, King George VI of England, a fitting reward for a monumental contribution to the problems of bacterial infection not only in the armed forces but also in the civilian population.

CONTRIBUTIONS OF AMERICAN INVESTIGATORS TO THE DEVELOPMENT OF PENICILLIN

I hope I have sufficiently emphasized the epochal character of the work of the British investigators in the development of penicillin. On the other hand, I would not be satisfied with my attempt to review the historical development of penicillin if I failed to correct the impression, which prevails to some degree, that scientists in this country were not intensely interested in penicillin before our government agencies, stimulated by Florey's visit, became actively engaged in sponsoring its development.

In 1935, Roger D. Reid, of Pennsylvania State College, whose work has been mentioned earlier in this chapter, reported in the "Journal of Bacteriology"[9] on the properties of a bacterial inhibiting substance produced by a mold. The mold was a strain of Penicillium and he was working with broth filtrates which contained penicillin. A 1:100 dilution of the filtrate was found to inhibit sensitive micro-organisms. In his studies on the broth filtrates containing penicillin he included observations on the effect of light, gases and temperature on the active substance. He also attempted to isolate the active substance by distillation at low temperatures.

Five years later, in 1940 (the same year in which the Oxford reports appeared) Bornstein,[10] whose work, also mentioned earlier, was carried out in the bacteriologic laboratories of Beth Israel Hospital, New York, reported on the antibacterial action of penicillin in broth cultures. The strain of Penicillium notatum which he used to produce penicillin was supplied by Fleming. Neither of these early American investigators was working with the purified substance but they made observations which were in agreement with the reports from Britain.

In May, 1941, at the meeting of the American Society for Clinical Investigation, the first American report[14] on studies of penicillin as a chemotherapeutic agent was made. According to this report, fairly active penicillin had been prepared at Columbia University in New York City. This report was the result of work carried out in the laboratories of

Martin H. Dawson and Karl Meyer. Collaborating in this report were Gladys L. Hobby and Eleanor Chaffee. It is proper, indeed, to recognize the significance of this work because it stimulated interested investigators to study penicillin further. Dawson, Meyer and their colleagues made brief mention of the use of penicillin against infections in human beings; however, data on its clinical use were not published at that time. Subsequent work by this group of investigators was most important in the development of penicillin in America.

Experimental studies on the antibacterial activity of penicillin were begun at the Mayo Clinic in the early part of 1941. Through the kindness of Dawson, we had received a transfer of Fleming's culture of the mold Penicillium notatum. My colleague, Dorothy H. Heilman, and I continued our studies on antibiotic agents at the Institute of Experimental Medicine. Without her help the early work on gramicidin and penicillin at the Mayo Clinic could not have been accomplished. I have already mentioned to what extent our studies had progressed by the time Florey visited our laboratories in August, 1941. In November, 1941, Heilman and I consulted with Florey's colleague, Heatley, and with Coghill and Moyer and their associates at the Northern Regional Research Laboratory in Peoria. The helpful suggestions we received from this group in connection with our early studies on penicillin are here acknowledged. Heatley discussed in detail with us the Oxford cup method for assay of penicillin, which he had devised. The results of the experimental observations made by Heilman and me on the antibacterial activity of penicillin were reported at the meeting of the Society of American Bacteriologists in Baltimore in December, 1941.[15] Subsequent to this time, Heilman and I were able to prepare and to obtain small quantities of penicillin for our investigations.

The work at the Mayo Clinic continued actively although the supplies of penicillin were exceedingly small. Our early clinical results, as was true also of those reported from Britain, were enough to inspire our continued investigation. As far as I know, the first published data on the systemic clinical use of more or less purified penicillin to appear in the American literature was the article published in December, 1942.[16] Simultaneously, there appeared another report[17] describing attempts to use penicillin clinically. The latter report dealt merely with the local irrigation of wounds with filtrates containing penicillin. It is understandable that results so dramatic as those seen following treatment with penicillin could not but stimulate intensive interest in this agent. When enough penicillin could be produced for further clinical trials, it was obvious that some mechanism for control of clinical investigation was necessary in order that complete information might be obtained and made available to the armed forces and to civilian physicians alike.

On January 17, 1942, a conference on antibiotic agents was called at the request of the Committee on Medical Research of the Office of Scientific Research and Development. It was my privilege to attend this conference in Washington. By this time, plans had been made for a more intensified study of penicillin, as well as of other antibotic agents, including gramicidin. Because the reports of this conference were classified as restricted, comments on the results of the conference are withheld. Suffice to say, however, it was already evident that the full weight of scientific and industrial ingenuity was to be imposed on the problem of penicillin and other agents which might be of value for the treatment of susceptible bacterial infections which could occur in the armed forces.

It became the charge of the Committee on Chemotherapeutic and Other Agents, a committee of the Division of Medical Sciences of the National Research Council, to supervise these studies. This committee was composed of Chester S. Keefer, Chairman, Massachusetts Memorial Hospitals, Boston; Francis G. Blake, Yale University School of Medicine, New Haven; John S. Lockwood, University of Pennsylvania School of Medicine, Philadelphia; E. K. Marshall, Jr., Johns Hopkins University School of Medicine, Baltimore; and W. Barry Wood, Jr., Washington University School of Medicine, St. Louis. In August, 1943, enough data had been collected by the Committee on Chemotherapeutic and Other Agents to justify the publication of a comprehensive report on the clinical use of penicillin in America.[18] This report was published by Chester S. Keefer and the other members of his committee. The results clearly confirmed and extended the experience obtained and previously reported by the Oxford investigators[13] and by my colleagues and me[16, 19] on the systemic use of penicillin. This report by Keefer and others did much to crystallize ideas on the clinical value of penicillin and made available to the armed forces and to civilians alike the necessary information for the successful and intelligent use of penicillin. The report was made possible only by the efforts of a group of American investigators working in a number of medical centers. Their contributions are of such importance that their names should be listed individually. The list of accredited investigators who served the Committee on Chemotherapeutic and Other Agents is as follows: W. A. Altemeier, University of Cincinnati; A. L. Bloomfield, Stanford University; Martin H. Dawson, Columbia University, New York; Robert Elman, Washington University School of Medicine, St. Louis; John Hirschfield, Wayne University College of Medicine, Detroit; Frank L. Horsfall, Jr., Rockefeller Institute, New York; Adolph Hutter, Bethesda, Maryland; Champ Lyons, Massachusetts General Hospital, Boston; J. F. Mahoney, U. S. Public Health Service, Staten Island; Roy D. McClure, Henry Ford Hospital, Detroit; C. F. McKhann, University of Michigan, Ann Arbor; Frank L. Meleney, Columbia University, New York; R. A. Nelson, Johns Hopkins Hospital, Baltimore; E. A. Park, Johns Hopkins Hospital, Baltimore; D. W. Richards, Jr., Columbia University, New York; Major George Robb, Washington, D. C.; David T. Smith, Duke University, Durham; Wesley W. Spink, University of Minnesota, Minneapolis; W. S. Tillett, New York University College of Medicine, New York.

A host of other American investigators were actively engaged in fundamental researches on penicillin which, although experimental, had much to do with its successful clinical application.

REFERENCES

1. Pasteur and Joubert: Quoted by Chain, E. and Florey, H. W.: The discovery of the chemotherapeutic properties of penicillin. Brit. M. Bull. 2:5-7 (No. 1) 1944.

2. Florey, H. W.: Penicillin: its development for medical uses. Nature. 153:40-42 (Jan. 8) 1944.

3. Emmerich and Loew: Quoted by Florey, H. W.[2]

4. Fleming, Alexander: The discovery of penicillin. Brit. M. Bull. 2:4-5 (No. 1) 1944.

5. Fleming, Alexander: On a remarkable bacteriolytic element found in tissues and secretions. Proc. Roy. Soc. London. 93:306-317 (May 1) 1922.

6. Gratia and Dath: Quoted by Chain, E. and Florey, H. W.: Penicillin. Endeavour. vol. 3, no. 9 (Jan.) 1944.

7. Fleming, Alexander: On the antibacterial action of cultures of a penicillium, with special reference to their use in the isolation of B. influenzae. Brit. J. Exper. Path. 10:226-236 (June) 1929.

8. Clutterbuck, P. W., Lovell, Reginald and Raistrick, Harold: Studies in the biochemistry of micro-organisms. XXVI. The formation from glucose by members of the Penicillium chrysogenum series of a pigment, an alkali-soluble protein and penicillin—the antibacterial substance of Fleming. Biochem. J. 26:1907-1918, 1932.

9. Reid, R. D.: Some properties of a bacterial-inhibitory substance produced by a mold. J. Bact. 29:215-221 (Feb.) 1935.

10. Bornstein, Siegbert: Action of penicillin on enterococci and other streptococci. J. Bact. 39:383-387 (Apr) 1940.

11. Chain, E., Florey, H. W., Gardner, A. D., Heatley, N. G., Jennings, M. A., Orr-Ewing, J. and Sanders, A. G.: Penicillin as a chemotherapeutic agent. Lancet. 2:226-228 (Aug. 24) 1940.

12. Dubos, R. J.: Studies on a bactericidal agent extracted from a soil bacillus. I. Preparation of the agent. Its activity in vitro. J. Exper. Med. 70:1-10 (July) 1939.

13. Abraham, E. P., Chain, E., Fletcher, C. M., Gardner, A. D., Heatley, N. G., Jennings, M. A. and Florey, H. W.: Further observations on penicillin. Lancet. 2:177-188; 189 (Aug. 16) 1941.

14. Dawson, M. H., Hobby, Gladys L., Meyer, Karl and Chaffee, Eleanor: Penicillin as a chemotherapeutic agent. (Society Report) J. Clin. Investigation. 20:434 (July) 1941.

15. Heilman, Dorothy H. and Herrell, W. E.: Comparative antibacterial activity of penicillin and gramicidin: tissue culture studies. Proc. Staff Meet., Mayo Clin. 17:321-327 (May 27) 1942. (Abstr.) Comparative bacteriostatic activity of penicillin and gramicidin. J. Bact. 43:12-13 (Jan.) 1942.

16. Herrell, W. E., Heilman, Dorothy H. and Williams, H. L.: The clinical use of penicillin. Proc. Staff Meet., Mayo Clin. 17:609-616 (Dec. 30) 1942.

17. Bordley, J. E., Crowe, S. J., Dolowitz, D. A. and Pickrell, K. L.: The local use of sulfonamides, gramicidin (tyrothricin) and penicillin in otolaryngology. Ann. Otol., Rhin. & Laryng. *51*:936–944 (Dec.) 1942.

18. Keefer, C. S., Blake, F. G., Marshall, E. K., Jr., Lockwood, J. S. and Wood, W. B., Jr.: Penicillin in the treatment of infections; a report of 500 cases. J. A. M. A. *122*:1217–1224 (Aug. 28) 1943.

19. Herrell, W. E.: Further observations on the clinical use of penicillin. Proc. Staff Meet., Mayo Clin. *18*:65–76 (Mar. 10) 1943.

CHAPTER II

METHODS OF PREPARING PENICILLIN

In general, three methods have been employed for the production of penicillin. They are the surface culture, submerged culture and bran culture methods. While Penicillium notatum is the species of mold most commonly used in the production of penicillin, it is now well established that other molds elaborate the material. Coghill[1] has pointed out that when large numbers of cultures are examined, there exists a continuous, graded series of strains capable of producing penicillin, ranging between and including typical Penicillium notatum and Penicillium chrysogenum. According to Coghill, one of the best producers of penicillin is Penicillium chrysogenum. Penicillium notatum NRRL 1249.B21 is the strain most commonly used for the production of penicillin by the surface culture method. This stems directly from Fleming's original strain. For the production of penicillin in submerged cultures, which will be mentioned subsequently, the strain commonly used is Penicillium notatum NRRL 832. This organism was found in the culture collection at the Northern Regional Research Laboratory at Peoria, Illinois. Both of these strains can be obtained from the American Type Culture Collection, Washington, D. C.

THE MEDIA

It is natural that many different media have been employed in which to grow penicillin, always with the idea of seeking the conditions which are most favorable for its growth and which, at the same time, will result in increasing yields of penicillin. In his early production of penicillin, Fleming[2,3] was of the opinion that a trypsin digest broth was the best medium in which to grow the mold. It was later found by Abraham and his colleagues[4] that Clutterbuck, Lovell and Raistrick's[5] modification of synthetic Czapek-Dox medium was more satisfactory. The medium contains the following ingredients:

Sodium nitrate ($NaNO_3$)	3.00 gm.
Potassium acid phosphate (KH_2PO_4)	1.00
Potassium chloride (KCl)	0.50
Magnesium sulfate ($MgSO_4.7H_2O$)	0.50
Ferrous sulfate ($FeSO_4.7H_2O$)	0.01
Glucose	40.00
Distilled water, q.s.	1,000 c.c.

13

Different investigators have modified this medium to some degree. For example, McKee and Rake[6] suggested that brown sugar be substituted for glucose; in other words, 40 gm. of brown sugar was employed. Subsequently, Hobby and her associates[7] recommended that the quantity of brown sugar be reduced to 20 gm. Later it was found by Foster, Woodruff and McDaniel[8] also that media made by the formula which included brown sugar gave the best results, but they suggested doubling the amount of sodium nitrate. Foster and his associates further demonstrated that the presence of zinc was of considerable importance both in promoting growth of the mold and in increasing the yield of penicillin. It was found that the optimal concentration of zinc for production of penicillin lies somewhere between 1 and 3 mg. of zinc sulfate ($ZnSO_4$.$7H_2O$) per liter. Foster and his associates were of the opinion that zinc acts as a catalyst to the oxidation and utilization of glucose by the mold and thereby prevents accumulation of gluconic acid, which is largely responsible for the fall in the pH of the medium. Many modifications have been made in the basic medium. It also has been found that ferrous sulfate and potassium chloride could be eliminated entirely and that the amount of potassium and phosphate could be lowered without reducing production of penicillin. However, the addition of monohydrogen phosphates and dihydrogen phosphates for the purpose of buffering the medium was thought desirable and was advocated by Challinor.[9] I have mentioned previously that Moyer discovered, in the course of his early studies, that the addition of corn-steep liquor to the medium increased the yield tenfold. This contribution by Moyer, together with the development of new strains of organisms, resulted in increase in the yields of penicillin from 2 to 40 Oxford units per cubic centimet r Although on the proper medium it was later possible to obtain yields of as much as 200 Oxford units per cubic centimeter, Moyer's contribution was an important step forward in connection with the efforts to increase the yields of penicillin.

Another medium which has been found satisfactory for the growth of Penicillium notatum and which, according to Taylor[10] resulted in better growth than any other is amigen. This is a trade name for a medium consisting of an enzyme digest of purified casein and pork pancreas in which the proteins have been hydrolyzed to amino acids 75 per cent and dipeptides and tripeptides together 25 per cent. For the production of crude penicillin, Fisher[11] used a fairly simple medium recommended by White. The medium consisted of the following: Bactotryptone (Difco) 20 gm., glucose 3 gm. and sodium chloride 5 gm. in 1,000 c.c. of distilled water. The pH of the medium is adjusted to 6.8 and it is then autoclaved. Pearl and Appling,[12] in certain experiments in which they used corn-steep liquor, found that starch dextrin can be substituted for lactose to give equally high quantities of penicillin. The advantage of this appears to be in the fact that starch dextrin is more plentiful and more readily available than lactose.

In studying a large number of different strains, ranging between and including Penicillium notatum and Penicillium chrysogenum, Waksman and Reilly[13] compared the production of penicillin by organisms of the various groups, as this was influenced by the composition of the different media. It seemed evident from their report that the media which contained corn-steep liquor and zinc resulted in production of considerably greater amounts of penicillin than did Czapek-Dox or brown sugar medium (table 1). The medium of choice in a given instance is the one

TABLE 1

INFLUENCE OF COMPOSITION OF MEDIUM UPON THE PRODUCTION OF PENICILLIN BY DIFFERENT ORGANISMS, AS MEASURED BY AGAR-TUBE METHOD

5-day incubation, top layer, mm. of zone produced on *B. subtilis* inoculated plate

Organism No.	Composition of medium			
	Czapek-Dox	Brown sugar[a]	Corn steep[b]	Zinc[c]
41	19.0	21.0	40.0	41.0
50	19.5	23.0	39.5	39.5
136	0	23.0	36.0	38.0
161	18.0	19.0	26.0	26.0

Brown sugar in place of glucose.
b Supplementary to above, 1.5 per cent.
c $ZnSO_4.7H_2O$, 0.001 per cent, supplementary to above.
From article by Waksman and Reilly, Proceedings of the National Academy of Sciences, May, 1944.

which is most readily available and most easily handled by the investigator who sets out to produce penicillin. Presumably he will make the attempt only if supplies of the material from commercial sources are not already available to him. Once the medium has been selected, spores from the master culture of the strain of Penicillium to be used are sown on the medium. The stock culture of the mold can be grown on a slope of Sabouraud's medium and a suspension of spores can be made from this culture by shaking with sterile water. This suspension of spores is then used for implantation.

PRODUCTION OF PENICILLIN FROM SURFACE CULTURE

Practically all of the penicillin used in the early studies was produced by means of the surface culture method. In this method, the spores of the mold are seeded on the surface of a layer of culture medium which is 1.5 to 2 cm. in depth. A convenient procedure is to use approximately 50 c.c. of medium in a 200 c.c. Erlenmeyer flask. Figure 2 is a photograph of such a preparation. Milk bottles or even large pans can be used. Use of metal containers should be avoided unless they are enameled or lined with glass because of the destructive effect of heavy metals on penicillin. This destruction of penicillin by heavy metals has been mentioned before and it will be taken up more fully in a subsequent section (p. 24). The

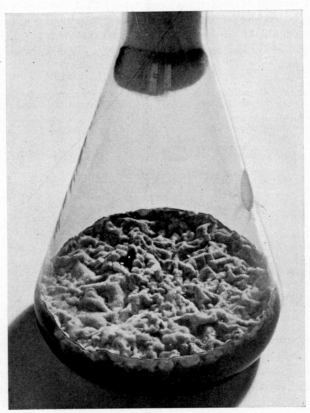

Fig. 2.—Surface culture of penicillin, growing in a flask.

medium having been seeded with the spores, the mold will be found to grow most satisfactorily at a temperature between 22° C. and 25° C. It fails to grow at 37° C. A delicate growth usually will appear twenty-four hours after the seeding, on the bottom of the vessel in which the cultures are made. By the third day, a white growth is present on the surface. This growth becomes coalesced and on about the fifth day the growth becomes green and somewhat rigid. After four or five days, samples with which to make tests for changes in pH and for the development of anti-bacterial potency are obtained by pipetting off a few cubic centimeters of the broth that lies beneath the surface growth, using sterile precautions. In most of the surface culture preparations the pH of the medium, which starts around 3.5 to 4.5, remains essentially the same for three or four days. As the growth of the mold becomes more profuse, a rise in pH will occur. This rise in pH is accompanied by a rather rapid development of antibacterial activity which usually reaches a peak when the pH approaches the neutral point. Beyond the neutral point, to a pH of 8, the medium rapidly will lose antibacterial activity. As a rule, after seven days many deep yellow drops of fluid are present on the surface. It is about this time that the material will be found to have its maximal antibacterial titer. To preserve the antibacterial titer it is important to filter off the mold about this time and to adjust the pH of the medium to 6.5 to 7. This crude broth filtrate which contains the active principle then can be stored. If the filtrate is kept at icebox temperature, it may remain active for as long as seven weeks, provided the pH is kept adjusted to 6.5 to 7. If the crude penicillin broth is frozen, it can be preserved for several months. The unfrozen or the melted crude filtrate, if still potent, is suitable for local application in clinical use.

The method described has several advantages over methods to be mentioned later if an investigator is attempting to prepare his own material. The yields are fairly high and the equipment necessary is not elaborate. One important advantage of growing penicillin by this method in individual small units is that if contamination occurs in one unit or bottle, it does not destroy the whole plant. If bacterial contamination occurs, serious trouble develops. Certain gram-negative bacteria such as Escherichia coli, Bacillus subtilis or Pseudomonas produce enzymes which rapidly will inactivate all of the penicillin present. It is necessary, therefore, that all contaminants be avoided.

EXTRACTION OF PENICILLIN FROM CULTURE MEDIUM

In the extraction or recovery of penicillin, as in the process of growing the mold, the same care must be exercised to protect the material from contamination and from conditions which destroy the active substance. After the mycelium has been removed from the cultures by filtration or centrifugation, the resulting filtrate is usually a clear yellow to brown solution. Since this broth filtrate still contains some of the nutrients, contaminating organisms will grow in the broth. To protect the broth from growth of contaminating organisms, aseptic handling or the addition of some disinfecting substance is essential. The broth also can be protected by immediate storage at low temperatures. Depending on the success of the procedure, the amount of penicillin present in these crude

2

broth filtrates may vary from 30 to 100 Oxford units per cubic centimeter. The free penicillin present exists in the form of an organic acid which reacts chemically to form various salts and esters.

It was evident from the work of the Oxford investigators[4] that penicillin could be extracted from broth filtrates by use of a solvent such as ether, amyl acetate or certain other organic solvents. This is best accomplished by adjusting the pH of the broth to between 2 and 3. (Penicillin is much more soluble in ether at pH 2 than at neutrality.) It must be remembered, however, that penicillin is very unstable at this low pH and for that reason the extraction must be done as rapidly as possible and at as low a temperature as is feasible.

In a search for solvents which would extract penicillin from aqueous solutions at a pH not harmful to the substance, Berger[14] found that a large portion of the substance could be extracted by n-butyl alcohol from culture filtrates adjusted to pH 6.4, at which penicillin is most stable. Furthermore, when ammonium sulfate was added to the filtrate, penicillin was almost completely extracted, according to him, by butyl alcohol. The addition of ammonium sulfate was also found to precipitate the greater part of the inactive pigments. Once the penicillin is extracted by butyl alcohol it can be brought back into the aqueous solution by adding light petroleum ether and shaking the mixture into dilute aqueous sodium bicarbonate solution. The advantages of this method, according to Berger, lie in the fact that there is no loss of penicillin during the extraction which is carried out at the pH of its greatest stability. The extraction is almost complete and considerable concentration is achieved by the same process. Furthermore, the extraction can be carried out at room temperature and only relatively small quantities of solvent are required.

In preparation of the sodium salt of penicillin (which was most commonly used in the early experimental and clinical studies) the penicillin present in the solvent that is used for extraction is obtained by shaking the solution with aqueous sodium bicarbonate. Following the extraction, the pH should be quickly readjusted to 6.5 to 7. Since the sodium salt of penicillin is hygroscopic, since sodium penicillin in aqueous solution is rather unstable and since heat destroys the material, it is essential in the drying operation to keep the penicillin frozen and to dry it in this state. This drying operation is best accomplished by a lypholyzing process similar to that used in the preparation of dried plasma. In general, the more nearly water-free that the sodium salt can be obtained, the more stable the preparation will be. In the process of drying the material from the water phase, the entire batch of the material can be used or the material can be dried in small individual ampules which are sealed after the drying operation has been completed. The final product is a powder which ranges from pale yellow to brown. The amount of penicillin present in such preparations may vary from 100 to 500 or more Oxford units per milligram. It is not a purified product but contains, in addition to penicillin, a mixture of certain organic acids that were present in the broth in which the mold was grown.

Obviously, many refinements and modifications of the early method of extracting penicillin have been made. It should be thoroughly emphasized that the foregoing description of the steps necessary to produce penicillin are outlined with the sole purpose of making available to the reader some general idea of a method which could be used if necessary in the production of small amounts of the material. Its large-scale production is a commercial and manufacturing problem and does not come within the scope of this book.

PRODUCTION OF PENICILLIN FROM SUBMERGED CULTURES

I have mentioned the problem of the production of penicillin on a large scale. One procedure for large-scale production of penicillin is the submerged culture method. The primary problem involved in the submerged culture is whether or not the strain of the mold used will grow beneath the surface of the medium and, therefore, whether large tanks or vats, in which penicillin can be produced on a large scale, can be used. This problem of submerged culture was extensively studied in the United States Department of Agriculture and certain commercial companies. In order to obtain submerged growth, it is necessary to aerate and agitate the culture by some means. This is done in order to prevent surface growth. Agitation can be effected by shaking the flasks and aeration by equipping vats and other storing devices with aerators. At Peoria, as Coghill has pointed out, rotary drum fermenters, equipped with aerators and agitators, were used. In such cultures the mold grows as small pellets rather than as a heavy pellicle. It was pointed out by Coghill that the strain of Penicillium notatum which grows well in surface cultures is not suitable for submerged culture work. On the other hand, the strain NRRL 832 is much more suitable for submerged culture than for surface culture. In these large vat cultures, yields as high as 80 units of penicillin per cubic centimeter have been obtained in two days, according to Coghill. The obvious advantage of this submerged method is the saving in time and labor. Its use, however, as has been indicated, is most adapted for large-scale and commercial production. It should be pointed out again, moreover, that when contamination occurs in such a system, the penicillin present in the entire batch may be lost.

PRODUCTION OF PENICILLIN ON BRAN

The bran method consists of growing suitable strains of Penicillium notatum on moist bran which is spread thinly in suitable trays or processed in a rotary drum. The bran first must be sterilized and then inoculated with the culture. After growth has continued for several days, it has been possible to produce as much as 200 to 400 units of penicillin per gram of dried bran. The penicillin is extracted by use of a suitable solvent. Coghill has pointed out the difficulties of this method; namely, that bran is a very poor conductor of heat and, as a result, it is extremely difficult to sterilize bran before it is inoculated, which in turn naturally results in loss of activity owing to contamination. The second difficulty mentioned by Coghill is that when the bran that has been inoculated with penicillin is incubated at 24° C. a great deal of heat is produced during the fermentation and some provision is required for dissipation of this heat. Likewise, Elder[15] has pointed out that the amount of equipment and the difficulties of temperature control and sterilization connected with this method have been troublesome.

For small-scale production of penicillin on bran, the procedure reported by Srinivasa Rao[16] may be useful. Thirty gm. of wheat bran (particles of large size preferred) are placed in 750 c.c. conical flasks. The bran is moistened with an equal weight of water and the water and bran are mixed well. The flasks are then plugged and autoclaved at 15 pounds of pressure for one hour. The sterile flasks are then inoculated with 1 c.c. of a suspension of spores of Penicillium notatum. The inoculated material is well shaken and incubated at 24° C. for two days. The flasks are shaken once at the end of twenty-four hours of incubation. One strain of Penicillium notatum grown under these conditions was said to result in an activity of 150 units per gram. The crude extract has been used for local application to surface wounds; however, fairly purified penicillin can be recovered by taking the penicillin up in a suitable solvent.

REFERENCES

1. Coghill, R. D.: Penicillin, science's Cinderella. Chem. & Eng. News. 22:588–593 (Apr. 25) 1944.

2. Fleming, Alexander: On the antibacterial action of cultures of a penicillium, with special reference to their use in the isolation of B. influenzae. Brit. J. Exper. Path. 10:226–236 (June) 1929.

3. Fleming, A.: On specific antibacterial properties of penicillin and potassium tellurite; incorporating method of demonstrating some bacterial antagonisms. J. Path. & Bact. 35:831–842 (Nov.) 1932.

4. Abraham, E. P., Chain, E., Fletcher, C. M., Gardner, A. D., Heatley, N. G., Jennings, M. A. and Florey, H. W.: Further observations on penicillin. Lancet. 2:177–188; 189 (Aug. 16) 1941.

5. Clutterbuck, P. W., Lovell, Reginald and Raistrick, Harold: Studies in the biochemistry of micro-organisms. XXVI. The formation from glucose by members of the

Penicillium chrysogenum series of a pigment, an alkali-soluble protein and penicillin—the antibacterial substance of Fleming. Biochem. J. *26*:1907–1918, 1932.

6. McKee, Clara M. and Rake, Geoffrey: Biological experiments with penicillin. J. Bact. *43*:645 (May) 1942.

7. Hobby, Gladys L., Meyer, Karl and Chaffee, Eleanor: Activity of penicillin in vitro. Proc. Soc. Exper. Biol. & Med. *50*:277–280 (June) 1942.

8. Foster, J. W., Woodruff, H. B. and McDaniel, L. E.: Microbiological aspects of penicillin. III. Production of penicillin in surface cultures of Penicillium notatum. J. Bact. *46*:421–433 (Nov.) 1943.

9. Challinor, S. W.: Production of penicillin. Nature. *150*:688 (Dec. 12) 1942.

10. Taylor, H. G.: Growth of Penicillium notatum on various media and the development of an antibacterial substance. Proc. Soc. Exper. Biol. & Med. *52*:299–301 (Apr.) 1943.

11. Fisher, A. M.: Antibacterial properties of crude penicillin. Bull. Johns Hopkins Hosp. *73*:343–378 (Nov.) 1943.

12. Pearl, I. A. and Appling, J. W.: Penicillin production. Science. n.s. *100*:51 (July 21) 1944.

13. Waksman, S. A. and Reilly, H. C.: Strain specificity and production of antibiotic substances. III. Penicillium notatum—chrysogenum group. Proc. Nat. Acad. Sc. *30*:99–105 (May) 1944.

14. Berger, F. M.: Extraction and purification of penicillin. Nature. *154*:459 (Oct. 7) 1944.

15. Elder, A. L.: Penicillin. Scient. Monthly. *58*:405–409 (June) 1944.

16. Srinivasa Rao, S.: Production of penicillin. Nature. *154*:83 (July 15) 1944.

CHAPTER III

PHYSICAL AND CHEMICAL PROPERTIES OF PENICILLIN

PENICILLIN AND ITS VARIOUS SALTS

I have mentioned in the previous chapter that free penicillin exists as an organic acid and reacts chemically to form various salts and esters. It was pointed out by Abraham and Chain[1] that the strongly dibasic acid is extremely unstable, probably because of the presence of labile, free carboxyl groups. Penicillin or its salts rapidly lose their activity on exposure to air and when heated. It is known that even air bacteria which contaminate preparations of penicillin will destroy the material. According to Abraham and Chain, free penicillin is very soluble in ether, alcohol, acetone, ethyl acetate, amyl acetate, cyclohexanon and dioxane. It is less soluble in benzene, chloroform and carbon tetrachloride. In water, free penicillin is soluble to the extent of 5 mg. per cubic centimeter.[2] The earthy salts of penicillin show the peculiarity of being readily soluble in absolute methyl alcohol but insoluble in absolute ethyl alcohol at room temperature. Penicillin is unstable under treatment with dilute acid, alkalies, primary alcohols, oxidizing agents and heavy metals. It is less sensitive to reducing agents. Below a pH of 5 and above a pH of 7 it is unstable.

The two salts of penicillin which have been most widely investigated are the sodium and the calcium salts.[3-6] Both have been obtained in highly purified crystalline form. The general configuration of the crystals of the highly purified sodium salt of penicillin is shown in figure 3. These crystals look somewhat like fence pickets. One end is pointed and the other is straight. The calcium salt which was examined by Nichols and me[5] contained approximately 146 Oxford units of penicillin per milligram. The calcium content of this preparation was approximately 5.6 per cent. Unlike the sodium salt, the calcium salt is not hygroscopic. Furthermore, in the dry state, in sealed ampules, it can be stored at room temperature for as long as six months without evidence of loss of activity. A more detailed comparison of these two salts with regard to stability and toxicity is further considered in the chapter on preparations of penicillin for clinical use (p. 102).

The other salts of penicillin which have been prepared include barium, potassium, magnesium, ammonium, silver and strontium salts. The barium salt, prepared by Abraham and Chain,[1] was reported to be stable for an indefinite period when obtained in the dry state. It is a non-hygroscopic white powder. Catch, Cook and Heilbron[7] prepared a highly purified yellow strontium salt of penicillin which possessed an activity of as much as 750 Oxford units per milligram. The ammonium salt of penicillin was prepared by Meyer, Hobby and their associates.[8,9] This ammonium salt was obtained in crystalline form and its activity was equivalent to 240 to 250 Oxford units per milligram. Like the potassium and sodium salts, the ammonium salt is very hygroscopic.

Methyl, ethyl, n-butyl and benzohydryl esters of penicillin were prepared by Meyer, Hobby and Chaffee,[10] and Meyer, Hobby and Dawson[11] who provided for reaction of the free acid of penicillin with the corres-

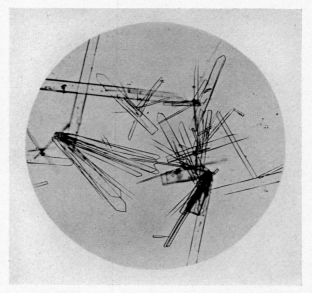

Fig. 3.—Crystals of sodium salt of penicillin. (Courtesy E. H. Volwiler, Ph.D.)

ponding diazo compounds. In contrast to the free acid, the esters were found to be insoluble in neutral or slightly alkaline buffers. The esters were found to be very soluble in benzene and could not be precipitated from chloroform-benzene solutions by dry ammonia. Although the aliphatic esters were considerably less active in vitro than the original penicillin, they were found to have considerable activity in vivo. This is probably due to hydrolysis of the esters, with subsequent liberation of active penicillin. Their importance lies in the fact that they are not destroyed by the gastric juices and therefore, experimentally, they can be administered by mouth. On the other hand, the dose of the methyl and ethyl esters required to protect experimental animals against certain infections rather closely approaches LD$_{50}$.* If higher esters can be prepared and prove less toxic, and at the same time retain their antibacterial activity, it may be possible yet to obtain a form of penicillin suitable for oral administration.

EFFECT OF HEAVY METALS AND VARIOUS OTHER AGENTS ON PENICILLIN

It was evident from the report of Abraham and Chain[1] that penicillin is inactivated by contact with various heavy metals. Copper, lead, zinc and cadmium resulted in the greatest inactivation of penicillin; however, other metals, such as nickel, mercury and uranium exerted some degree of inactivation. On the other hand, penicillin does not appear to be inactivated by certain bases such as ammonia, aniline and quinine in the ionized state. Penicillin does not reduce Fehling's solution but the blue color changes to green, probably from the formation of various complexes. This slight change in color may occur, therefore, when urine which contains penicillin is subjected to tests in which Fehling's solution is employed. Contact with potassium permanganate and hydrogen peroxide results in fairly rapid and complete oxidation of penicillin when it exists in the form of either the acid or its salts. This oxidation of penicillin results in loss of its antibacterial action. Penicillin is less sensitive to reducing agents. For example, Abraham and Chain carried out hydrogenation experiments on penicillin, using the Warburg apparatus at 37° C. The reduced material was found to retain its activity. When penicillin is incubated for three hours at a pH of 7, in the presence of an excess of hydrazine, antibacterial activity is lost.

ANALYSIS

Unfortunately, but for reasons of national safety, few data have been published dealing with recent studies on further purification, synthesis and analysis of penicillin. Therefore, little can be said concerning the chemistry in this present volume. What has been published and therefore is not in any sense secret will be summarized.

The empirical formula which was suggested by Abraham and Chain,[1] who analyzed the barium salt, was as follows: $C_{24}H_{32}O_{10}N_2Ba$ (M.W. 645) or $C_{23}H_{30}O_9N_2Ba$. In the discussion of their results they suggested that there was evidence to indicate the presence of one ketonic, two acetylatable and one latent carboxylic group. At any rate, it was evident from the beginning that penicillin possessed an exceptionally unstable chemical configuration. The spectrographic examination of preparations of penicillin by Holiday[1] yielded certain suggestions as to the structure of

* LD$_{50}$ designates the dose that will kill 50 per cent of a group of animals to which it is administered.

penicillin if it could be assumed that the barium salt with which he was working was almost pure. He concluded that it had a polysubstituted hydroaromatic ring structure, that the acidic groups (probably carboxyl) were not conjugated with the chromophore responsible for the absorption, and that a trisubstituted alpha-beta unsaturated ketone grouping was possibly present. Holiday stated that the basic structure indicated was R_2 R_1 and suggested that R_1 and R_2 and R_2 and R_3

$$R_2 \diagdown \quad R_1 \diagdown \diagup$$
$$C = C - C = O$$
$$\diagup$$
$$R_3$$

might each be cyclically combined or not. Subsequently Catch, Cook and Heilbron[7] conducted investigations on the purification and chemistry of penicillin. They used a strontium salt which was considered to be fairly pure for that stage of the development of penicillin. The preparation they examined contained 500 units of penicillin per milligram and some batches were of a potency as high as 750 units per milligram. As a result of their analysis of this form of penicillin, the following formula was suggested: $C_{24}H_{34}O_{11}NSr$. This agreed fairly closely with the formula previously suggested by Abraham and Chain. Further analysis reported by Catch and his associates indicated that the following substances were formed when the molecule was broken down: (1) a colorless water-soluble acid which on further hydrolysis appeared to be a simple peptide, (2) varying amounts of a yellow insoluble pigment ($C_{16}H_{20}O_6$ or $C_{16}H_{18}O_5H_2O$), and (3) acetaldehyde, which is accompanied by a minute quantity of an alpha-beta unsaturated aldehyde. According to Catch and his associates,[7] no carbon dioxide was liberated during the analysis of their preparation. It was suggested by them, on the basis of further studies of the pigment, that it was not a quinone. These authors further suggested that although the material titrated as a monobasic acid, it was more probably enolic in character.

Meyer and his associates[9] reported on studies dealing with the analysis of an ammonium salt of penicillin. The ammonium salt as studied by them was considered to be fairly stable. A considerable increase in stability was obtained by acetylation of the ammonium salt. The free acids of the acyl derivatives formed fine needles which possessed about the same activity in vitro as did the mother substances. According to Meyer and his associates, the analysis of penicillin best fitted the formula $C_{14}H_{19}NO_6$ or $C_{14}H_{17}NO_5 + H_2O$. This penicillin was found to be strongly dextrorotatory and had an absorption maximum on spectrographic examination of 2750A°. The potency of this penicillin was not as high as that analyzed by Catch and his associates. Its Oxford unit value was reported as 240 units per milligram.

REFERENCES

1. Abraham, E. P. and Chain, E.: Purification and some physical and chemical properties of penicillin; with a note on the spectrographic examination of penicillin preparations by E. R. Holiday. Brit. J. Exper. Path. *23*:103–115 (June) 1942.

2. Chain, E.: Discussion. Biochem. J. *36*:4–5, 1942.

3. Chain, E., Florey, H. W., Gardner, A. D., Heatley, N. G., Jennings, M. A., Orr-Ewing, J. and Sanders, A. G.: Penicillin as a chemotherapeutic agent. Lancet. *2*:226–228 (Aug. 24) 1940.

4. Abraham, E. P., Chain, E., Fletcher, C. M., Gardner, A. D., Heatley, N. G., Jennings, M. A. and Florey, H. W.: Further observations on penicillin. Lancet. *2*:177–188; 189 (Aug. 16) 1941.

5. Herrell, W. E. and Nichols, D. R.: The calcium salt of penicillin. Proc. Staff Meet., Mayo Clin. *18*:313–319 (Sept. 8) 1943.

6. Herrell, W. E.: The clinical use of penicillin; an antibacterial agent of biologic origin. J. A. M. A. *124*:622–627 (Mar. 4) 1944.

7. Catch, J. R., Cook, A. H. and Heilbron, I. M.: Purification and chemistry of penicillin. Nature. *150*:633–634 (Nov. 28) 1942.

8. Hobby, Gladys L., Meyer, Karl and Chaffee, Eleanor: Activity of penicillin in vitro. Proc. Soc. Exper. Biol. & Med. *50*:277–280 (June) 1942.

9. Meyer, Karl, Chaffee, Eleanor, Hobby, Gladys L., Dawson, M. H., Schwenk, Erwin and Fleischer, G.: On penicillin. Science. n.s. *96*:20–21 (July 3) 1942.

10. Meyer, Karl, Hobby, Gladys L. and Chaffee, Eleanor: On esters of penicillin. Science, n.s. *97*:205–206 (Feb. 26) 1943.

11. Meyer, K., Hobby, G. L. and Dawson, M. H.: The chemotherapeutic effect of esters of penicillin. Proc. Soc. Exper. Biol. & Med. *53*:100–104 (June) 1943.

CHAPTER IV

ANTIBACTERIAL ACTIVITY OF PENICILLIN IN VITRO

SELECTIVE ANTIBACTERIAL ACTION

Among the many properties exhibited by penicillin, one of the most interesting is its selective antibacterial activity. With a few exceptions, its antibacterial power has been shown to be against gram-positive micro-organisms, regardless of whether these organisms are aerobic or anaerobic. Its action is feeble against most gram-negative pathogens. On the other hand, not all gram-positive pathogens are highly susceptible to its action and some very important gram-negative micro-organisms are not resistant.

This selective antibacterial activity was evident to Fleming,[1] who was the first to test the action of the substance which he had named "penicillin" and which was present in the broth filtrates of cultures of Penicillium notatum with which he worked. From Fleming's studies it was evident that an inhibitory effect occurred against various staphylococci, Diplococcus pneumoniae, Streptococcus pyogenes, Neisseria gonorrhoeae, Neisseria intracellularis and Corynebacterium diphtheriae. Penicillin was found by Fleming to be somewhat inhibitory for Bacillus anthracis. In the studies on the so-called green-producing streptococci there was considerable variation, some strains being found to be sensitive and others resistant. It was further evident from Fleming's investigations that penicillin was relatively ineffective against members of the colon-typhoid group of micro-organisms. In addition, Pseudomonas aeruginosa (Bacillus pyocyaneus), Proteus vulgaris (Bacillus proteus), and Vibrio comma were found to be insensitive. Enterococci, Klebsiella pneumoniae (Friedländer's bacillus) and Hemophilus influenzae were also found to be insensitive. This selective action stimulated Fleming[2, 3] to consider the possible uses of penicillin, which in 1932 he listed as (1) the isolation of insensitive bacteria from the midst of large numbers of sensitive organisms; (2) the demonstration of some bacterial inhibitions, and (3) the treatment of infections by sensitive organisms. It seemed evident further from Fleming's work that penicillin was primarily bacteriostatic, a finding which was corroborated by Reid in 1935.[4]

Further intensive studies[5] on the selective nature of the antibacterial activity of penicillin were begun at Oxford and elsewhere following the isolation of fairly purified penicillin by the Oxford investigators. The

TABLE 2

DILUTIONS OF PENICILLIN AT WHICH VARIOUS INHIBITORY EFFECTS HAVE BEEN OBSERVED

Bacterial species	No. of strains	Dilutions at which inhibitory effects were observed		
		Complete	Partial	None
Neisseria gonorrhoeae[1]	6	2,000,000	>2,000,000	>2,000,000
Neisseria meningitidis	1	1,000,000	2,000,000	4,000,000
Staphylococcus aureus	4	1,000,000	2,000,000	4,000,000
Streptococcus pyogenes	3	1,000,000	2,000,000	4,000,000
Bacillus anthracis	1	1,000,000	2,000,000	4,000,000
Actinomyces bovis (hominis)	1	1,000,000	2,000,000	4,000,000
Clostridium tetani[2]	1	1,000,000	......	......
Clostridium welchii	1	1,500,000	......	......
Clostridium septique	1	300,000	1,500,000	7,500,000
Clostridium oedematiens	1	300,000	......	1,500,000
Streptococcus viridans[3]	2	625,000	......	3,125,000
Pneumococcus[3]	6	250,000	500,000	1,000,000
C. diphtheriae (mitis)	1	125,000	......	625,000
C. diphtheriae (gravis)	1	32,000	64,000	128,000
Salmonella gärtneri	1	20,000	40,000	80,000
Salmonella typhi	2	10,000	30,000	90,000
Pneumococcus[3]	3	9,000	......	27,000
Anaerobic streptococcus[3]	1	4,000	8,000	16,000
Proteus	3	4,000	32,000	60,000
Streptococcus viridans[3]	1	4,000	8,000	16,000
Pasteurella pestis	2	1,000	100,000	500,000
Salmonella typhimurium	1	<1,000	8,000	16,000
Salmonella paratyphi B.	2	<1,000	5,000	10,000
Bact. dysenteriae Shiga	1	2,000	4,000	8,000
Brucella abortus	1	2,000	4,000	8,000
Brucella melitensis	1	<1,000	2,500	10,000
Anaerobic streptococcus	1	<4,000	<4,000	4,000
Vibrio cholerae	1	<1,000	1,000	2,000
Bact. coli	5	<1,000	<1,000	1,000
B. friedländeri	1	<1,000	<1,000	1,000
Pseudomonas pyocyanea	2	<1,000	<1,000	1,000
Mycobacterium tuberculosis	1	<1,000	<1,000	1,000
Leptospira icterohaemorrhagiae	1	<3,600	<3,600	3,600

[1]Another strain was inhibited only up to 32,000.
[2]Grown in Lemco broth. In beef broth complete inhibition only reached 100,000.
[3]In Pneumococcus, Strep. viridans, and anaerobic streptococci, different strains appear at different levels in the table.
From article by Abraham, Chain, Fletcher Gardner, Heatley, Jennings and Florey, Lancet, August 16, 1941.

early studies carried out by the Oxford investigators[6] on the effectiveness of penicillin against a wide variety of micro-organisms is reproduced in table 2. These studies were carried out with what would now be considered relatively crude preparations of penicillin. Subsequent investigations, in which more nearly pure and more potent products were used, indicated some slight variation from these results; however, in general, results of comparative studies have been for the most part in agreement with the data published from Oxford; variations will be mentioned later.

Susceptible Organisms.—Based on the results of studies carried out by a host of investigators in vitro, it can be stated that, according to present knowledge, penicillin appears to be effective against the following organisms: Diplococcus pneumoniae, Streptococcus pyogenes, Streptococcus salivarius, microaerophilic streptococci, Staphylococcus aureus, Staphylococcus albus (some strains), Neisseria gonorrhoeae, Neisseria intracellularis, Actinomyces bovis, Bacillus anthracis, Bacillus subtilis, Clostridium botulinum, Clostridium tetani, Clostridium perfringens (Clostridium welchii), Clostridium septicum, Corynebacterium diphtheriae, micrococci (some strains), Streptobacillus moniliformis, Erysipelothrix rhusiopathiae and Treponema pallidum.

Insusceptible Organisms.—On the basis of studies made in vitro, the organisms which have been found insusceptible to the action of penicillin include the following: Eberthella typhosa, Salmonella paratyphi, Salmonella enteritidis, Shigella dysenteriae, Proteus vulgaris, Pseudomonas aeruginosa (Bacillus pyocyaneus), Pseudomonas fluorescens, Serratia marcescens (Bacillus prodigiosus), Klebsiella pneumoniae, Hemophilus influenzae, Hemophilus pertussis, Escherichia coli, Staphylococcus albus (some strains), Monilia albicans, Monilia candida, Monilia krusei, blastomycetes, Mycobacterium tuberculosis, Streptococcus faecalis, Brucella melitensis and Vibrio comma. It is now evident that certain pathogenic organisms may be rather insensitive on the basis of studies made in vitro, and yet penicillin has been found to be effective in vivo in the control of infections owing to some of these micro-organisms. Details of such studies are discussed in the chapter on the antibacterial activity of penicillin in vivo (Chapter V).

FACTORS WHICH INFLUENCE ANTIBACTERIAL ACTION

Studies of factors which influence antibacterial activity of penicillin have value, not only from the standpoint of certain laboratory procedures, but also in connection with the treatment of a variety of infections.

Variations in Sensitivity of Strains.—The original reports of the Oxford investigators[6] made evident that considerable difference in sensitivity was manifested by different strains of the same organism; for example, three strains of pneumococci examined by them were inhibited at a dilution of only 1:9,000, whereas six other strains were inhibited at a dilution of 1:250,000. Furthermore, the pneumococci tested by the Oxford investigators were much less sensitive than Staphylococcus aureus and certain other highly sensitive micro-organisms. On the other hand, three strains of pneumococci examined by Dorothy Heilman and me[7] were of approximately the same order of sensitivity as were strains of Staphylococcus aureus. From our studies it also was evident that this difference in sensitivity of strains was especially marked in the group of organisms commonly referred to as "Streptococcus viridans." For example, three different strains of Streptococcus salivarius were found by us to be fairly sensitive to the action of penicillin in vitro (tissue culture). On the other hand, three different strains of Streptococcus faecalis were found to be relatively insensitive to the action of penicillin. This was in agreement with the reports of Fleming[1] and also with the reports of Abraham and his associates.[6]

Bornstein[8] also recognized this variation in sensitivity of strains in his early studies in which he used the crude broth filtrates containing penicillin. His experiments demonstrated a rather sharp difference in sensitivity between enterococci and Streptococcus lactis on the one hand and, on the other, the so-called Streptococcus viridans. This suggested to him that the degree of sensitivity to penicillin might be used as an aid in the identification of related bacterial strains. The practical significance of these early observations is adequately demonstrated in the variations which occur in the response to treatment with penicillin in different cases of bacterial endocarditis. The treatment of endocarditis owing to Streptococcus faecalis, for example, presents an entirely different and more difficult problem than the treatment of a similar condition owing to one of the sensitive green-producing streptococci, such as Streptococcus salivarius. Dawson, Hobby and Lipman,[9] for example, recently have studied fifty different strains of streptococci isolated in cases of subacute bacterial endocarditis and they pointed out further the importance of consideration of the difference in sensitivity of strains as a guide to the appropriate clinical use of the material. A comparison of sensitivity of the so-called Streptococcus viridans with Streptococcus pyogenes more clearly brings out this difference in sensitivity of strains, which is of considerable importance in connection with factors which influence the antibacterial action of penicillin. Robinson[10] found, for example, that two different strains of Streptococcus pyogenes were completely inhibited at a dilution of 1:2,000,000, whereas so-called Streptococcus viridans was only partially inhibited at a dilution of 1:128,000.

While staphylococci appear to be more uniform than streptococci in their sensitivity to the action of penicillin, minor variations occur with this organism, which is generally considered to be rather highly sensitive. The studies on this subject reported by Dorothy Heilman and me[7] in 1942 indicate to some degree this difference. It was found, for example, that 10 micrograms of penicillin per cubic centimeter in tissue culture preparations was necessary to produce total inhibition of one strain, whereas two other strains were completely inhibited at 2.5 micrograms

TABLE 3

AMOUNTS OF BACTERICIDAL SUBSTANCE CAUSING TOTAL INHIBITION OF GROWTH OF BACTERIA

Organism	Strain number	Penicillin, micrograms per c.c.	
		Tissue present	No tissue present
Diplococcus pneumoniae Type I	1	5	2.5, 5
Type III	1	5	5
Type VII	1	5	5
Streptococcus pyogenes (Group A Lancefield)	2	2.5	2.5
	4	2.5	
	6	2.5	2.5
Streptococcus salivarius	1	40	40
	2	40	20
	3	40	40
Streptococcus faecalis	1	—*	—*
	2	—*	—*
	5	—*	—*
Staphylococcus aureus	1	2.5	2.5
	2	2.5	2.5
	7	10.0	10.0

* Not inhibited by 200 micrograms per c.c. of bactericidal substance.

per cubic centimeter (table 3). The report of Rammelkamp and Maxon,[11] in 1942, further suggested that this variation in sensitivity was sufficiently wide to necessitate the use of a standard strain of organisms for assay work. Likewise, Spink and his associates[12] found considerable variation in sensitivity of strains of pathogenic staphylococci.

Size of the Inoculum.—Other studies concerning factors which influence the action of penicillin would tend to indicate that the number of organisms in the initial inoculum affects somewhat the activity of penicillin. This was evident from the report of Rantz, Kirby and Randall,[13] whose studies were carried out on the action of penicillin against staphylococci in vitro, using photo-electric turbidimetric methods. Hobby and her associates[14] also have investigated this factor in connection with the action of penicillin and have concluded that the size of the inoculum is significant.

The pH of the Medium.—I have mentioned already the effect of the pH of the medium on production of penicillin. The pH also may be of some importance in connection with the bacteriostatic action of penicillin. It was found by Foster and Woodruff[15] that when reduction occurred in the pH of the medium from 7 to 5.5, there appeared to be a threefold increase in bacteriostatic action. When these observations were made, the plate method was used. From subsequent experiments,[16] however, it appeared that the changes in pH were the result rather than the cause of the changes in bacteriostatic action.

Inhibitors of Penicillin.—In connection with the factors which influence antibacterial activity of penicillin, in the previous chapter I have mentioned the effect of acids, alkalies, certain alcohols, gastric acidity, heat, heavy metals, oxidation and reduction, as well as bacterial contamination, which influence markedly the antibacterial activity of penicillin.

Certain other substances which occur naturally have been classified as inhibitors of penicillin. For example, Abraham and Chain,[17] as early as 1940, by grinding suspensions of Escherichia coli, produced an enzyme-like substance which completely inhibited the action of penicillin. To this substance was given the name "penicillinase." It appeared from their studies that this substance was intracellular, since penicillinase was not found in filtrates of cultures of Escherichia coli. Likewise Kirby,[18] in studying this phenomenon, found no inactivator of penicillin in filtrates of culture fluids of seven coagulase-positive strains of Staphylococcus aureus, from which micro-organisms he was able, nevertheless, to extract the substance which inactivates penicillin. These strains were naturally penicillin resistant. No inactivator of penicillin was found in seven other strains which were sensitive to penicillin. I might elaborate somewhat on these observations by pointing out that penicillin is destroyed in urine which contains Escherichia coli and that if penicillinase is intracellular and does not destroy penicillin when the Escherichia coli is in the actively growing stage, as reported by Abraham and his associates,[6] the destruction of penicillin must, therefore, occur when the organisms present in the urine die and disintegrate, which accomplishes the same thing as grinding the bacteria in a mill. Abraham and his associates were unable to demonstrate the presence of, or to extract, a substance which would inactivate penicillin either from sensitive staphylococci or from staphylococci rendered insensitive to penicillin by repeated subcultures in the presence of this agent. It was evident from their studies,[17] also, that a substance inhibitory to penicillin may, however, be elaborated by certain other micro-organisms (an extracellular substance) since the inhibitory substance could be found in culture medium containing a gram-negative rod found as a contamination in some cultures of Penicillium. This gram-negative rod, just as is true of Escherichia coli, also was insensitive to the action of penicillin.

Of further interest, however, is the fact that this enzyme which inhibits penicillin also can be found in certain organisms which are sensitive to the action of penicillin. It must be deduced from these studies, therefore, that the presence or absence of the enzyme, with reference to a certain micro-organism, is not the sole factor which determines the antibacterial action of penicillin against that organism. That this appears to be true was further indicated by the report of Bondi and Dietz,[19] who pointed out that the inability of an organism to produce penicillinase is not the determining factor in the sensitivity of the organism. It did appear to them, however, that bacteria which produce penicillinase are not likely to be highly susceptible to penicillin. Further, it was evident that the development of resistance to penicillin by a bacterium is not associated with acquired ability of the organism to produce the enzyme. This is in contrast to the synthesis of para-aminobenzoic acid by certain organisms that develop resistance to sulfonamides. In other words, penicillinase does not hold a relationship to penicillin fastness that is analogous to the relationship between para-aminobenzoic acid and sulfonamide fastness.

Harper[20] succeeded in isolating a powerful inhibitor of penicillin which was elaborated by a paracolon bacillus. The living cultures, the culture filtrates and the dried preparation of the paracolon organism all appeared to destroy penicillin. The enzymatic nature of this inhibitor at the time of Harper's publication was not definitely proved. At any rate, the practical value of this substance was apparent to Harper, who suggested that if the dried bacterial powder were added to cultures of the blood of patients who had been given penicillin, the possibility of obtaining false negative cultures probably would be eliminated. As a matter of fact, it was evident from the reports of Bondi and Dietz[21] and Ungar[22] that this would be the effect. These observers used filtrates of cultures containing penicillinase with moderate success in securing positive cultures of body fluids which contained penicillin. They pointed out that penicillinase should be as valuable for culturing such fluids as is para-amino-benzoic acid for culturing specimens containing sulfonamides.

This ability to produce substances which destroy or inactivate penicillin is widespread among different bacteria. Woodruff and Foster[23] have pointed out that the enzyme is formed whether or not a micro-organism is resistant to penicillin. This is in general agreement with the reports which appeared previously.

It was suggested in a report by Lawrence[24] that the enzyme, clarase, would inactivate the antibacterial effects of penicillin in two hours or less when incubated in the presence of the agent in a water bath at 40° C. It appeared that taka-diastase also was effective under these conditions at pH 6.0 and 8.0. As a result of these studies, a method for routine tests of sterility of penicillin powder was suggested, in which use was made of the fact that the antibacterial activity of penicillin could be blocked by the presence of clarase. From subsequent reports by this same author,[25] it appeared that the demonstrated power of clarase and taka-diastase to inactivate penicillin was due to bacterial end products which these preparations contained. On the other hand, it was evident from the report of Stanley[26] that observations on the ability of clarase to inactivate penicillin are open to considerable question, since only one of five samples of clarase tested by him produced inactivation.

MODE OF ACTION

While the mode of action of penicillin is still not clear, a host of investigators have presented evidence that penicillin may act as a bacteriostatic agent and, under certain conditions, may behave as a bactericidal agent. It was evident from the tissue culture studies reported from the Mayo Clinic[7] that penicillin apparently killed bacteria in a majority of cultures containing Diplococcus pneumoniae, Streptococcus pyogenes, and Staphylococcus aureus. Among strains of Streptococcus salivarius, however, there was a greater survival than occurred in the tests in which the former three organisms were used, as measured by subcultures of what appeared to be negative clots. It should be emphasized, also, that the character of the bacteriologic medium may influence such results. That this is so is apparent from the report of Miller and Foster[27] on studies concerning the action of penicillin. In a study of the action of penicillin on meningococci in vitro, for example, it appeared that the presence of inactivated serum frequently reduces the activity of penicillin and that penicillin acts on bacteria in an environment which promotes their multiplication.

Hobby and her associates[14] have reported observations on the mechanism of action of penicillin. Under the conditions of their experiments it was found that the number of surviving organisms decreased by geometric units as the time increased by arithmetic units. They further found that the rate of killing of a strain of Streptococcus pyogenes decreased as the number of organisms present in the original inoculum was increased. Within certain limits it also was found that the rate of killing increased when increasing concentrations of penicillin were present. Subsequent studies by Hobby and Dawson[28] indicated that the rate at which penicillin acts is increased under conditions which increase the rate of growth of bacteria. Also, there appeared to be a decrease in the rate at which penicillin acts under conditions which decrease the rate of growth of the bacteria. Penicillin appeared to be most effective when active multiplication was taking place. Conditions which increased the rate of growth of Streptococcus pyogenes included the addition of serum, para-aminobenzoic acid and dextrose. The addition of sulfadiazine to broth which contained penicillin did not appear additionally to decrease the rate of growth of hemolytic streptococci. Under the conditions of Hobby and Dawson's experiment, it appeared that during the first five to seven hours, the combination of penicillin with sulfadiazine killed bacteria at the same rate as occurred when penicillin was used alone. After five to seven hours, the combination of penicillin and sulfadiazine destroyed the remaining organisms even more slowly than did penicillin alone. This is at variance with some reports which suggest that synergism exists between sulfonamides and penicillin.

In connection with studies on the action of penicillin, Dorothy Heilman and I[7] have reported observations which suggest that considerable time is necessary for penicillin to act on certain bacteria. Subcultures of preparations containing bacteria and penicillin, made at various intervals, revealed that bacterial inhibition is not complete until some time between four and six hours of contact between the antibacterial agent and the organisms (table 4). The practical significance of this observation lies in the fact that if penicillin is to be used as a local agent, conditions must be such that the agent is allowed to remain in contact with the organism for a considerable time and that merely irrigating surfaces with the agent is not likely to be followed by success. This will be mentioned again in connection with the local application of penicillin (p. 107).

Observations made by Hobby and her associates[14] suggest that penicillin apparently is not absorbed or destroyed in the process of bacterial inhibition. When Streptococcus pyogenes was incubated in penicillin broth, it was found that the penicillin titer remained the same after inhibition had occurred. In this same report it was suggested that penicillin probably exerted its antibacterial effect only against organisms in their active phase of growth.

From the studies reported by Dorothy Heilman and me,[29] it appears further that penicillin does not behave as a detergent which detergent like action probably, in part, explains the mode of action of at least one other antibiotic agent (gramidicin). Furthermore, unlike sulfonamides, the action of penicillin is not inhibited in the presence of pus, products of breakdown of tissue, or para-aminobenzoic acid. Studies reported by the Oxford investigators,[6] by Hobby and her associates,[30] and by my colleagues and me[7, 31] are in agreement concerning the effect of these substances on the action of penicillin. Likewise, the presence of whole blood and serum does not appear to have any appreciable antagonistic effect.

TABLE 4
TIME FACTOR IN BACTERICIDAL EFFECT OF GRAMICIDIN AND PENICILLIN

Substance	Penicillin		
Amount	10 micrograms per c.c.*	5 micrograms per c.c.*	200 micrograms per c.c.*
Organism	D. pneumoniae, type VII	Staph. aureus	Staph. aureus
Time, hours	Positive subcultures †		
0	10	10	9
½	10	10	9
1	9	9	3
1½	10	9	0
2	6	2	2
4	2	0	0
6	0	0	0
8	0	0	—
12	0	0	—

* Twice the minimal effective amount required to inhibit growth of bacteria.
† Number positive in ten brain broth subcultures of original tissue culture preparations.

There seems to be general agreement that the mode of action of penicillin differs from that of the sulfonamides. In studying the mechanism of action of penicillin, Hobby and her colleagues[14] presented data which seemed to suggest that the action of penicillin may be somewhat similar to the action of other antibiotic agents, such as gramicidin and tyrocidine, although it appeared from their report that penicillin acts more slowly than either gramicidin or tyrocidine.

It is my opinion that the most likely approach to the problem is in study of the ability of penicillin to block certain enzyme systems or the utilization of certain nutrients essential for the growth and multiplication of bacteria.

EFFECT OF OTHER ANTIBACTERIAL AGENTS AND PENICILLIN COMBINED

It was evident from the studies of Ungar[32] that another antibacterial agent, sulfapyridine, produced an enhancing effect on the action of penicillin. According to his studies made in vitro, which were confirmed in mice, the action of penicillin was said to be at least doubled in the presence of sulfapyridine. He pointed out that the increased activity when the two substances were applied simultaneously might be due to synergistic action between them or, less probably, to a chemical reaction which may have occurred between the sulfonamide and the penicillin. Some later work by Hobby and Dawson[33] on this subject, on the other hand, led them to conclude that there was no evidence of synergistic action between either sulfapyridine or sulfadiazine and penicillin.

Further evidence to support the belief that the action of penicillin was considerably enhanced by sulfonamides is the work of T'ung,[34] in which he found that the combination of penicillin with small amounts of sodium sulfathiazole resulted in a considerably greater antibacterial action than penicillin had alone. This synergistic action was more noticeable on certain strains than on others. That the degree of synergism existing between penicillin and sulfathiazole varied with the strain of organism also seemed apparent in the report of Bigger[35] on the synergistic action of penicillin and sulfonamides. It was evident from his report furthermore, that, in association with penicillin, sulfathiazole was more effective than either sulfanilamide or sulfapyridine. This was true not only for Staphylococcus aureus but for Streptococcus pyogenes, in studies of which there appeared to be considerable reinforcement of the action of penicillin by the presence of sulfathiazole. The fact that the investigators T'ung and Bigger used sulfathiazole rather than sulfadiazine may explain the apparent variation of their results from those obtained by Hobby and Dawson,[28] which were mentioned on p. 35. Bigger also concluded that not only was the simultaneous administration of sulfathiazole and penicillin as effective as double the dose of penicillin alone, but also that the simultaneous administration would prevent multiplication of bacteria at those periods when the concentration of penicillin in the blood fell to a low level prior to the next injection in cases in which penicillin was being administered by the intermittent intravenous or intramuscular method.

Some reports are available on the combined action of penicillin with other antibiotic agents. Dorothy Heilman and I[7, 29] have reported observations which suggest that the activity of penicillin was not interfered with nor enhanced by the presence of at least one antibiotic; namely, gramicidin. When the two substances were added to tissue cultures in which Diplococcus pneumoniae, type VII, was growing, it was found necessary to use almost a full inhibiting dose of each substance to produce total inhibition. While there is no antagonism between the two substances, these results suggest that together their antibacterial action is only slightly additive.

The effect of combining penicillin with another antibiotic, streptothricin, has been reported by Foster and Woodruff.[36] Unlike the results obtained by us with gramicidin, it appeared from their studies that there was a considerable additive effect between penicillin and streptothricin. They found that the combined inhibiting action of these two substances was almost quantitatively the sum of inhibitions of both substances acting separately. Such studies on the effect of other antibacterial agents in combination may prove of considerable importance in their future use for clinical purposes.

CYTOTOXICITY OF PENICILLIN

It was evident to Fleming,[1] in the very beginning of his studies, that the amount of penicillin which completely inhibited the growth of staphylococci in vitro did not interfere with leukocytic function any more than would the presence of ordinary broth. It was subsequently evident from the reports made by the Oxford investigators[5] on a more or less purified preparation of penicillin that even the leukocytes of man remained active for at least three hours in the presence of a 1:1,000 dilution of penicillin. All subsequent investigations are in agreement with the declaration that antibacterial amounts of penicillin do not appear to embarrass or interfere with leukocytic activity in vitro.

Furthermore, studies on tissue cultures reported by Florey and his associates,[6] and by Dorothy Heilman and me,[29] seem to indicate that the presence of penicillin in antibacterial amounts does not seriously interfere with the growth and migration of tissue elements such as lymphocytes, fibroblasts or macrophages. In fact, penicillin is noted for its low degree of cytotoxicity as compared with practically all of the commonly employed germicides available at the time of the introduction of penicillin.

MORPHOLOGIC CHANGES IN BACTERIA AND TUMOR CELLS

It appears that Gardner[37] was the first investigator to describe the morphologic changes which occurred in different bacteria when the organisms came in contact with slightly less than inhibitory amounts of penicillin. It was evident from his studies that microscopic examination of bacteria such as Clostridium welchii in contact with penicillin revealed that these organisms underwent extreme elongation and took the form of unsegmented filaments ten or more times longer than the average normal cell. Similar changes were found to occur in other bacterial forms, including gram-negative rods which were relatively resistant to the action of penicillin; Escherichia coli, for example, often took on grotesque giant forms under these conditions. The morphologic changes which occur in staphylococci take the form of spherical enlargement of the cells, with imperfect fission. However, Neisseria intracellularis, an organism which is very sensitive to the action of penicillin, has been found to undergo no such changes when in contact with the agent. It is of some interest to point out that changes similar to those which have been recounted in this paragraph were observed by Walker and Murray[38] as early as 1904 in experiments in which certain dye substances were allowed to act on the colon-typhoid group of bacteria. In 1939, a similar phenomenon was reported by Tunnicliff[39] in connection with studies in which Streptococcus viridans was acted on by sulfanilamide.

Certain facts become obvious from examination of these results. First, the morphologic changes which are produced in bacteria do not take place because of a property limited to penicillin, since various other antibacterial agents have been found to produce the same phenomenon. Second, the phenomenon occurs following contact with penicillin in the case of bacteria which are insensitive as well as in the case of bacteria which are known to be sensitive. Third, organisms known to be sensitive to penicillin at times do not show this phenomenon. While the direct action of penicillin may be of some significance, it appears, therefore, that the peculiar changes in micro-organisms which have been pointed out do not explain that property of penicillin which accounts entirely for its antibacterial activity.

Morphologic changes in coccal forms present in the blood of patients who were receiving penicillin intravenously have been observed by my colleagues and me.[31] Further observations on morphologic changes which occur in bacteria during the course of administration of penicillin to human beings, have been reported by Miller, Scott and Moeller.[40] Two to three hours after penicillin was administered to patients for gonococcal infections, microscopic examinations of urethral secretions were made. By this time the gonococci were swollen and irregular in shape. The bacteria were stained irregularly and were surrounded by clear areas.

Smith and Hay[41] noted these morphologic changes in certain strains of Staphylococcus aureus cultured in penicillin broth. The penicillin used in their studies was obtained from Penicillium chrysogenum. They were inclined to interpret these findings as indicating that penicillin either had some direct action on the cell wall or that it interferes with assimilation of growth factors necessary for actual fission.

Another example of the action of penicillin on cellular formation was the observation by Cornman[42] concerning the effect of penicillin on normal, as compared with malignant cells. These studies were carried out on rat and mouse sarcoma cells. It appeared from his studies that certain types of malignant cells may be affected by the action of penicillin. To cause damage to normal cells, two or three times as much penicillin was required as was required to cause damage to malignant cells. When cultures of these malignant cells had showed marked damage as a result of contact with penicillin, Cornman was unable to produce tumors in rats by implantation of this tissue. The untreated control tumor cultures, however, regularly produced tumors. This is, indeed, an interesting observation. However, it must be emphasized that many other agents will interfere with the normal metabolism and growth of malignant cells. Whether or not subsequent studies will lead to possible relevant clinical use of penicillin is a matter of pure conjecture.

The report by Lewis[43] on the general subject of the effect of penicillin on the growth of grafts of sarcoma is at variance with the report by Cornman. Using purified penicillin, Lewis was unable to demonstrate any retardation of the growth of grafts of sarcoma in mice. From her studies, therefore, it would appear that the inhibition previously claimed for penicillin was probably lost from the highly purified product.

DEVELOPMENT OF RESISTANCE TO PENICILLIN

Those interested in the problems of chemotherapy of bacterial infections are constantly challenged in their studies on each new chemotherapeutic agent introduced. The question is always present, "Will microorganisms develop resistance to the antibacterial agent?" It is not surprising, therefore, that immediately following the introduction of penicillin a number of investigators have attempted to determine whether or not organisms develop resistance or whether the organisms can be made to develop such resistance experimentally. The Oxford investigators[6] were able to increase resistance to penicillin in a strain of Staphylococcus aureus 1,000 times by subculturing the organism in the presence of increasing amounts of penicillin over a period of nine weeks. As I have mentioned concerning bacteria in general, however (p. 33), there was no evidence that the adaptation of Staphylococcus aureus to penicillin depended on the acquired ability of Staphylococcus aureus to produce a penicillin-destroying enzyme. Rammelkamp and Maxon[11] also carried out studies which indicate that strains of Staphylococcus aureus would develop resistance in the presence of gradually increasing concentrations of penicillin.

Further studies on the general subject were reported by McKee and Houck,[44] who found that the resistance of staphylococci could, under the conditions of their experiments, be markedly increased. On the other hand, penicillin fastness was not so easily accomplished in the case of Diplococcus pneumoniae or Streptococcus pyogenes. These investigators further pointed out that as resistance to penicillin increased, virulence of the organism declined. This development of resistance and loss of virulence, once established, appeared to be permanent characteristics of the organism. It is of further interest that when these characteristics developed in organisms, their susceptibility to other antibiotic agents remained unchanged. This, therefore, may be of considerable practical significance in clinical chemotherapy.

Similarly, the investigations of Powell and Jamieson,[45] McKee and Rake,[46] and Tillett, Cambier and Harris[47] suggest that resistance to sulfonamides and resistance to penicillin are not interrelated. Spink and his associates[12] have carried out studies which further confirm these earlier observations and which suggest a possible difference in the mechanism of resistance developed by certain organisms to sulfonamides and to penicillin. From their studies it was evident, also, that when staphylococci have been allowed to become resistant to penicillin they were many more times susceptible to the antibacterial action of human blood than the parent strain of staphylococci from which they were derived. Such an observation suggests that while strains of staphylococci that have become resistant to penicillin may still act as pathogens, they become of less danger to the patient.

That the development of resistance to penicillin varies significantly with different strains of pneumococci was evident from the studies reported by Schmidt and Sesler.[48] However, when resistance was developed in vitro, there appeared to be a simultaneous increase in resistance to the drug in vivo. From their studies it also was evident that the therapeutic effectiveness of sulfonamides against pneumococci was not altered by the development of resistance to penicillin. That resistance to penicillin might occur among patients who were under treatment with penicillin seemed evident from the reports of Rammelkamp and Maxon[11] as well as from the report of Lyons.[49]

The question of the development of resistance is indeed a fundamental one. It is my conviction, however, that although resistance on the part of the causative organism occasionally may develop among patients who are under treatment, poor therapeutic results are too often ascribed to this development of resistance on the part of different pathogenic organisms. All too often the actual difficulty encountered is explainable on another basis and the actual resistance of the organism to the chemotherapeutic agent, as measured by studies in vitro, has not been examined adequately.

REFERENCES

1. Fleming, Alexander: On the antibacterial action of cultures of a penicillium, with special reference to their use in the isolation of B. influenzae. Brit. J. Exper. Path. *10:*226–236 (June) 1929.

2. Fleming, Alexander: Penicillin for selective culture and for demonstrating bacterial inhibitions. Brit. M. Bull. *2:*7–8 (No. 1) 1944.

3. Fleming, Alexander: On the specific antibacterial properties of penicillin and potassium tellurite; incorporating a method of demonstrating some bacterial antagonisms. J. Path. & Bact. *35:*831–842 (Nov.) 1932.

4. Reid, R. D.: Some properties of bacterial-inhibitory substance produced by a mold. J. Bact. *29:*215–221 (Feb.) 1935.

5. Chain, E., Florey, H. W., Gardner, A. D., Heatley, N. G., Jennings, M. A., Orr-Ewing, J. and Sanders, A. G.: Penicillin as a chemotherapeutic agent. Lancet. *2:*226–228 (Aug. 24) 1940.

6. Abraham, E. P., Chain, E., Fletcher, C. M., Gardner, A. D., Heatley, N. G., Jennings, M. A. and Florey, H. W.: Further observations on penicillin. Lancet. *2:*177–188; 189 (Aug. 16) 1941.

7. Heilman, Dorothy H. and Herrell, W. E.: Comparative antibacterial activity of penicillin and gramicidin: tissue culture studies. Proc. Staff Meet., Mayo Clin. 17:321–327 (May 27) 1942. (Abstr.) Comparative bacteriostatic activity of penicillin and gramicidin. J. Bact. *43:*12–13 (Jan.) 1942.

8. Bornstein, Siegbert: Action of penicillin on enterococci and other streptococci. J. Bact. *39:*383–387 (Apr.) 1940.

9. Dawson, M. H., Hobby, Gladys L. and Lipman, Miriam O.: Penicillin sensitivity of strains of non-hemolytic streptococci isolated from cases of sub-acute bacterial endocarditis. Proc. Soc. Exper. Biol. & Med. *56:*101–102 (June) 1944.

10. Robinson, H. J.: Toxicity and efficacy of penicillin. J. Pharmacol. & Exper. Therap. *77:*70–79 (Jan.) 1943.

11. Rammelkamp, C. H. and Maxon, Thelma: Resistance of *Staphylococcus aureus* to the action of penicillin. Proc. Soc. Exper. Biol. & Med. *51:*386–389 (Dec.) 1942.

12. Spink, W. W., Ferris, Viola and Vivino, Jean J.: Comparative *in vitro* resistance of staphylococci to penicillin and to sodium sulfathiazole. Proc. Soc. Exper. Biol. & Med. *55:*207–210 (Mar.) 1944.

13. Rantz, L. A., Kirby, W. M. M. and Randall, Elizabeth: The action of penicillin on the staphylococcus in vitro. J. Immunol. *48:*335–343 (June) 1944.

14. Hobby, Gladys, Meyer, Karl and Chaffee, Eleanor: Observations on the mechanism of action of penicillin. Proc. Soc. Exper. Biol. & Med. *50:*281–285 (June) 1942.

15. Foster, J. W. and Woodruff, H. B.: Microbiological aspects of penicillin. I. Methods of assay. J. Bact. *46:*187–202 (Aug.) 1943.

16. Foster, J. W. and Wilker, B. L.: Microbiological aspects of penicillin. II. Turbidimetric studies on penicillin inhibition. J. Bact. *46:*377–389 (Oct.) 1943.

17. Abraham, E. P. and Chain, E.: An enzyme from bacteria able to destroy penicillin. Nature. *146:*837 (Dec. 28) 1940.

18. Kirby, W. M. M.: Extraction of a highly potent penicillin inactivator from penicillin resistant staphylococci. Science. n.s. *99:*452–453 (June 2) 1944.

19. Bondi, Amedeo, Jr. and Dietz, Catherine C.: Relationship of penicillinase to the action of penicillin. Proc. Soc. Exper. Biol. & Med. *56:*135–137 (June) 1944.

20. Harper, G. J.: Inhibition of penicillin in routine culture media. Lancet. *2:*569–571 (Nov. 6) 1943.

21. Bondi, Amedeo, Jr. and Dietz, Catherine C.: Production of penicillinase by bacteria. Proc. Soc. Exper. Biol. & Med. *56:*132–134 (June) 1944.

22. Ungar, J.: Penicillinase from B. subtilis. Nature. *154*:236–237 (Aug. 19) 1944.

23. Woodruff, H. B. and Foster, J. W.: Bacterial penicillinase. (Abstr.) J. Bact. 47: 425–426 (May) 1944.

24. Lawrence, C. A.: Sterility test for penicillin. Science. n.s. *98*:413–414 (Nov. 5) 1943.

25. Lawrence, C. A.: Action of clarase upon penicillin. Science. n.s. *99*:15–16 (Jan. 7) 1944.

26. Stanley, A. R.: Clarase inactivation of penicillin. Science. n.s. *99*:59 (Jan. 21) 1944.

27. Miller, C. P. and Foster, Alice Z.: Studies on the action of penicillin. III. Bacterial action of penicillin on meningococcus *in vitro*. Proc. Soc. Exper. Biol. & Med. *56*:205–208 (June) 1944.

28. Hobby, Gladys L. and Dawson, M. H.: Effect of rate of growth of bacteria on action of penicillin. Proc. Soc. Exper. Biol. & Med. *56*:181–184 (June) 1944.

29. Herrell, W. E. and Heilman, Dorothy H.: Tissue culture studies on cytotoxicity of bactericidal agents. III. Cytotoxic and antibacterial activity of gramicidin and penicillin; comparison with other germicides. Am. J. M. Sc. *206*:221–226 (Aug.) 1943.

30. Hobby, Gladys L., Meyer, Karl and Chaffee, Eleanor: Activity of penicillin *in vitro*. Proc. Soc. Exper. Biol. & Med. *50*:277–280 (June) 1942.

31. Herrell, W. E., Heilman, Dorothy H. and Williams, H. L.: The clinical use of penicillin. Proc. Staff Meet., Mayo Clin. *17*:609–616 (Dec. 30) 1942.

32. Ungar, J.: Synergistic effect of para-aminobenzoic acid and sulphapyridine on penicillin. Nature. *152*:245–246 (Aug. 28) 1943.

33. Hobby, Gladys L. and Dawson, M. H.: Relationship of penicillin to sulfonamide action. Proc. Soc. Exper. Biol. & Med. *56*:184–187 (June) 1944.

34. T'ung, Tsun: *In vitro* action of penicillin alone, and in combination with sulfathiazole, on *Brucella* organisms. Proc. Soc. Exper. Biol. & Med. *56*:8–11 (May) 1944.

35. Bigger, J. W.: Synergic action of penicillin and sulphonamides. Lancet. *2*:142–145 (July 29) 1944.

36. Foster, J. W. and Woodruff, H. B.: Microbiological aspects of streptothricin. II. Antibiotic activity of streptothricin. Arch. Biochem. *3*:241–255 (Dec.) 1943.

37. Gardner, A. D.: Morphological effects of penicillin on bacteria. Nature. *146*:837–838 (Dec. 28) 1940.

38. Walker, E. W. A. and Murray, W.: The effect of certain dyes upon the cultural characters of the Bacillus typhosus and some other micro-organisms. Brit. M. J. *2*:16–18 (July 2) 1904.

39. Tunnicliff, Ruth: The action of prontosil-soluble and sulfanilamide on the phagocytic activity of leukocytes and on the dissociation of streptococci. J. Infect. Dis. *64*:59–65 (Jan.-Feb.) 1939.

40. Miller, C. P., Scott, W. W. and Moeller, Velma: Studies on the action of penicillin. I. The rapidity of its therapeutic effect on gonococcic urethritis. J. A. M. A. *125*:607–610 (July 1) 1944.

41. Smith, L. D. and Hay, Thelma: The effect of penicillin on the growth and morphology of Staphylococcus aureus. J. Franklin Inst. *233*:598 (June) 1942.

42. Cornman, Ivor: Survival of normal cells in penicillin solutions lethal to malignant cells. Science. n.s. *99*:247 (Mar. 24) 1944.

43. Lewis, Margaret R.: The failure of purified penicillin to retard the growth of grafts of sarcoma in mice. Science. n.s. *100*:314–315 (Oct. 6) 1944.

44. McKee, Clara M. and Houck, Carol L.: Induced resistance to penicillin of cultures of staphylococci, pneumococci and streptococci. Proc. Soc. Exper. Biol. & Med. *53*:33–34 (May) 1943.

45. Powell, H. M. and Jamieson, W. A.: Response of sulfonamide-fast pneumococci to penicillin. Proc. Soc. Exper. Biol. & Med. *49*:387–389 (Mar.) 1942.

46. McKee, Clara M. and Rake, Geoffrey: Activity of penicillin against strains of pneumococci resistant to sulfonamide drugs. Proc. Soc. Exper. Biol. & Med. *51*:275–278 (Nov.) 1942.

47. Tillett, W. S., Cambier, Margaret J. and Harris, W. H., Jr.: Sulfonamide-fast pneumococci. A clinical report of two cases of pneumonia together with experimental studies on the effectiveness of penicillin and tyrothricin against sulfonamide-resistant strains. J. Clin. Investigation. *22*:249–255 (Mar.) 1943.

48. Schmidt, L. H. and Sesler, Clara L.: Development of resistance to penicillin by pneumococci. Proc. Soc. Exper. Biol. & Med. *52*:353–357 (Apr.) 1943.

49. Lyons, Champ: Penicillin therapy of surgical infections in the U. S. Army; a report. J. A. M. A. *123*:1007–1018 (Dec. 18) 1943.

CHAPTER V

ANTIBACTERIAL ACTIVITY OF PENICILLIN IN VIVO

In general it appears that results of studies on the activity of penicillin in vivo coincide fairly well with the results obtained from studies on its activity in vitro. There are a few exceptions to this general statement, however, which will be mentioned subsequently.

STAPHYLOCOCCAL INFECTIONS

The first attempt to employ penicillin in the treatment of infections in vivo was that reported by Chain and his associates[1] in 1940. They used the mouse as the experimental animal and reported on the effectiveness of penicillin against staphylococci as well as against streptococci and certain pathogenic anaerobes.

Although the penicillin used by Chain and his associates was relatively impure, they met with notable success in the treatment of staphylococcal infections in mice. Infections were established in these animals by injecting intraperitoneally twenty to twenty-four hour broth cultures of virulent staphylococci. The inoculum varied from 200,000,000 to 760,000,000 cocci. The infections were of lethal intensity. In the final experiment reported by these investigators, twenty-four of twenty-four control mice died and twenty-one of twenty-four of the treated group survived. Penicillin was administered subcutaneously every three hours for four days. The total amount of penicillin used per mouse for treatment in this experiment was 11.5 mg. Treatment was begun one hour after inoculation with staphylococci. Thus, from these original observations in 1940, the therapeutic possibility of penicillin became evident. When more thoroughly purified penicillin became available, studies on its effectiveness against staphylococcal infections naturally were extended.

Robinson[2] later reported that mice could be completely protected by the subcutaneous administration of penicillin when these animals had received intraperitoneally from 10,000 to as much as 100,000 lethal doses of Staphylococcus aureus. In Robinson's studies, treatment was begun almost immediately after the bacterial inoculation, and penicillin was given every three hours night and day for five days. The amount of penicillin necessary to afford complete protection was 60 Oxford units per day, or a total dose of 300 units. In these experiments, Robinson compared the effectiveness of penicillin with that of sulfathiazole. To

45

afford complete protection, 4 mg. of sulfathiazole per day were required as compared with 1 mg. of penicillin. It was obvious from these experiments, therefore, that a considerably smaller quantity of penicillin than of sulfonamides was required for equally effective treatment of experimental staphylococcal infections.

Powell and Jamieson[3] also studied the protective effect of penicillin when given orally to mice infected with Staphylococcus aureus. In these experiments, again, the effectiveness of penicillin was compared with that of sulfathiazole. The survival rate among the animals which received penicillin by mouth was approximately 60 per cent and this was double the survival rate which obtained among the group of animals which received sulfathiazole by mouth. In these studies, in which penicillin was administered orally, sodium bicarbonate was given simultaneously to neutralize the gastric acids and thereby to protect penicillin from them. I suspect that the death rate of 40 per cent probably was due to the fact that in many instances adequate therapeutic levels of penicillin never were reached in the blood stream because of destruction of penicillin by gastric acids.

Further studies in vivo on the effectiveness of penicillin against Staphylococcus aureus were reported by Robson and Scott.[4] They produced ulceration of the cornea of the eye of the rabbit by using extremely virulent strains of staphylococci. The lesions were treated locally with penicillin every hour, starting one hour after inoculation and continuing for forty-eight hours. Lesions were produced in both eyes of individual rabbits and one eye was treated, the other serving as a control. There appeared to be a definite beneficial effect on the development of these lesions following local application of penicillin. If twenty-four hours were allowed to elapse between the inoculation and the beginning of treatment, no benefit followed application of penicillin. However, the staphylococci were eliminated from the flora of the conjunctival sac. Robson and Scott pointed out the importance, therefore, of early treatment if clinical use of penicillin for these conditions was to be made on the basis of their experiments. In these studies it again was evident that penicillin was far superior to the other agents used by the investigators, including sulfathiazole.

Further work of a similar nature was then reported by von Sallmann.[5] Experimental staphylococcal infections were produced in the anterior chamber of the eye of the rabbit. The effectiveness of sulfadiazine, given orally and topically, was compared with the effectiveness of penicillin applied topically. Beneficial effects were obtained in 21.7 per cent of the eyes treated, orally or topically, with sulfadiazine, whereas the infection was controlled in between 62.5 and 75 per cent of the eyes in which penicillin was used topically. In these experiments, six to seven hours were allowed to elapse between inoculation and onset of treatment. Purulent endophthalmitis was present in all of these eyes.

Further experimental studies on the effectiveness of penicillin in vivo against staphylococcal infections were reported by Pilcher and Meacham.[6] Experimental staphylococcal meningitis was produced in dogs. The animals then received penicillin intravenously in single large doses of 2,500 to 3,000 Oxford units in one experiment and in another series the animals received repeated intravenous injections of 500 units each five times a day. The infection was not controlled by this form of treatment. On the other hand, this fact does not discredit the effectiveness of penicillin in vivo against the Staphylococcus aureus. When penicillin was administered by the intrathecal route, a reduction in mortality occurred among these animals. These results are best explained on the basis that when penicillin is administered intravenously it does not appear sufficiently to diffuse into the normal or the diseased cerebrospinal structures. Studies which confirm this interpretation are discussed in the section on absorption, diffusion and excretion of penicillin.

These fundamental studies made in vivo leave little doubt that penicillin is superior to any other agent available to date in the treatment of experimental staphylococcal infections.

STREPTOCOCCAL INFECTIONS

Chain and his associates[1] established lethal infections in mice with Streptococcus pyogenes. The inoculum varied between 350,000,000 and 450,000,000 cocci, living and dead. In their final experiment, reported in 1940, two hours were allowed to elapse between inoculation and institution of treatment. Treatment was continued for forty-five hours and each mouse received a total dose of 7.5 mg. of penicillin. The animals were observed for ten days. Of twenty-five untreated animals, all were dead within twenty-four hours following inoculation. Twenty-four of the twenty-five animals which received penicillin were alive and well at the end of the ten days of observation. Here, again, it became evident that penicillin was an exceedingly effective agent against another serious pyogenic infection.

Subsequently, Hobby and her associates[7] examined the effectiveness of penicillin against overwhelming infections with Streptococcus pyogenes in mice. These animals received at least 1,000,000 lethal doses of a virulent strain of the organism. Using a sample of penicillin, the potency of which varied between 150 and 200 Oxford units per milligram, it was found that 1.5 mg. of this material was sufficient to protect animals so infected. This protective effect of penicillin could be obtained by giving the drug either intravenously, intraperitoneally or subcutaneously. Implantations of dry pellets of penicillin, or injections of penicillin in sesame oil, also yielded a high degree of protection to nearly two-thirds of the animals inoculated with 1,000 lethal doses of Streptococcus pyogenes. These investigators used both the ammonium and the sodium salts of penicillin.

Karl Meyer and his associates[8] also investigated the possible value of the esters of penicillin in treatment of hemolytic streptococcal infections of mice. The methyl, ethyl, and n-butyl esters of penicillin used in these studies were prepared by Meyer. While these esters possessed very feeble activity in vitro, marked protection was afforded experimental animals by a total dose of 1.5 mg. of the ethyl ester and 2.5 mg. of the methyl ester of penicillin. These amounts of the esters of penicillin were found to afford complete protection against as much as 100,000 lethal doses of the organism. As was pointed out in a previous chapter (p. 23), the value of such preparations of penicillin lies primarily in the fact that these esters are stable at the pH of the gastric juice and, therefore, can be administered by mouth. It seems likely that the protection afforded by these preparations is due to hydrolysis of the ester within the body, by which active penicillin is freed. Approximately ten times as much of the material must be administered by mouth as by the subcutaneous route. As I have mentioned earlier also (p. 24), it is unfortunate that the dose of the methyl and ethyl esters of penicillin which afforded protection to these animals rather closely approached LD_{50}. If the higher esters of penicillin prove less toxic and at the same time retain their antibacterial activity, it may yet be possible to prepare penicillin that will be suitable for oral administration.

The studies of Robinson[2] further established the effectiveness of penicillin against experimental infections due to Streptococcus pyogenes. A comparison also was made by Robinson between the effectiveness of penicillin and that of sulfanilamide. According to his studies, 120 Oxford units of penicillin per day (2 mg.) was sufficient to protect 100 per cent of the animals against streptococcal infections produced by intraperitoneal inoculation. To afford the same degree of protection it was necessary, on the other hand, to administer 16 mg. of sulfanilamide per day as compared with a dose of 2 mg. of penicillin. None of the untreated mice survived as long as twenty-four hours. Here again is emphasized that penicillin is exceedingly more effective against certain coccal infections than is sulfanilamide. Robinson gave penicillin subcutaneously and began treatment immediately after inoculation. Treatment was continued for five days and penicillin was administered every three hours day and night.

PNEUMOCOCCAL INFECTIONS

I already have indicated that there appeared to be some variation in the sensitivity of different strains of pneumococci to penicillin as measured by tests made in vitro (p. 30). However, most of the reports to date on the effectiveness of penicillin against pneumococci in vivo are in agreement that penicillin is fairly effective against this group of organisms. The first report on the general subject was that of Powell and Jamieson,[9] who examined the effectiveness of penicillin against Diplococcus pneumoniae. They used different strains of types I, II and III, including sulfapyridine-fast strains. Penicillin was given to mice orally, with soda, at different intervals for several days. Their results indicated that penicillin was highly effective against both the parent strains and the sulfonamide-fast strains of types I and II. Penicillin also was found to be moderately effective against both parent and sulfonamide-fast strains of Diplococcus pneumoniae, type III.

The report of McKee and Rake[10] on the effectiveness of penicillin against sulfonamide resistant pneumococci is in agreement with the above mentioned studies. It was evident that the development of resistance to sulfonamides, therefore, does not interfere with the activity of penicillin. In the experiments carried out by McKee and Rake, penicillin was administered simultaneously with the inoculum into the peritoneum. Eighty-four per cent of the treated mice could be protected with as little as 1 unit of penicillin. Likewise, Hobby and her associates[7] reported that mice could be satisfactorily protected against severe infections owing to virulent pneumococci, type II, following subcutaneous administration of penicillin. In a subsequent report on the general subject, Robinson[2] compared the effectiveness of penicillin and sulfadiazine in overwhelming infections due to Diplococcus pneumoniae, type I. He found that 120 units (2 mg.) of penicillin daily for five days completely protected the mice against these infections. Under similar conditions, eight times as much sulfadiazine (16 mg.) per day did not afford complete protection. For example, of the twenty animals which received sulfadiazine, only three survived for ten days. It was further evident from Robinson's studies that penicillin would protect these animals even when six or seven hours had been allowed to elapse between inoculation and onset of treatment. In contrast, when the same interval elapsed between inoculation and institution of treatment of the animals with sulfonamide, there was no protective effect whatever. It can be concluded from these reports, therefore, that penicillin is superior to sulfonamides in the treatment of infections due to at least some strains of Diplococcus pneumoniae.

Further experimental studies on the effectiveness of penicillin against Diplococcus pneumoniae were reported by von Sallmann.[11] Experimental intra-ocular infections were produced in rabbits with Diplococcus pneumoniae, types III, VII and X. Both the sodium and the ammonium salts of penicillin were applied locally to the infected eyes for two to four days. The solutions used contained 0.25 and 0.1 per cent of penicillin. In check-

3

ing these infections, penicillin proved effective even when treatment was started as long as twelve or thirteen hours after the infection had been produced. Even when the infection was accompanied by injury to the capsule of the lens, penicillin was effective against infections caused by types III and X. In this investigation a comparison also was made between the effectiveness of penicillin and sulfadiazine. Under the conditions of the experiment, sulfadiazine was found ineffective. This is in general agreement with the findings of Robinson, mentioned above.

Von Sallmann[11] reported that Diplococcus pneumoniae, types VI, XIV, XIX and XXIII also were found to be equally as sensitive to penicillin in vitro as were types III and VII, which were used to produce these experimental infections in the eyes of rabbits. I am inclined to believe that practically all strains of pneumococci are sufficiently sensitive to penicillin to justify its clinical use against infections with the organism.

MENINGOCOCCAL INFECTIONS

It is evident from all the reports available on studies in vitro that Neisseria intracellularis (meningococcus) is extremely sensitive to the action of penicillin. The first report on the effectiveness of penicillin in vivo against meningococcal infections was that of Dawson and his associates.[12] Infections were established in mice; two strains of Neisseria intracellularis were used. The treated animals received a total of 1,800 Oxford units given in sesame oil, subcutaneously, a half hour, eighteen hours and twenty-four hours after inoculation. This amount of penicillin afforded almost complete protection against the infection while all of the control animals died within twenty-four hours.

Miller and Foster[13] likewise carried out studies which clearly indicate that penicillin is effective in the treatment of experimental meningococcal infections of mice. Mice were inoculated with 100,000 minimum lethal doses. The animals received single injections of 100 Oxford units each at varying intervals following the infection. Not all of the animals could be protected. However, of one group of thirteen mice to which a smaller inoculum (10,000 minimum lethal doses) was administered, and which were treated at the same intervals, all survived except one. In this instance treatment was given a half hour after inoculation. These authors also pointed out that the method of producing experimental meningococcal infections in the mouse involves the use of mucin, without which meningococci, even the most virulent strains according to them, will not initiate a genuine infection. They wrote that penicillin was found equally effective if administered intravenously, subcutaneously or intramuscularly.

INFECTIONS DUE TO ANAEROBES

In their original studies, the Oxford investigators[1] examined the effectiveness of penicillin in vivo against certain pathogenic anaerobic organisms. While they encountered some difficulty in establishing infections in mice with Clostridium welchii, they were successful in their experiments in which the organism of infection was Clostridium septicum. In their preliminary experiments it was found that the administration of penicillin for two days did not prevent the development of the infection after administration of penicillin had been discontinued. In their final experiment, however, in which fifty mice were used, the twenty-five controls all died within seventeen hours after the inoculation. To the twenty-five treated mice, penicillin was administered by subcutaneous injection for ten days. At the end of the experiment, twenty-four of the twenty-five treated mice had survived. From these studies it became evident that penicillin might prove of value in the treatment of infections due to certain anaerobes responsible for gas gangrene.

McIntosh and Selbie[14, 15] were successful in producing lethal infections in mice with Clostridium welchii and were, therefore, able to examine the effectiveness of penicillin against this organism in vivo. Since most animals which survived three days lived indefinitely, the study was based primarily on the survival rate in the first three days. When infections produced with 100 lethal doses of Clostridium welchii were followed immediately by one injection of 34 Oxford units of penicillin into the site of inoculation, the infections were controlled in all of the animals. When treatment was withheld for three to six hours after inoculation, the animals died although their lives were slightly prolonged. Penicillin proved much superior to other therapeutic agents studied, including the sulfonamides, against infections owing to Clostridium welchii. The investigators also confirmed the value of penicillin in treatment of experimental infections due to Clostridium septicum, which had been reported previously by Chain and his associates. McIntosh and Selbie also were aware of the additive effect of antitoxin combined with chemotherapy in the treatment of these anaerobic infections. The practical significance of this will be discussed in the section on the clinical use of penicillin in the treatment of gas gangrene.

Hac and Hubert[16] further investigated the effectiveness of penicillin against Clostridium welchii. They had shown previously that sulfadiazine and sulfathiazole would protect approximately half of the animals infected with Clostridium welchii. However, in none of these animals was the infection completely eradicated. Using a single subcutaneous injection of 50 units of penicillin administered at the same time that the infection was established, they could protect 98 per cent of the infected animals. Repeated small doses were equally effective if the first dose was given immediately after inoculation. If three or more hours elapsed between inoculation and beginning of treatment, decrease in survival rate resulted. In addition to these studies carried out on mice, Hac and Hubert also reported equally satisfactory results in the treatment of these infections in guinea pigs. Using larger doses in a subsequent study, Hac[17] found that 100 per cent of animals could be protected by administration of penicillin in the presence of infections owing to Clostridium welchii. In addition to establishing the fact that penicillin was effective in vivo, their studies definitely indicated that penicillin is far superior to the sulfonamides in treatment of these infections.

Dawson and his associates[12] carried out studies which indicate that rather large amounts of penicillin are essential in the treatment of anaerobic infections. It appeared from their studies that in order to afford complete protection to guinea pigs against infections with spores of Clostridium welchii (equivalent to half the minimal lethal dose) 666 units of penicillin was necessary. Their studies also indicated that relatively large amounts of penicillin were required to protect mice infected with Clostridium septicum.

McKee, Hamre and Rake[18] reported studies in which penicillin was found to be effective in the treatment of infections owing to Clostridium perfringens. Mice were infected intramuscularly and penicillin was used locally for treatment. When guinea pigs were infected through established wounds, these investigators were unsuccessful in treatment of this infection. According to them, the failure was due to the frequency of intercurrent infections and to toxicity of penicillin for guinea pigs when it was necessary to give repeated doses of the drug.

Von Sallmann[5] was unsuccessful in his attempt to control destructive endophthalmitis of rabbits, produced by intralenticular injections of Clostridium welchii. It seems likely that the long period (six hours) which elapsed between establishment of the infection and beginning of treatment explains this failure.

It is evident that penicillin is effective against the anaerobic organisms commonly associated with gas gangrene. The experimental results reported to date, however, are somewhat irregular due in part to the difficulty associated with establishing uniform infections. The irregularity in the reports may be explainable in part also on the basis of the wide variations in the amounts of penicillin used in the early studies. At any rate, the evidence is definitely in favor of penicillin over many other therapeutic agents available up to the time that penicillin was introduced. Obviously, penicillin has no neutralizing effect against the toxin produced by these organisms. It is understandable, therefore, that a combination of penicillin with antitoxin must be considered in treatment of established infections due to these microbes.

ANTHRAX INFECTIONS

It was evident from the studies in vitro reported by Fleming[19] and by the Oxford investigators[20] that Bacillus anthracis was fairly sensitive to the action of penicillin. Until penicillin became available, the chemo-therapeutic agents used experimentally to combat anthrax infections produced in small animals were limited, for the most part, to neoars-phenamine and sulfonamides. According to Gold,[21] the published reports on neoarsphenamine for treatment of experimental anthrax have not been encouraging. Cruickshank[22] reported results which seemed to indicate that the sulfonamides possess some effect against experimental anthrax. Others, including May and Buck,[23] however, found no reduction in mortality following use of these drugs but did find that the lives of animals which received sulfonamides were somewhat prolonged.

In order to determine the possible effectiveness of penicillin against experimental infections due to Bacillus anthracis, F. R. Heilman and I[24] carried out experiments. In the initial experiments the animals received at least 10,000 lethal doses of Bacillus anthracis and sixteen hours were

TABLE 5

EFFECT OF PENICILLIN ON MORTALITY RATE AMONG MICE INOCULATED
WITH BACILLUS ANTHRACIS

Number	Mice that died each day after inoculation										Number of mice that died	Mortality rate, per cent
	Days after inoculation											
	1	2	3	4	5	6	7	8	9	10–26		
Treated (20 mice)	0	0	0	0	0	0	0	0	0	0	0	0
Untreated (20 mice)	0	8	8	4	0	0	0	0	0	0	20	100

allowed to elapse between the time of inoculation and the beginning of treatment. The mice received 1,000 units of penicillin every twenty-four hours. Both the sodium and the calcium salts of penicillin were used for treatment; 125 Oxford units of penicillin were administered in physiologic saline solution at 9 a. m., 12 noon, 3 p. m. and 6 p. m. At 9 p. m. 500 units of penicillin suspended in sesame oil was administered, to last through the night. Even though the mice received so overwhelming an infection and were allowed to remain without treatment for sixteen hours, we were able to protect more than half (55 per cent) of them. By using a smaller inoculum, and starting treatment with penicillin one hour after injection, the results were even more striking. In the final experiment, in which forty mice were concerned, the twenty untreated controls all died within ninety-six hours after they had received the inoculation. All twenty of the animals that were treated with penicillin survived and all appeared well at the end of the experiment. These animals were observed for a period of twenty-six days (table 5).

SPIROCHETAL INFECTIONS

One of the most interesting phases in connection with intensive studies on the selective antibacterial action of penicillin was the discovery by Mahoney, Arnold and Harris[25] that penicillin exhibited at least spirochetostatic action. A report of these studies on the effectiveness of penicillin against Treponema pallidum, together with the first attempts to treat syphilis of man with penicillin, was made by Mahoney at the seventy-second annual meeting of the American Public Health Association in New York City, October 12–14, 1943.

Experimental Syphilis.—Mahoney and his associates mentioned that limited animal experiments indicated that penicillin possessed some spirocheticidal activity. The results of their studies on the effectiveness of the substance against experimental syphilis of rabbits were sufficiently encouraging to cause them to proceed with treatment of human beings who were suffering with acute syphilis. The results of the clinical studies will be considered later in the section on the clinical use of penicillin.

Subsequent studies by Dunham and his associates[26] were carried out to test the effectiveness of penicillin against experimental syphilis of rabbits. It appeared from their studies that penicillin did exert at least some protection against syphilis. In the studies on prophylaxis of syphilitic skin infections of rabbits it was noted, however, that some chancres developed late, although the lesions were smaller than usual. Dunham and his associates further reported that rabbits which received insufficient amounts of penicillin were found to harbor strains of the spirochete which were more resistant to the action of penicillin than was the Nichols strain used to produce the experimental infections. If such resistance develops through subeffective doses, the practical significance of these findings is, of course, far reaching.

In the opening part of this chapter it was pointed out that the activity of penicillin in vivo coincides fairly well with its activity in vitro. However, it also was pointed out that there were some exceptions to this general statement. The antispirochetal action of penicillin is one of these exceptions. For example, in the preliminary tests in vitro reported by Dunham and his associates, 240 Oxford units per 0.8 c.c. of culture failed to reveal any action on the spirochetes of syphilis. There was, however, some activity when concentrations of penicillin as high as 800 to 1,600 units were present per 0.8 c.c. of culture. These findings suggest a rather feeble action of penicillin against spirochetes of syphilis in vitro; yet studies in vivo clearly indicate that penicillin is rather effective.

Experimental Relapsing Fever.—The report of Mahoney and his associates stimulated investigators to test further the possible effectiveness of penicillin against other pathogenic spirochetes. The next spirochetal infection to be studied in vivo was that produced by a strain of the spirochete of relapsing fever. In spite of the fact that there appeared to be no evident effect in vitro on the motility of the spirochete of relapsing fever (Borrelia novyi), F. R. Heilman and I[27] examined the possible effectiveness of penicillin against this infection in vivo.

Mice were heavily inoculated with Borrelia novyi by intra-abdominal injection of 0.3 c.c. of rat blood containing great numbers of the organisms. The course of the infection was followed by daily examination of thick smears of blood from the tail, stained with Giemsa's stain. Twenty-two hours after inoculation, treatment with penicillin was begun and was continued for four days. In the blood of the treated animals, the number of organisms was markedly reduced and, in some instances, they were totally absent after twenty-four hours of treatment with penicillin.

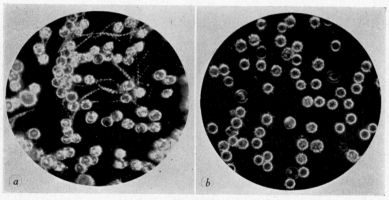

Fig. 4.—*a*, Dark field of blood of untreated mouse, containing spirochetes of relapsing fever, forty-eight hours after inoculation; *b*, dark field of blood of treated mouse, free of spirochetes, forty-eight hours after inoculation and twenty-four hours after beginning of treatment with penicillin.

At the same time, in the blood of untreated mice the degree of infection was severe. As is evident in figures 4 and 5, penicillin exhibited a rather marked antispirochetal action in vivo.

The infections produced in these studies were sufficiently severe to cause the death of 75 per cent of the untreated animals. Only 4 per cent of the treated mice failed to recover and those animals that did die did not have spirochetes in their blood and did not harbor the other pathologic changes commonly found in animals which die of this infection. In addition to suggesting that penicillin would be of value in the treatment of relapsing fever, these studies lend considerable confirmation to the spirochetostatic action of penicillin.

Almost immediately following the reports from the Mayo Clinic on experimental relapsing fever, Lourie and Collier[28] reported studies which were in agreement with our results. It was evident from their studies that the blood of mice infected with another strain of the spirochete of relapsing fever (Spirochaeta recurrentis) could be cleared of the spirochetes within twenty-four hours by subcutaneous injection of 250 units of penicillin.

Likewise, Augustine, Weinman and McAllister[29] succeeded in sterilizing, within twenty-seven hours, the blood streams of mice inoculated with Borrelia novyi. That penicillin eliminated the spirochete from the blood stream of these experimental animals was evident from the fact that inoculation of the blood from treated animals into fresh mice in an attempt to convey the infection was unsuccessful.

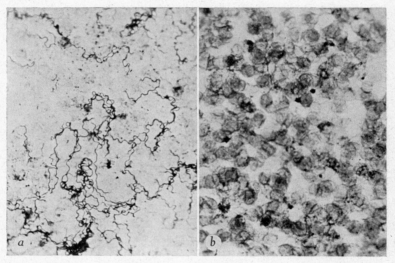

Fig. 5.—a, Thick smear of blood of untreated mouse containing spirochetes of relapsing fever forty-eight hours after inoculation; b, thick smear of blood of treated mouse free of spirochetes, forty-eight hours after inoculation and twenty-four hours after beginning of treatment with penicillin (Giemsa's stain, × 1000).

Further confirmation of the effectiveness of penicillin against infections with Borrelia novyi was the report of Eagle, Magnuson and Musselman.[30] Their studies were carried out on both mice and rats.

Experimental Weil's Disease.—The next disease of spirochetal origin in which the effectiveness of penicillin was tested was experimental leptospirosis icterohaemorrhagica (Weil's disease). These studies were reported from the Mayo Clinic by F. R. Heilman and me.[31] Previous to the introduction of penicillin, none of the chemotherapeutic agents, including arsenicals and sulfonamides, had been found to be effective against this infection. It is of some interest, also, that the Oxford investigators[20] concluded from in vitro tests that Leptospira icterohaemorrhagiae was relatively insensitive to the action of penicillin. Here is another example of the feeble action of penicillin in vitro, and yet studies made in vivo clearly indicate a fairly high degree of effectiveness. This difference between results of studies in vivo and in vitro seems to be characteristic of the spirochetes.

In the experiments reported by Heilman and me, guinea pigs received lethal infections with the spirochete of Weil's disease. In the final experiment, sixty-four guinea pigs were infected. Seventeen to twenty-four hours were allowed to elapse between inoculation and the beginning of treatment. The treated animals received only 800 units of the calcium salt of penicillin per day. Treatment was continued for seven days. Of the thirty-two untreated animals, twenty-nine (91 per cent) died of Weil's disease (table 6). Examination of these animals revealed the

TABLE 6

Effect of Penicillin (Calcium) on Mortality Among Guinea Pigs Inoculated with Leptospira Icterohaemorrhagiae

| | Guinea pigs that died each day after inoculation | | | | | | | Number of guinea pigs that died | Mortality rate, per cent |
| | Days after inoculation | | | | | | | | |
	1 to 4	5	6	7	8	9	10		
Treated (32 guinea pigs)	0	2*	1*					3	9
Untreated (32 guinea pigs)	0	2	7	13	3	1	3	29	91

* Died from toxic effects of penicillin.

presence of typical lesions of experimental Weil's disease, including multiple hemorrhagic lesions in the lungs which impart to the lungs the appearance commonly described as "butterfly lung" (fig. 6). The untreated animals also ran a fever which persisted for several days. Rectal temperatures as high as 104.5° F. were recorded among the untreated guinea pigs (fig. 7).

Of the thirty-two animals treated with penicillin, none died of the disease although three died from the toxic effects of penicillin that commonly are encountered among guinea pigs, especially if these animals receive 800 or more units of penicillin per day. This intolerance for penicillin is a peculiarity of guinea pigs and is of some importance to the investigator who attempts to use this animal for studies in vivo. The treated animals, in none of which Weil's disease developed, were later killed and examined. None were found to have the lesions of leptospirosis icterohaemorrhagica. It was evident from these studies that penicillin might be of value in the treatment of Weil's disease.

Subsequent studies on the general subject were reported by Augustine, Weinman and McAllister[32] which seemed to indicate that penicillin

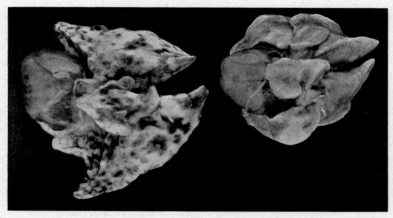

Fig. 6.— Lung and heart of two guinea pigs inoculated with Leptospira icterohaemor-rhagiae. *Left*, lung of untreated guinea pig killed seven days after inoculation. Note multiple hemorrhages, so-called butterfly lung. *Right*, entirely normal heart and lung of animal treated with penicillin.

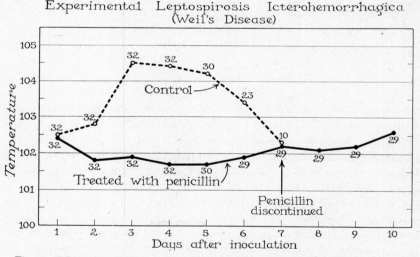

Fig. 7.—Effect of penicillin on experimental leptospirosis icterohaemorrhagica (Weil's disease); mean temperatures of control animals and animals treated with penicillin. Numbers represent surviving animals on respective days of experiment.

might prove effective in the treatment of Weil's disease. Their experiment also brought out two other significant points. Penicillin is not likely to save young guinea pigs if treatment is delayed until these animals are moribund. Their experiment also confirmed the previously established fact that penicillin in large doses is toxic for guinea pigs.

RAT-BITE FEVER

It is now fairly well established that the disease known as rat-bite fever has been recognized for many centuries. It is established, also, that two different pathogens may be associated with the disease: Spirillum minus or Streptobacillus moniliformis. While the disease usually follows the bite of a rat, infections apparently due to the latter organism also may occur in epidemic form without the bite of a rat being the source of infection. Arsenical preparations have been found to be of some value against infections owing to Spirillum minus. On the other hand, neither arsenical drugs nor sulfonamides have proved of value in the treatment of experimental infections known to be due to Streptobacillus monilifor-mis or in clinical infections apparently due to this organism.

F. R. Heilman[33] studied the effect of gold sodium thiomalate in the treatment of mice experimentally infected with Streptobacillus monilifor-mis. A single injection of the preparation of gold was found to protect these animals against otherwise rapidly fatal infections. On the other hand, the hazards attending the use of gold therapy are well known to all. In the search for a more suitable therapeutic agent in the treatment of rat-bite fever, studies were carried out by Heilman and me[34] to test the effect of penicillin against both Spirillum minus and Streptobacillus moniliformis.

While these studies were in progress, Lourie and Collier[28] reported results obtained by them, which definitely suggested that penicillin would be effective against infections of mice with Spirillum minus. These investigators found that 250 units of penicillin administered intravenously fifteen minutes after inoculation of the animals with Spirillum minus prevented the development of disease. In one experiment carried out by them seven to ten days were allowed to elapse between the time of inoculation and the onset of treatment. At that time, a few spirochetes were still present in the blood of these animals. The investigators then compared the results obtained in a group of animals treated with neoarsphenamine and in another group treated with penicillin. It was evident from their studies that penicillin was more effective than neoarsphenamine. They did not examine the effectiveness of penicillin against the other pathogenic organism which apparently can be responsible for rat-bite fever (Streptobacillus moniliformis).

In the experiments reported by Heilman and me, fifty mice were inoculated with Spirillum minus by intra-abdominal injection of 0.4 c.c. of infected, citrated mouse blood. Treatment of twenty-five of the mice with penicillin was begun ten days after inoculation. The blood of both

the control and the treated animals was examined throughout the course
of the experiment, which extended for thirty days. At the time that
treatment with penicillin was begun, all of the blood films of the treated
mice revealed spirilla. After twenty-four hours' treatment with penicillin,
the blood films were all negative for spirilla and remained negative
throughout the entire experiment. While this infection is not usually
fatal to mice, five of the untreated, and one of the treated, mice died
during the course of the experiment.

After Heilman and I had determined that complete inhibition of
growth of Streptobacillus moniliformis was obtained in vitro in the
presence of 0.1 unit of penicillin per cubic centimeter, and that partial
inhibition occurred in tubes containing 0.01 unit per cubic centimeter,
we inoculated eighty-six mice with Streptobacillus moniliformis. When
animals are so infected, acute septicemic infections may develop, from
which they may die in from one to several days. In some instances a
more chronic disease may develop, characterized by polyarthritis and
periarticular swellings of the feet and legs. The type of infection varies
with the dose and virulence of the organism. Half (forty-three) of the
animals infected with Streptobacillus moniliformis were treated. The
other half served as controls. Forty-two of the forty-three untreated
mice died, a mortality rate of 98 per cent. Most of these deaths took
place within the first forty-eight hours after inoculation. In the group
which received penicillin, treatment was started two to four and a half
hours after inoculation and was continued for five and a half to seven
days. At the end of thirty days' observation all of the treated animals
were alive and well (table 7).

TABLE 7

EFFECT OF PENICILLIN ON MORTALITY AMONG MICE INOCULATED WITH
STREPTOBACILLUS MONILIFORMIS

Group	Mice that died each day after inoculation										Number of mice that died	Mortality, per cent
	1	2	3	4	5	6	7	8	9	10 to 30		
Treated (43 mice)	0	0	0	0	0	0	0	0	0	0	0	0
Untreated (43 mice)	22	12	0	1	0	0	2	0	1	4	42	98

These studies, as well as those of the other investigators mentioned,
amply suggest that penicillin should prove useful in the treatment of
infections owing to either Spirillum minus or Streptobacillus moniliformis.

ERYSIPELOTHRIX RHUSIOPATHIAE

It is well established that the organism Erysipelothrix rhusiopathiae
is responsible for the disease erysipeloid in man. Until penicillin became
available, no form of treatment except administration of antiserums had

proved effective either experimentally or clinically. Sulfonamides are entirely ineffective.

F. R. Heilman and I[35] reported experiments which tend to indicate that penicillin is exceedingly effective in vivo against this organism. From tests made in vitro it had become evident that all three strains of the organism examined were completely inhibited in the presence of 0.1 Oxford unit of penicillin per cubic centimeter. Partial inhibition also had occurred in tubes containing 0.01 unit per cubic centimeter. Eighty mice were inoculated with a virulent strain of Erysipelothrix rhusiopathiae. In mice infected with this organism, septicemia usually develops and the mice die in a few days. Forty of the mice received penicillin and forty served as controls. Treatment of some of the animals with penicillin was begun immediately after inoculation but treatment of one group was not begun until twenty-one hours after inoculation. Of the forty untreated mice, all were dead at the end of the eighth day of the experiment, a mortality rate of 100 per cent. More than half of them died in the first four days. Of the forty animals that received penicillin only two died, a mortality rate of 5 per cent (table 8).

TABLE 8

EFFECT OF PENICILLIN ON MORTALITY AMONG MICE INOCULATED WITH
ERYSIPELOTHRIX RHUSIOPATHIAE

	Mice that died each day after inoculation										Total mice that died	Mortality rate, per cent
	Days after inoculation											
	1	2	3	4	5	6	7	8	9	10 to 14		
Treated (40 mice)	0	0	0	0	0	0	0	1	0	1	2	5
Untreated (40 mice)	0	6	12	8	6	4	3	1	0	0	40	100

These results justify the speculation that penicillin may prove effective in the treatment of this disease in man. Eventually it may be possible to examine the effect of penicillin in the treatment of the disease in swine.

VIRUS AND RICKETTSIAL INFECTIONS

Based on studies made in vivo, there appears to be general agreement among virologists that penicillin is not exceedingly effective against most small viruses. Results of certain studies made in vivo on several larger viruses, however, are somewhat more encouraging. This is possibly explainable on the basis that these larger viruses more nearly approach in their behavior and in certain other characteristics the pathogenic bacteria. F. R. Heilman and I[36, 37] have published reports dealing with the effectiveness of penicillin against the virus of ornithosis and the virus of psittacosis.

It is fairly well established that no therapeutic agent has proved of any significant value in the past in the treatment of experimental infections produced by the virus of ornithosis. In the studies reported by Heilman and me,[36] eighty mice were inoculated with this virus. Of the forty untreated mice, thirty-five died, a mortality rate of 88 per cent. Of the forty mice that received penicillin only two died, a mortality rate of 5 per cent (table 9). The possibility that bacterial infections were

TABLE 9

EFFECT OF PENICILLIN (SODIUM) ON MORTALITY AMONG MICE
INOCULATED WITH THE VIRUS OF ORNITHOSIS

	Mice that died each day after inoculation										Number of mice that died	Mortality, per cent
	Days after inoculation											
	1	2	3	4	5	6	7	8	9	10 to 30		
Treated (40 mice)	0	0	0	0	0	0	0	0	0	2	2	5
Untreated (40 mice)	0	0	7	8	5	5	2	1	2	5	35	88

present to account for the difference in mortality in the two groups[38] was adequately excluded by suitable cultural methods. These results are particularly encouraging since treatment with penicillin was not begun until seventeen hours after inoculation, at which time the infection had become well established. Treatment was continued for seven days and the animals were observed for thirty to thirty-five days. While the animals were protected against otherwise generally fatal infections, it was evident from these studies that penicillin did not completely eliminate the virus from the bodies of the treated mice. On the other hand, a fairly good protective effect against these usually fatal infections was obtained.

Similar studies were reported by Heilman and me[37] in which a highly virulent strain of psittacosis virus of parakeet origin was used to establish experimental infection in mice. In this experiment, 104 mice received lethal doses of the virus of psittacosis. Of the fifty-two untreated mice, all were dead at the end of the sixth day after inoculation, a mortality rate of 100 per cent. Of the fifty-two mice that received penicillin, only four failed to survive the thirty days of observation, a mortality rate of 8 per cent (table 10). In one experiment, sixteen hours were allowed to elapse between the time of inoculation and the beginning of treatment. Treatment was continued for twelve days. It seems certain, therefore, that the virus had become well established in the cells of the mice before treatment was begun and still these animals were protected against lethal infections by the use of penicillin. As in the case of ornithosis, the virus of psittacosis could be recovered from the organs of the mice that survived. In spite of the fact that the virus could not be completely eradicated from the bodies of the animals, the results are encouraging enough to justify the use of penicillin in the treatment of infections owing to these viruses in man.

Greiff and Pinkerton[39] have reported studies which suggest that penicillin is effective against certain rickettsial infections. They found that penicillin exerted a striking inhibitory action on the multiplication of the Rickettsia which causes murine typhus. Their studies were carried out by injecting penicillin in three doses at intervals of forty-eight hours, into the yolk sac of the fetal hen's egg. They suggested that their observations indicated that penicillin probably penetrated the cells as well as exerting a direct effect on extracellular organisms. It was also evident from their studies that while a striking inhibitory action was exerted on rickettsiae, the rickettsiae were not completely eliminated from the infected egg. Sulfonamides were found to have no such inhibitory effect.

TABLE 10

EFFECT OF PENICILLIN (SODIUM) ON MORTALITY AMONG MICE
INOCULATED WITH THE VIRUS OF PSITTACOSIS

	Mice that died each day after inoculation										Total mice that died	Mortality rate, per cent
	Days after inoculation											
	1	2	3	4	5	6	7	8	9	10 to 30		
Treated (52 mice)	0	0	0	0	1	0	0	1	0	2	4	8
Untreated (52 mice)	0	0	8	21	21	2	0	0	0	0	52	100

Moragues, Pinkerton and Greiff[40] extended these studies on rickettsiae to therapeutic trials of penicillin in the treatment of experimental infections of dba mice with murine typhus. When the inoculum was relatively small; namely, when it approached the minimal lethal dose, and when penicillin was administered in relatively large amounts, the survival rate among the treated mice was greatly increased. As a result of these studies, the investigators concluded that the results were sufficiently encouraging to justify thorough clinical trial of penicillin in the treatment of this infection.

From the studies of Robinson,[2] it appeared that penicillin was completely ineffective in the treatment of experimental infections of mice due to the virus PR8 of epidemic influenza. Likewise, penicillin was found ineffective against this virus by the investigators of Naval Laboratory Research Unit No. 1[41] and by Andrewes, King and van den Ende[42] at the National Institute for Medical Research in London.

According to the reports of Andrewes and his associates, the virus of lymphogranuloma venereum was found to be resistant to the action of penicillin. This negative result is not surprising in view of the rather small amount of penicillin used against these experimental infections in mice. I am inclined to the opinion that possibly larger concentrations of penicillin might be effective.

In the studies of Andrewes and his associates, again, it was found that penicillin exhibits little or no activity against the virus of vaccinia.

All are aware of the handicaps and difficulties involved in the chemotherapy of virus infections. Many claims for success against certain viruses have failed to be substantiated, with the possible exception of the effectiveness of the sulfonamides against such larger viruses as those of lymphogranuloma venereum and trachoma. It is my opinion that penicillin does possess some virostatic activity against at least some of the larger viruses. I am further of the opinion that it is possible that penicillin in rather large amounts may prove of value in the treatment of some of these infections.

DIPHTHERIA

Although Corynebacterium diphtheriae has been found to be susceptible to the action of penicillin in vitro, results of studies of its effectiveness made in vivo have not appeared to be very striking. This is another example of some variability between activity in vitro and in vivo. F. R. Heilman[43] established fatal infections in guinea pigs and hamsters with gravis strains of Corynebacterium diphtheriae. Penicillin in quantities usually effective against susceptible organisms failed to protect either of these experimental animals against diphtheria.

MISCELLANEOUS

Experimental Tuberculosis.—The Oxford investigators, as a result of their studies in vitro, were led to conclude that penicillin was relatively ineffective against Mycobacterium tuberculosis. Several other investigators, including Robinson[2] as well as Smith and Emmart,[44] have reported negative results in their attempts to treat experimental tuberculosis of mice and guinea pigs with penicillin. Robinson's studies were made on avian tuberculosis whereas Smith and Emmart used a single strain of Mycobacterium tuberculosis of human origin.

Trypanosomes.—Mice were inoculated intraperitoneally with lethal doses of Trypanosoma equiperdum and were treated with 1,000 units of penicillin daily by Robinson.[2] No effect on the course of the infection was noted among the animals treated with penicillin whereas tryparsamide protected these animals under the conditions of the experiment. Augustine and his colleagues[29] reported that penicillin was of little or no value in the treatment of infections owing to Trypanosomas lewisi.

Pleuropneumonia-like Organisms, So-called.—Powell and Rice[45] were unable to demonstrate any beneficial effect of penicillin on arthritic rats infected with pleuropneumonia-like organisms.

Toxoplasma.—It appears from the reports of Augustine and others,[29] furthermore, that penicillin is ineffective in the treatment of experimental infections produced by toxoplasma.

Infections with Gram-negative Bacteria.—Certain studies have been reported on the treatment with penicillin of infections owing to some gram-negative bacteria. Robinson,[2] for example, produced experimental infections in mice with Salmonella aertrycke, Salmonella schottmülleri and Bacterium shigae. Penicillin was found to afford no protection whatever against these infections.

SUSCEPTIBLE AND INSUSCEPTIBLE ORGANISMS

Based on present knowledge from in vitro (Chapter IV) and in vivo studies, it appears that the organisms which are susceptible and those which are insusceptible to the action of penicillin are essentially those listed in table 11.

TABLE 11

ANTIBACTERIAL ACTION OF PENICILLIN IN VITRO AND IN VIVO

Susceptible organisms	Insusceptible organisms
Diplococcus pneumoniae	Eberthella typhosa
Streptococcus pyogenes	Salmonella paratyphi
Streptococcus salivarius	Salmonella enteritidis
Micro-aerophilic streptococci	Shigella dysenteriae
Staphylococcus aureus	Proteus vulgaris
Staphylococcus albus (some strains)	Pseudomonas aeruginosa (Bacillus pyocyaneus)
Neisseria gonorrhoeae	Pseudomonas fluorescens
Neisseria intracellularis	Serratia marcescens (Bacillus prodigiosus)
Actinomyces bovis	Klebsiella pneumoniae
Bacillus anthracis	Hemophilus influenzae
Bacillus subtilis	Hemophilus pertussis
Clostridium botulinum	Escherichia coli
Clostridium tetani	Staphylococcus albus (some strains)
Clostridium perfringens (welchii)	Monilia albicans
Clostridium septicum	Monilia candida
Corynebacterium diphtheriae	Monilia krusei
Micrococci (some strains)	Blastomyces
Streptobacillus moniliformis	Mycobacterium tuberculosis
Erysipelothrix rhusiopathiae	Streptococcus faecalis
Borrelia novyi (spirochete of relapsing fever)	Brucella melitensis
Treponema pallidum	Plasmodium vivax
Leptospira icterohaemorrhagiae	Trypanosoma equiperdum
Spirillum minus	Toxoplasma
Psittacosis virus	Virus of influenza
Ornithosis virus	Vibrio comma

TOXICITY OF PENICILLIN FOR CERTAIN ANIMALS

Fairly purified penicillin is well tolerated by most laboratory animals. In fact, little difficulty has been encountered in administering adequate therapeutic amounts of penicillin to such laboratory animals as mice, rats, rabbits, cats or dogs.

Of some importance to those interested in experiments on laboratory animals is the apparent toxicity of penicillin for the commonly used laboratory animal, the guinea pig. It has been found that even fairly purified preparations of penicillin will at times prove toxic for these animals. For example, it was evident from the studies of Hamre and her associates[46] that guinea pigs did not tolerate well the subcutaneous administration of penicillin over a period of days. In the experiment reported by them, 7,000 to 12,000 Oxford units per kilogram per day of penicillin, as prepared for clinical use, given subcutaneously over a period of several days caused death. On the other hand, a similar amount did not cause death of mice or rabbits. Guinea pigs did tolerate, however, doses approximating those used clinically (1,000 units per kilogram of body weight) when given subcutaneously for twenty days. The observations by this group of investigators were made on normal, healthy guinea pigs.

In the treatment of animals harboring serious infections, the range of safety of penicillin with relation to the guinea pig appears to be even less than that reported by Hamre and her associates. In the studies reported by F. R. Heilman and me[31] on experimental Weil's disease, in which we used the guinea pig, it was evident that 800 Oxford units per day of either the sodium or the calcium salt was the largest amount of penicillin well tolerated by these animals. Although toxic effects of penicillin have not been observed in mice which receive 1,000 units of sodium penicillin subcutaneously in divided doses each day for periods up to seven days, it soon was found that penicillin could cause toxic effects in guinea pigs. Young guinea pigs which received from 1,000 to 5,000 units of penicillin daily in divided doses frequently died after several days. Death was preceded for a day or two by a state of apathy during which anorexia, loss of weight, ruffled fur and rectal temperature at the lower limits of normal were noted. Examination of such animals revealed only a state of generalized vasodilatation. They gave no evidence of scurvy. This toxic effect was noted on use of both sodium and calcium penicillin from four different sources. In sections of brain, liver and kidney the only significant finding was markedly dilated capillaries throughout the tissues. Animals which received injections of penicillin frequently had pronounced erythema of the skin at the site of, and adjacent to the point of, injection. This reaction was most severe in animals which later died from treatment with the substance and, in some cases, appeared to affect to some degree much of the surface of the body. The reaction was much more evident among albino animals than among those of which the coat was colored. The susceptibility of individual animals of similar weights to the toxicity of penicillin varied greatly. Toxic effects also varied with the dose of the substance. What we observed concerning toxic effects appeared to be identical with what was described by Hamre and others.

Since the normal bacterial intestinal flora of the guinea pig is predominantly gram-positive, the inclination is to suspect that penicillin may seriously interfere with this flora and, thereby, with the metabolism of certain substances, perhaps vitamins, that are essential to the health of these animals. Herein may lie certain fundamental factors concerned not only with the toxicity but perhaps with the action of penicillin. In this connection, it is interesting that Hamre and her associates were unable to protect guinea pigs from the toxicity of penicillin by administration of large doses of sodium ascorbate although this does not exclude the possibility of some other essential nutrient being absent. At any rate, those interested in studies made in vivo, in which the guinea pig is used as the experimental animal, will do well to be aware of this toxicity, which might interfere with the interpretation of results.

REFERENCES

1. Chain, E., Florey, H. W., Gardner, A. D., Heatley, N. G., Jennings, M. A., Orr-Ewing, J. and Sanders, A. G.: Penicillin as a chemotherapeutic agent. Lancet. *2:*226–228 (Aug. 24) 1940.

2. Robinson, H. J.: Toxicity and efficacy of penicillin. J. Pharmacol. & Exper. Therap. *77:*70–79 (Jan.) 1943.

3. Powell, H. M. and Jamieson, W. A.: Penicillin chemotherapy of mice infected with Staphylococcus aureus. J. Indiana M. A. *35:*361–362 (July) 1942.

4. Robson, J. M. and Scott, G. I.: Local chemotherapy in experimental lesions of the eye produced by *Staph. aureus.* Lancet. *1:*100–103 (Jan. 23) 1943.

5. von Sallmann, Ludwig: Penicillin and sulfadiazine in treatment of experimental intraocular infections with Staphylococcus aureus and Clostridium welchii. Arch. Ophth. *31:*54–63 (Jan.) 1944.

6. Pilcher, Cobb and Meacham, W. F.: The chemotherapy of intracranial infections. III. The treatment of experimental staphylococcic meningitis with intrathecal administrations of penicillin. J. A. M. A. *123:*330–332 (Oct. 9) 1943.

7. Hobby, Gladys L., Meyer, Karl and Chaffee, Eleanor: Chemotherapeutic activity of penicillin. Proc. Soc. Exper. Biol. & Med. *50:*285–288 (June) 1942.

8. Meyer, Karl, Hobby, Gladys L. and Chaffee, Eleanor: On esters of penicillin. Science. n.s. *97:*205–206 (Feb. 26) 1943.

9. Powell, H. M. and Jamieson, W. A.: Response of sulfonamide-fast pneumococci to penicillin. Proc. Soc. Exper. Biol. & Med. *49:*387–389 (Mar.) 1942.

10. McKee, Clara M. and Rake, Geoffrey: Activity of penicillin against strains of pneumococci resistant to sulfonamide drugs. Proc. Soc. Exper. Biol. & Med. *51:*275–278 (Nov.) 1942.

11. von Sallmann, Ludwig: Penicillin and sulfadiazine in the treatment of experimental intraocular infection with pneumococcus. Arch. Ophth. *30:*426–436 (Oct.) 1943.

12. Dawson, M. H., Hobby, Gladys L., Meyer, Karl and Chaffee, Eleanor: Penicillin as a chemotherapeutic agent. Ann. Int. Med. *19*:707–717 (Nov.) 1943.

13. Miller, C. P. and Foster, Alice Z.: Studies on the action of penicillin. II. Therapeutic action of penicillin on experimental meningococcal infection in mice. Proc. Soc. Exper. Biol. & Med. *56*:166–169 (June) 1944.

14. McIntosh, James and Selbie, F. R.: Zinc peroxide, proflavine and penicillin in experimental *Cl. welchii* infections. Lancet. *2*:750–752 (Dec. 26) 1942.

15. McIntosh, James and Selbie, F. R.: Combined action of antitoxin and local chemotherapy on *Cl. welchii* infection in mice. Lancet. *2*:224–225 (Aug. 21) 1943.

16. Hac, Lucille R. and Hubert, Agnes C.: Penicillin in treatment of experimental *Clostridium welchii* infection. Proc. Soc. Exper. Biol. & Med. *53*:61–62 (May) 1943.

17. Hac, Lucille R.: Experimental *Clostridium welchii* infection. IV. Penicillin therapy. J. Infect. Dis. *74*:164–172 (Mar.-Apr.) 1944.

18. McKee, Clara M., Hamre, Dorothy M. and Rake, Geoffrey: The action of antibiotics on organisms producing gas gangrene. Proc. Soc. Exper. Biol. & Med. *54*:211–213 (Nov.) 1943.

19. Fleming, Alexander: On the antibacterial action of cultures of a penicillium, with special reference to their use in the isolation of B. influenzae. Brit. J. Exper. Path. *10*:226–236 (Jan.) 1929.

20. Abraham, E. P., Chain, E., Fletcher, C. M., Gardner, A. D., Heatley, N. G., Jennings, M. A. and Florey, H. W.: Further observations on penicillin. Lancet. *2*:177–188; 189 (Aug. 16) 1941.

21. Gold, Herman: Anthrax; a review of 60 cases with a report on the therapeutic use of sulfonamide compounds. Arch. Int. Med. *70*:785–821 (Nov.) 1942.

22. Cruickshank, J. C.: Chemotherapy of experimental anthrax infection. Lancet. *2*:681–684 (Sept. 23) 1939.

23. May, H. B. and Buck, S. C.: Action of the sulphonamides in experimental anthrax. Lancet. *2*:685–686 (Sept. 23) 1939.

24. Heilman, F. R. and Herrell, W. E.: Unpublished data.

25. Mahoney, J. F., Arnold, R. C. and Harris, Ad: Penicillin treatment of early syphilis; a preliminary report. Am. J. Pub. Health. *33*:1387–1391 (Dec.) 1943; also Ven. Dis. Inform. *24*:355–357 (Dec.) 1943.

26. Dunham, W. B., Hamre, Dorothy M., McKee, Clara M. and Rake, Geoffrey: Action of penicillin and other antibiotics on *Treponema pallidum*. Proc. Soc. Exper. Biol. & Med. *55*:158–160 (Mar.) 1944.

27. Heilman, F. R. and Herrell, W. E.: Penicillin in the treatment of experimental relapsing fever. Proc. Staff Meet., Mayo Clin. *18*:457–467 (Dec. 1) 1943.

28. Lourie, E. M. and Collier, H. O. J.: The therapeutic action of penicillin on *Spirochaeta recurrentis* and *Spirillum minus* in mice. Ann. Trop. Med. *37*:200–205 (Dec. 31) 1943.

29. Augustine, D. L., Weinman, David and McAllister, Joan: Rapid and sterilizing effect of penicillin sodium in experimental relapsing fever infections and its ineffectiveness in the treatment of trypanosomiasis (Trypanosomas lewisi) and toxoplasmosis. Science. n.s. *99*:19-20 (Jan. 7) 1944.

30. Eagle, Harry, Magnuson, H. J. and Musselman, Arlyne D.: The therapeutic efficacy of penicillin in relapsing fever infections in mice and rats. Pub. Health Rep. *59*:583–588 (May 5) 1944.

31. Heilman, F. R. and Herrell, W. E.: Penicillin in the treatment of experimental leptospirosis icterohaemorrhagica (Weil's disease). Proc. Staff Meet., Mayo Clin. *19*:89–99 (Feb. 23) 1944.

32. Augustine, D. L., Weinman, David and McAllister, Joan: Penicillin sodium therapy in experimental Weil's disease. New England J. Med. *231*:358–359 (Sept. 7) 1944.

33. Heilman, F. R.: Chemotherapy in experimental infections caused by Streptobacillus moniliformis. Science. n.s. *91:*366–367 (Apr. 12) 1940.

34. Heilman, F. R. and Herrell, W. E.: Penicillin in the treatment of experimental infections with Spirillum minus and Streptobacillus moniliformis (rat-bite fever). Proc. Staff Meet., Mayo Clin. *19:*257–264 (May 17) 1944.

35. Heilman, F. R. and Herrell, W. E.: Penicillin in the treatment of experimental infections due to Erysipelothrix rhusiopathiae. Proc. Staff Meet., Mayo Clin. *19:*340–345 (June 28) 1944.

36. Heilman, F. R. and Herrell, W. E.: Penicillin in the treatment of experimental ornithosis. Proc. Staff Meet., Mayo Clin. *19:*57–65 (Feb. 9) 1944.

37. Heilman, F. R. and Herrell, W. E.: Penicillin in the treatment of experimental psittacosis. Proc. Staff Meet., Mayo Clin. *19:*204–207 (Apr. 19) 1944.

38. Editorial: Penicillin in experimental viral and rickettsial diseases. New England J. Med. *231:*164–165 (July 27) 1944.

39. Greiff, Donald and Pinkerton, Henry: Inhibition of growth of Typhus rickettsiae in the yolk sac by penicillin. Proc. Soc. Exper. Biol. & Med. *55:*116–119 (Feb.) 1944.

40. Moragues, Vicente, Pinkerton, Henry and Greiff, Donald: Therapeutic effectiveness of penicillin in experimental murine typhus infection in dba mice. J. Exper. Med. *79:*431–437 (Apr. 1) 1944.

41. Personnel of Naval Laboratory Research Unit No. 1: Attempts to protect against influenza virus with various sulfonamides, acridines and antibiotics. Science. n.s. *98:*348–349 (Oct. 15) 1943.

42. Andrewes, C. H., King, H. and van den Ende, M.: Chemotherapeutic experiments with viruses of influenza A, Lymphogranuloma venereum and vaccinia. J. Path. & Bact. *55:*173–181 (Apr.) 1943.

43. Heilman, F. R.: Personal communication to the author.

44. Smith, M. I. and Emmart, E. W.: The action of penicillium extracts in experimental tuberculosis. Pub. Health Rep. *59:*417–423 (Mar. 31) 1944.

45. Powell, H. M. and Rice, R. M.: Ineffective penicillin chemotherapy of arthritic rats infected with pleuropneumonia-like organisms. J. Lab. & Clin. Med. *29:*372–374 (Apr.) 1944.

46. Hamre, Dorothy M., Rake, Geoffrey, McKee, Clara M. and MacPhillamy, H. B.: The toxicity of penicillin as prepared for clinical use. Am. J. M. Sc. *206:*642–652 (Nov.) 1943.

CHAPTER VI

ABSORPTION, DIFFUSION AND EXCRETION OF PENICILLIN

In view of the rather high degree of solubility of penicillin in most solvents, it is not surprising that penicillin is rather readily absorbed and diffuses fairly well into most body fluids and tissues. There are, of course, exceptions to this statement which will be dealt with separately.

ABSORPTION

When administered by the intramuscular, intravenous or subcutaneous routes, penicillin is rather rapidly absorbed and its presence in blood or other tissues can be determined by various means. While penicillin may be absorbed following subcutaneous infusion, its absorption following this method of administration is erratic and variable.

Florey and his associates[1] studied the distribution or concentration of penicillin in the blood following its administration by various routes. As evidence of penicillin activity they used the ring test (Oxford method) which is described in the following chapter (p. 85). It was evident from their studies that penicillin disappeared rather rapidly from the blood after a single intravenous injection although an initial high level was obtained in the blood following administration by this route. When penicillin was given by subcutaneous injection, the concentration in the blood was less but detectable amounts were found to be present for a longer period than after a single intravenous injection.

These observations of Florey and his colleagues were extended to human subjects by Rammelkamp and Keefer,[2, 3] by Rammelkamp and Helm[4, 5] and also by Dawson and his associates.[6] To determine the presence of penicillin in the body fluids these investigators used a tube method such as the one described by Rammelkamp[7] (p. 93). From the reports of all these investigators it was evident that, when the drug was administered by a single intravenous injection, the concentration in the blood reached its peak very soon after the injection and thereafter fell at a rather rapid rate. In general, when large doses were administered, the peak concentration was higher, and detectable amounts of penicillin remained in the blood slightly longer, than when the doses were small. In spite of the concentrations attainable, however, all of the reports seemed to indicate that inhibitory amounts of penicillin in the serum were no longer present three hours after a single injection. The same conditions obtained also when penicillin was administered by means of a single intramuscular injection, although there was some evidence that the intramuscular administration resulted in a slight prolongation of the time during which inhibitory amounts of penicillin were present, that is, in comparison with a single intravenous injection.

My colleagues and I[8] also have carried out studies on the absorption of penicillin and the maintenance of concentration in the blood. As much as 50,000 units of penicillin were administered in a single dose by the intramuscular route. With these comparatively large amounts of penicillin being administered, the blood obtained one hour after injection

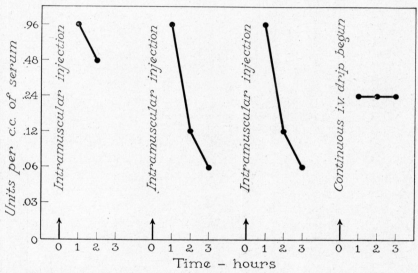

Fig. 8.—The falling serum concentration of penicillin in three hours when 50,000 units is administered by intramuscular injection and the approximately constant serum concentration when the same amount is given by continuous intravenous drip over the same period. (From article by Herrell, Nichols and Heilman, Journal of the American Medical Association, August 12, 1944.)

did not contain more than 1 unit of penicillin per cubic centimeter. Three hours after injection of penicillin by this route, no penicillin activity could be determined in the blood. These results were compared with the concentrations of penicillin which could be obtained in the blood following administration of penicillin by means of the continuous intravenous drip method. Using the same amount of penicillin as that which had been given in a single dose intramuscularly, it was possible, by continuous intravenous administration, to obtain a more or less constant level of penicillin activity in the blood (fig. 8). For determining the presence of penicillin activity in the serum we have, as a rule, used Fleming's adaptation of the Wright slide-cell technic. This method is described in the following chapter (p. 94). If patients received as little as 40,000 units of penicillin per day by the intravenous drip method, concentration of penicillin in their blood usually would be between 0.06 and 0.12 unit per cubic centimeter.

The results obtained in the studies just described are in complete agreement with those reported by Fleming,[9] who compared the bacteriostatic power of the patient's serum after the continuous intravenous drip

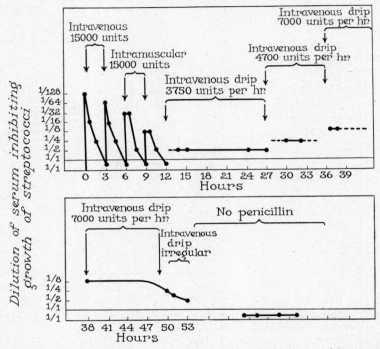

Fig. 9.—Bacteriostatic power of patient's serum after intravenous and intramuscular injections and a continuous intravenous drip at different rates. (From discussion by Fleming, Proceedings of the Royal Society of Medicine, January, 1944.)

method of administration and after intermittent intramuscular injection of penicillin. The results obtained by Fleming are shown in figure 9.

Not much absorption of penicillin will occur if the substance is administered orally under normal and unmodified conditions. The failure of penicillin to be absorbed from the gastro-intestinal tract is due primarily to its inactivation by the gastric acids. This observation was made by the Oxford investigators[1] at the beginning of their work. That the gastric hydrochloric acid is responsible for the inactivation of penicillin when the substance is administered by mouth was evident also from the studies of Rammelkamp and Helm.[5] They found that, following oral administration, therapeutic levels of penicillin were obtainable in the serum of patients suffering with pernicious anemia, in the gastric juice of whom, of course, no free hydrochloric acid was present. These results immediately suggest, therefore, that given a subject with achlorhydria, penicillin could be absorbed following its oral administration. In contrast to the reports just mentioned, it would appear from the studies of Free and his associates[10] that at least some penicillin reached the general circulation and was excreted in the urine following oral administration of large doses (100,000 Oxford units) of penicillin to human subjects who had fasted for three to six hours before the penicillin was administered. According to them, between 8 and 33 per cent of the quantity taken by mouth was excreted in the urine (p. 116).

It is possible, also, to obtain absorption of penicillin, with resulting therapeutic levels of penicillin in the blood, by giving large quantities of soda with orally administered penicillin. At least this appears to be true in experimental animals. Powell and Jamieson[11] reported on this subject in connection with the treatment of experimental pneumococcal infections in mice. Naturally, the combination of large amounts of soda with penicillin results in a somewhat erratic absorption of the material and, therefore, is not very practical from a clinical standpoint. Further studies on the general subject were reported by Free and others. When 10 gm. of bicarbonate of soda were given to human subjects along with 100,000 Oxford units of penicillin, the amount of penicillin excreted in the urine was definitely decreased as compared with the amount of penicillin excreted following its administration without soda. They were inclined to interpret these results on the basis that bicarbonate of soda may have decreased gastric emptying and therefore permitted more destruction of penicillin in the stomach. Another possibility which they suggested for this apparent decrease in excretion of penicillin in the urine was that an alkaline urine was excreted following the ingestion of bicarbonate of soda which permitted destruction of the compound to occur in the bladder.

Penicillin can be absorbed from the duodenum. Florey and his associates[1] reported that inhibitory levels could be obtained in the blood following absorption of penicillin from the duodenum (administration through a tube placed in the duodenum). According to their results, the levels in the blood obtained following absorption by this method were steadier, and persisted for a longer period of time, than when the material was administered intravenously or intramuscularly.

Little or no absorption of penicillin occurs when it is administered rectally. This is presumed to be due to the inactivation of penicillin by certain organisms present in the fecal stream.

Certain studies have been carried out which indicate that penicillin is absorbed, and can be detected in the blood, following its injection into inflamed body cavities such as knee joints, empyema cavities or the spinal canal. That this is true is evident from the studies reported by Rammelkamp and Keefer.[2, 3] Under such circumstances, absorption of penicillin is not rapid, as was indicated by the fact that the substance remained in the region where it had been injected for as long as twenty-four hours. In the matter of absorption from the spinal canal, there appeared to be some evidence that penicillin passed more rapidly from the cerebrospinal fluid into the blood when the meninges were inflamed than when they were not.

The studies of Bryson, Sansome and Laskin[12] revealed that penicillin was absorbed into the general circulation following its introduction into the bronchial tree by means of nebulization or aerosolization. Sixty per cent of the penicillin introduced by this route could be recovered in the urine. This amount compares favorably with the amount usually recoverable following intravenous administration or other systemic methods of administration.

In general, it may be stated that the ease and rapidity with which penicillin is absorbed are responsible for the difficulties encountered in maintaining more or less constant concentrations of the material in body tissues. The rather feeble absorption associated with enteral methods of administration, and the rapidity of absorption following parenteral administration, therefore, necessitate the use of frequent injections or continuous infusions. For this reason, efforts have been made to delay the absorption of penicillin following its subcutaneous and intramuscular administration. The most promising means of delaying absorption is by the combination of penicillin suspended in beeswax and oil mixtures (peanut oil or sesame oil) along the lines suggested by Romansky and Rittman.[13] This method will be discussed in further detail under methods of administration (p. 108).

DIFFUSION

When penicillin is given by the common methods of administration (subcutaneous, intramuscular or intravenous) experimental as well as clinical studies reveal that it diffuses fairly well into many body tissues, although there are exceptions to this general statement.

Diffusion into Erythrocytes.—Rammelkamp and Keefer[2] have reported on studies concerned with the determination of the concentration of penicillin in erythrocytes following administration of the drug by various routes. It was evident from their studies that exceedingly small amounts of the drug penetrate the erythrocytes. In the erythrocytes they found less than 10 per cent of the amount of penicillin that was present in the plasma. In general, therefore, studies referring to the diffusion and distribution of penicillin in the blood usually refer to the concentration in the plasma or serum.

Diffusion into Cerebrospinal Fluid.—Florey and his colleagues[1] made observations on the diffusion of penicillin into the cerebrospinal fluid of experimental animals. No penicillin activity could be demonstrated in the cerebrospinal fluid of cats following intravenous administration of the material. According to the reports of Rammelkamp and Keefer,[2, 3] also, following intravenous administration of penicillin to human subjects, no penicillin activity could be demonstrated in the cerebrospinal fluid. My colleagues and I[8] carried out similar studies, the results of which are in complete agreement with the findings of Rammelkamp and Keefer. The spinal fluid of patients who received as much as 100,000 units of penicillin per day by the continuous intravenous method of administration gave no evidence of penicillin activity while treatment was in progress. This was true not only of subjects who, on spinal puncture, were found to be free of disease involving the cerebrospinal structures, but was also true of patients who were suffering from disease (syphilis) involving these structures. When 10,000 units of penicillin were administered by the intrathecal route, the material remained in the spinal fluid for at least twenty-four hours. Forty-eight hours after intrathecal administration of 10,000 or 20,000 units of penicillin, no penicillin activity could be detected in the spinal fluid. It is evident from these studies, therefore, that if penicillin is to be used for treatment of infections of the cerebrospinal apparatus, the material should be administered by the intrathecal route at least every twenty-four hours in order to maintain adequate concentrations.

Rosenberg and Sylvester[14] have reported studies which suggest that under some conditions penicillin might diffuse into the cerebrospinal fluid following systemic administration alone. They reported that antibacterial amounts of penicillin may reach the spinal fluid when the meninges are acutely inflamed to the extent which obtains in the presence of acute meningococcal meningitis. If these findings are confirmed, it may not be entirely necessary to supplement systemic therapy in the treatment of acute meningitis. On the other hand, the intrathecal use of penicillin still seems desirable.

Diffusion into Ocular Tissues and Tears.—The Oxford investigators[1] reported that following the systemic administration of penicillin, tears were found to exert no antibacterial activity. Likewise, Rammelkamp and Keefer[2] were unable to demonstrate the presence of any penicillin activity in tears following the systemic administration of therapeutic doses.

The report of Struble and Bellows,[15] however, suggests that if large amounts of penicillin are administered, the substance can be demonstrated readily in the tears of experimental animals. The tears of dogs which received intravenously 12,800 units of penicillin per kilogram of body weight were found to contain as high as 3.19 units of penicillin per cubic centimeter fifteen minutes after the injection had been made. Penicillin activity was still demonstrable in the tears of these animals at the end of half an hour. The possible effect of lysozyme in the tears was excluded. Furthermore, following the administration of large doses of penicillin intravenously, these observers were able to demonstrate the presence of penicillin activity in the extra-ocular muscles, the sclera, the conjunctiva, the chorioretinal layer and the aqueous humor. The concentration of penicillin in the vitreous humor and the cornea usually was small and no penicillin could be demonstrated at any time in the lens. The observations recorded in the previous sentence are understandable · in view of the avascular nature of these tissues. When penicillin was administered in amounts which approximate clinical doses, detectable amounts of penicillin were not present in the tissues of the eye. This, however, does not exclude the possibility that traces of penicillin are present nor the possibility that some clinical effect might follow systemic administration of fairly large amounts. The results, however, do strengthen the recommendation that for the treatment of infections of the eye, penicillin should be applied locally as well as administered systemically.

Diffusion into Saliva.—Regardless of the method of administration, the Oxford investigators[1] were able to demonstrate penicillin activity in the saliva although the concentrations as a rule were lower than those found in the blood at the same time. Struble and Bellows[15] also found small amounts of penicillin in the saliva following systemic administration of penicillin. Rammelkamp and Keefer,[2] on the other hand, were unable to confirm this finding. On the basis of clinical observations, however, I am inclined to believe that fairly adequate amounts of penicillin do reach the saliva following systemic administration.

Diffusion into Pancreatic Juice.—It is generally agreed that penicillin does not reach the pancreatic juice following systemic administration. However, observations to be mentioned presently seem to indicate that pancreatic tissue itself contains some penicillin following intramuscular administration of large doses of the material.

Diffusion into the Peritoneal Cavity.—It is evident from the reports of Miller and Foster[16] that penicillin diffuses fairly rapidly into the peritoneal cavity. Following intramuscular injection of penicillin into mice, it appeared that penicillin diffused into the peritoneal cavity within five minutes and that the concentration rose to a relatively higher level than that which obtained in the blood. Under the conditions of Miller and Foster's experiment, mucin had been placed in the peritoneal cavity to aid in the establishment of meningococcal infections and the investigators pointed out that the penetration of penicillin into the peritoneal cavity may or may not have been affected by the presence of the mucin.

Diffusion into the Pleural Space.—I already have pointed out that penicillin remains in the pleural space for a considerable time after its injection directly into this cavity (p. 74). Absorption is slow. Very little information is available concerning the amounts of penicillin which reach the normal and the inflamed pleural space following systemic injection. At all events, the amounts which reach this cavity are probably small and for that reason intrapleural instillations of penicillin are indicated in the treatment of infections which involve the pleural cavity.

Diffusion into Joint Fluid.—My colleagues and I[8] have reported studies which indicate that, following systemic administration of penicillin, antibacterial amounts of the material reach the fluid of inflamed joints. This is also true of the fluid of joints which are not inflamed. The amount of penicillin present in the joint fluid usually will be approximately half that found in the blood.

Diffusion into the Placenta (Placental Transmission).—In view of the possibility of the use of penicillin in treatment of prenatal infections, including syphilis, my colleagues and I[8] carried out studies to determine whether or not penicillin passed into the placental circulation following systemic administration and, therefore, became available to the fetus. On therapeutic indications, a fairly large amount of penicillin (100,000 units) was administered to patients by means of the intravenous drip method over a short period of time toward the end of the second stage of labor. At delivery, or shortly thereafter, blood was obtained from the umbilical cord and also from the mother for the determination of penicillin activity. The results of these studies are shown in figure 10. In some instances the umbilical cord contained an amount of penicillin which was approximately half the amount present in the mother's blood. This is true not only of the mother who is free of syphilis but also of the mother who has the disease. It is evident from these studies, therefore, that penicillin diffuses through the placenta and becomes available to the fetus.

The results reported by my colleagues and me on the placental transmission of penicillin have been confirmed in a subsequent report by Greene and Hobby.[17]

Concentrations Attainable in Various Body Tissues.—The studies of Struble and Bellows[15] added considerable information concerning the concentrations of penicillin which can be attained in various tissues of the body following intravenous injection of a rather large dose of the material. On the basis of clinical results obtained by many investigators in the treatment of a variety of infections, it seemed reasonable to suspect that penicillin would reach practically all of the tissues, at least in some concentration, with the possible exception of the structures of the central nervous system and the bone marrow.

Under the conditions of the experiment reported by Struble and Bellows it was apparent that penicillin activity could be demonstrated one

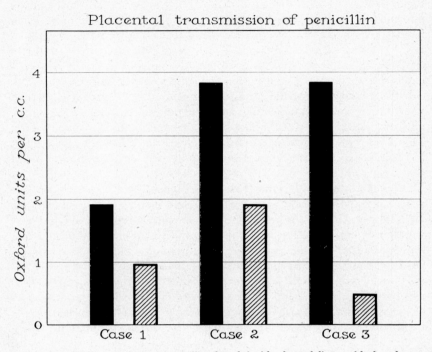

Placental transmission of penicillin

Fig. 10.—Columns represent penicillin found in blood at delivery: black columns, mother's blood; shaded columns, blood from umbilical cord. In the different cases 100,000 units of penicillin were administered at different intervals before delivery. In case 1 the interval was forty-five minutes, in case 2 fifteen minutes and in case 3 five minutes. In case 3 both mother's blood and blood from the umbilical cord gave positive complement fixation tests for syphilis. (From article by Herrell, Nichols and Heilman, Journal of the American Medical Association, August 12, 1944.)

hour after injection, in decreasing order of amounts, as follows: kidney, small intestine, lung, buccal mucosa, bile, skin, liver, adrenal glands, pancreas, heart, voluntary muscle and spleen. In their studies, even after massive injections of penicillin, none was found in nerve tissue or bone marrow. The brain and dura at times revealed very faint traces. It is further significant, as these investigators pointed out, that only faint traces of penicillin, or none, could be recovered from various tissues and fluids two hours after injection or later, with the exception that bile contained appreciable amounts even three hours after intravenous injection (table 12). It was further pointed out by the observers that their studies

TABLE 12

CONCENTRATION OF PENICILLIN IN BODY TISSUES AND FLUIDS AFTER A SINGLE MASSIVE INTRAVENOUS INJECTION

Tissue	Time in hours		
	1 Hour	2 Hours	3 Hours
	Units per gm. or c.c.	Units per gm. or c.c.	Units per gm. or c.c.
Liver	4.77	*	*
Bile	6.65	. .	4.99
Heart	2.41	. .	*
Kidney	17.38	*	*
Lung	8.91	*	*
Voluntary muscle	1.90	*	*
Skin	6.06	*	*
Nerve	0	0	0
Brain	0 to *	0	0
Dura	0 to *	. .	. .
Bone marrow	0	0	0
Pancreas	2.69	. .	*
Adrenal	2.72	0	0
Spleen	1.89	. .	*
Buccal mucosa	8.39	*	0
Small intestine	9.68	. .	0

Each figure represents two or more determinations.
* Equals trace of penicillin.
From article by Struble and Bellows, Journal of the American Medical Association, July 8, 1944.

lend substantial support to the clinical recommendation that penicillin be administered either by frequent intramuscular injection or by intravenous drip over a long period of time, a procedure advocated by my colleagues and me.

EXCRETION

Renal Excretion.—It was evident from the reports of the Oxford investigators[1] that penicillin was excreted fairly readily by the normal kidney. In fact, as was pointed out in an earlier chapter (Chapter I) these investigators were able to recover penicillin from the urine of patients who had received the substance. It is generally agreed among most investigators that between 50 and 60 per cent of penicillin is excreted fairly rapidly by the kidney. The amounts of penicillin recovered in the urine, however, have ranged from 40 to 99 per cent, according to different reports. Following a single intravenous injection, the urinary excretion of penicillin at times may be complete within the first hour. Following other methods of administration, however, the rate of excretion is somewhat slower. This variation in the amount of penicillin recovered from the urine probably can be explained on the basis of the volume of the urine excreted and the presence or absence of bacteria in the urinary tract. The presence of coliform bacteria in urine is accompanied by rapid loss of penicillin activity, particularly if the specimen is kept at room temperature. Observations on this subject have been reported by my colleagues and me.[8] On several occasions for example, urine which contained coliform bacteria and which was found to contain as much as 120 units of penicillin per cubic centimeter soon after being voided, completely lost its penicillin activity overnight, even after being kept in the icebox. At all events, however, there is ample evidence that a very large portion of the penicillin which is administered systemically is ultimately excreted in the urine.

Certain other factors influence excretion of penicillin in the urine. The presence of renal failure due to any cause delays excretion and, as a result, high concentrations of penicillin can be maintained in the blood due to this damming effect which results from renal failure or urinary suppression.

Attempts have been made to delay renal excretion of penicillin in man. For example, Rammelkamp and Bradley[18] reported that when penicillin was administered to normal subjects by constant intravenous drip, excretion of the material by the kidneys could be depressed by the addition of diodrast to the infusion. Whether this procedure could be adopted as a routine for increasing the concentration of penicillin in the blood is not established as this paragraph is written.

Further experiments have been reported in connection with the reduction of renal excretion of penicillin and consequent prolongation of retention of penicillin in the body. Beyer, Woodward, Peters, Verwey and Mattis,[19] for example, administered para-aminohippuric acid to experimental animals to which penicillin was being administered and thereby reduced considerably the renal excretion; this resulted in maintenance of higher levels in the plasma. They suggested that the combination of this acid with penicillin might make possible the maintenance of larger amounts of penicillin in the blood. Here again, however, unless supplies of penicillin were extremely small, it remains to be decided whether use of any agent designed primarily to reduce renal excretion would form an undesirable part of penicillin therapy.

Excretion in Bile.—The Oxford investigators[1] demonstrated that penicillin apparently was excreted in the bile of animals following its intravenous administration. Rammelkamp and Helm[4] likewise reported that penicillin could be found in greater concentration in the bile than in the serum which, of course, suggests that the material may be concentrated by the liver. That appreciable amounts of penicillin reach the liver following systemic administration was further evident from the studies of Struble and Bellows,[15] which have been discussed previously.

REFERENCES

1. Abraham, E. P., Chain, E., Fletcher, C. M., Gardner, A. D., Heatley, N. G., Jennings, M. A. and Florey, H. W.: Further observations on penicillin. Lancet. *2*:177–188, 189 (Aug. 16) 1941.

2. Rammelkamp, C. H. and Keefer, C. S.: Absorption, excretion and distribution of penicillin. J. Clin. Investigation. *22*:425–437 (May) 1943.

3. Rammelkamp, C. H. and Keefer, C. S.: Absorption, excretion and toxicity of penicillin administered by intrathecal injection. Am. J. M. Sc. *205*:342–350 (Mar.) 1943.

4. Rammelkamp, C. H. and Helm, J. D., Jr.: Excretion of penicillin in bile. Proc. Soc. Exper. Biol. & Med. *54*:31–34 (Oct.) 1943.

5. Rammelkamp, C. H. and Helm, J. D., Jr.: Studies on the absorption of penicillin from the stomach. Proc. Soc. Exper. Biol. & Med. *54*:324–327 (Dec.) 1943.

6. Dawson, M. H., Hobby, Gladys L., Meyer, Karl and Chaffee, Eleanor: Penicillin as a chemotherapeutic agent. Ann. Int. Med. *19*:707–717 (Nov.) 1943.

7. Rammelkamp, C. H.: Method for determining concentration of penicillin in body fluids and exudates. Proc. Soc. Exper. Biol. & Med. *51*:95–97 (Oct.) 1942.

8. Herrell, W. E., Nichols, D. R. and Heilman, Dorothy H.: Penicillin; its usefulness, limitations, diffusion and detection, with analysis of 150 cases in which it was employed. J. A. M. A. *125*:1003–1010 (Aug. 12) 1944.

9. Fleming, A.: Discussion on penicillin. Proc. Roy. Soc. Med. *37*:101–104 (Jan.) 1944.

10. Free, A. H., Leonards, J. R., McCullagh, D. R. and Biro, Barbara E.: The urinary excretion of penicillin after oral administration to normal human subjects. Science. n.s. *100*:431–432 (Nov. 10) 1944.

11. Powell, H. M. and Jamieson, W. A.: Response of sulfonamide-fast pneumococci to penicillin. Proc. Soc. Exper. Biol. & Med. *49*:387–389 (Mar.) 1942.

12. Bryson, Vernon, Sansome, Eva and Laskin, Sidney: Aerosolization of penicillin solutions. Science. n.s. *100*:33–35 (July 14) 1944.

13. Romansky, M. J. and Rittman, G. E.: A method of prolonging the action of penicillin. Science. n.s. *100*:196–198 (Sept. 1) 1944.

14. Rosenberg, D. H. and Sylvester, J. C.: The excretion of penicillin in the spinal fluid in meningitis Science. n.s. *100*:132–133 (Aug. 11) 1944.

15. Struble, G. C. and Bellows, J. G.: Studies on the distribution of penicillin in the eye; and its clinical application. J. A. M. A. *125*:685–690 (July 8) 1944.

16. Miller, C. P. and Foster, Alice Z.: Studies on the action of penicillin. II. Therapeutic action of penicillin on experimental meningococcal infection in mice. Proc. Soc. Exper. Biol. & Med. 56:166–169 (June) 1944.

17. Greene, H. J. and Hobby, Gladys, L.: Transmission of penicillin through human placenta. Proc. Soc. Exper. Biol. & Med. 57:282–283 (Nov.) 1944.

18. Rammelkamp, C. H. and Bradley, S. E.: Excretion of penicillin in man. Proc. Soc. Exper. Biol. & Med. 53:30–32 (May) 1943.

19. Beyer, K. H., Woodward, Roland, Peters, Lawrence, Verwey, W. F. and Mattis, P. A.: The prolongation of penicillin retention in the body by means of para-aminohippuric acid. Science. n.s. 100:107–108 (Aug. 4) 1944.

CHAPTER VII

METHODS OF STANDARDIZING PENICILLIN AND OF DETERMINING THE CONCENTRATION OF PENICILLIN IN BODY FLUIDS

Practically all of the methods used for standardizing or determining the potency of penicillin, or for determining the concentration of penicillin in various body fluids, are based on tests which measure the degree of bacteriostasis produced by the sample under assay. These microbiologic tests differ somewhat but, for the most part, the difference lies only in the means by which they are carried out.

The potency of a preparation of penicillin is expressed, therefore, in terms of units. This purely arbitrary value originally was defined by the Oxford investigators[1] and for that reason is called the Oxford unit. It is, therefore, a unit of antibacterial activity and is based on a comparison between the potency of any sample of penicillin and that of a standard. The Oxford unit as defined by its originators is that amount of penicillin which, when dissolved in 1 c.c. of water, gives the same inhibition as the original standard. By this is meant the same inhibition of growth against a known inoculum of the test organism. The test organism used by the Oxford investigators was a strain of Staphylococcus aureus (H). The test organism has varied from time to time, depending on the individual investigator. Some methods are available for testing penicillin which do not require the use of a standard.

METHODS OF STANDARDIZING

One of the various methods available for assay is commonly referred to as the "serial dilution method" which first was utilized by Fleming.[2] Liquid broth assays and cup or plate methods of assay are examples of the serial dilution method. In other words, the dilutions are made in either liquid, solid or semisolid medium. Another method of assay is referred to as the "turbidimetric method" and is based on the proportional inhibition of growth of the test organism in liquid medium as a function of the concentration of penicillin. This method was described by Foster.[3] Another method for standardizing penicillin, in which the tissue culture preparation is utilized, has been described by Dorothy Heilman.[4]

I propose to describe a few of the methods which at present are in use for assay of penicillin. The fact that so many methods and modifications have been made in these tests amply indicates that the ideal and completely accurate method has not yet evolved. Until chemical methods can be devised, the individual investigator must select that microbiologic test which is most adaptable to his laboratory routine. A comprehensive review of the merits and faults of the various methods of assay has been published by Foster and Woodruff.[5]

Modified Broth Dilution Method Described by Foster and Woodruff.[5]
—This broth dilution method was alleged to have an accuracy of 15 per cent and the details of the method were devised by Hoogerhide of the Squibb Biological Laboratories. The description of the method follows:

Two ml. amounts of beef-heart infusion broth containing 0.25 per cent glucose and inoculated with a 1 to 10 dilution of a six-hour culture of Staphylococcus aureus H are distributed in a series of ten small tubes. To one tube each is added respectively with a micro pipette, 0.10, 0.09, 0.08, 0.07, 0.06, 0.05, 0.045, 0.040, 0.035, and 0.030 ml. of a standard made up to contain 0.60 Florey units per ml. Similar amounts of the unknowns diluted to 0.60 units per ml. on the basis of predicted potency are added to other series of tubes. After overnight incubation, the endpoint is stated to be reproducibly clear-cut between two tubes. The endpoint is not necessarily that dilution which inhibits growth completely but, rather, that dilution in which growth is so retarded that the organism fails to develop a uniform turbidity throughout the broth, forming, instead, a sediment in the bottom of the tube leaving a clear supernatant. The endpoint on the unknown contains that amount of penicillin corresponding to the endpoint in the standard series. Samples would have to be reasonably free from contaminating bacteria. Aside from the tedium of making a large number of accurately measured pipettings, this would appear to be one of the most promising methods for practical application.

Quick Assay Method of Rake and Jones.[6]—In the method described by Rake and Jones, hemolysis is utilized as an indicator. According to the investigators, this method is fairly rapid. As described by the investigators, the method is as follows:

Optimal conditions for the test have been determined. Beef heart infusion broth has proven the best medium; for red blood cells, 1 per cent defibrinated rabbit's blood is better than any other concentration of the same or other blood; for incubation, most satisfactory results have been obtained by use of a water-bath at 37° C.

In performing the test a 2- to 3-hour culture in 1 per cent rabbit's blood broth of C-203 (i.e., one in which hemolysis is just appearing) subsequently stored overnight at 0° C., is used for the inoculation of a lot of 1 per cent rabbit's blood broth in volumes of 0.1 ml. of inoculum for each 2.0 ml. of blood broth. As soon as this fresh culture shows detectable hemolysis (i.e., within 2 hours), and the organisms are dividing rapidly, it is ready for use in the test. With such a culture, readings of potency can be read in 55 to 90 minutes. If it is desirable to test filtrates or other preparations without this 2-hour delay, the overnight culture may be used directly, but in this case it may be 2 hours before detectable hemolysin will be formed.

In carrying out the test, 2 ml. amounts of 1 per cent rabbit's blood beef heart infusion broth are placed in a series of 13 × 100 mm. tubes. To each tube is added 0.1 ml. of the appropriate dilution of penicillin standard or unknown filtrate. As a control of culture one tube receives 0.1 ml. of distilled water. As a control of preformed hemolysin one tube receives 0.7 Florey units in 0.1 ml., i.e., an amount of penicillin which will certainly inhibit growth of the streptococci. To each tube is now added 0.2 ml. of culture. Contents of tubes are well mixed before incubation.

With the test as set out above, between .03 and .05 of a Florey unit in a total volume of 2.3 ml. will prevent growth and production of hemolysin. In the standard the range used is from 0.08 to 0.01 Florey units (.08, .06, .04, .03, .02, .015, and .01). Filtrates are diluted and tested, according to their expected potency, in the following manner: 1/2, 1/3, 1/4, 1/6, 1/8, etc. up to 1/256.

In reading the test it has been found that the first signs of hemolysis can be most readily detected by whirling the tubes slightly and throwing a plume of red cells into the clear supernatant broth. In the presence of a trace of hemolysin this plume becomes rapidly hemolyzed. All tubes showing such commencing hemolysin are thoroughly mixed and replaced in the water-bath for 2 or 3 minutes by which time uniform hemolysis will have appeared. In most cases all tubes which are to show hemolysis will do so at almost the same time, and an end-point is obtained by taking the last tube in each series showing no hemolysis. Occasionally a tube shows hemolysis delayed by about 30 minutes over the others. Such a tube is given a ± reading and an interpolated potency.

The test can be set up rapidly and without sterile precautions. It can be performed with turbid or heavily contaminated samples. Potencies obtained by its use have been compared on many occasions with those obtained by more accurate 18-hour tests and a remarkably good correlation has been obtained.

The Oxford or Cup Method.—This method is probably the one which is most generally used for routine assay purposes. The test is based on the fact that when penicillin is allowed to diffuse into the medium of a plate previously seeded with the test organism, a zone of inhibition around the point of diffusion occurs. The diameter of this zone of inhibition is then taken as a measure of the concentration of penicillin. The method was devised by N. G. Heatley and has been described by the Oxford investigators[1] and later in more detail by Heatley.[7] The procedure is carried out as follows:

Ordinary nutrient agar plates are seeded with the test organism—Staphylococcus aureus has been used in this work—by allowing a broth culture of the organism to flow over the surface of the agar and draining off the excess broth. The plates are then dried for an hour in the incubator at 37° C. in a special rack which supports the lid of the Petri dish half an inch above the lower part. When dry the seeded plates are removed from the incubator and can be kept in the refrigerator for one or two days. Cylinders made from short lengths of glass tubing, the dimensions of which will be seen from the inset of fig. 1*, are placed on the agar. The lower edge of the cylinder is carefully ground level and has an internal bevel so that the thin edge tends to sink into the agar and make a water- and bacteria-tight seal. Vitreous porcelain cylinders of the same size and shape, coloured at the non-bevelled end to facilitate their orientation, have also proved satisfactory. The cylinders are filled with the fluid to be tested, and the plates, resting on a block of wood, are incubated for 12-16 hours at 37° C. (If placed directly on the warm incubator shelves moisture may condense on the lids of the Petri dishes and drop on the agar, thus obscuring the results.) By the end of incubation most of the fluid in the cylinders has disappeared and each cylinder is surrounded by a circular zone where no bacterial growth has occurred. The diameter of the zone depends on the concentration of the penicillin, the type of relation being shown in fig. 1.*

* Not reproduced here. W. E. H.

The possibilities and limitations of this method of assay have not yet been fully worked out but the following points may be noted.

1. The diameter in mm. of the zone of inhibition (which we have called the "assay value") is only slightly smaller (1-2 mm.) when the cylinder is half filled than when it is fully filled.

2. The assay value is unaffected by the pH of the fluid being tested, provided it is not strongly buffered and lies within the range pH 5–8.5.

3. No inhibition is produced by a saturated aqueous solution of ether or by water containing free droplets of chloroform.

4. Diffusion of penicillin seems to be practically complete in 2–3 hours, and assay values after 14 hours of incubation are only very slightly smaller (0.5–1 mm.) than after a further 8 hours at 37° C.

5. Provided the plate is not jarred the fluid cannot escape from the cylinders, and even if the fluid is not sterile the contaminating bacteria are confined to the inside of the cylinder.

6. The assay value is not affected by the thickness of the agar provided it is between the limits of 3 to 5 mm.

7. The assay value varies slightly with different batches of plates and with the density of bacterial population at the beginning of incubation. For this reason uneven seeding of the plates must be avoided.

8. Sometimes the clear zone of inhibition is surrounded by a halo of partial inhibition, which varies from a faint ghost to almost complete inhibition. So far no explanation for, or means of controlling, this phenomenon has been discovered.

9. When the antibacterial activity of blood is to be assayed, plasma or serum must be used, since red cells tend to form a layer immediately on top of the agar, which seriously impedes the diffusion of penicillin and leads to low values.

High accuracy cannot be claimed for this method of assay, but if it is done in triplicate (preferably on three different plates), and if the unknown solution is diluted so as to give an assay value of not more than 25 mm. (before the curve has flattened out), the error is probably not greater than ±25 per cent and may be considerably less. We have no evidence that under suitable conditions this method is inferior in accuracy to the serial dilution method and it is certainly many times quicker. In addition, less than 0.25 ml. of fluid is required for each test.

Various modifications of this method have been recommended. Vincent and Vincent,[8] for example, have substituted filter paper disks saturated with penicillin for the cylinders employed by the Oxford investigators. The Vincents claim that, by this substitution, time is saved in setting up the test. Another modification which has been suggested is substitution of Bacillus subtilis for Staphylococcus aureus as the test organism. This was recommended by Foster and Woodruff.[9] Their communication on this modification of the Oxford method is as follows:

A sensitive strain of Bacillus subtilis is used as the test organism and for inoculum is cultivated submerged in 100 ml. of nutrient broth on a shaking machine until maximum sporulation takes place (7 to 14 days). The culture is then pasteurized to destroy the vegetative cells and titrated under the conditions of the assay to determine the optimum amount of inoculum (usually 0.1 to 0.4 ml. per 200 ml. of agar). That amount is used thereafter as long as that culture lasts. The spore cultures are stored in the refrigerator and may be used indefinitely; practically complete standardization of the inoculum is thereby achieved and its daily preparation eliminated. The melted agar is seeded before it is apportioned into plates. With spores it is not necessary to cool the melted agar to 42° before seeding. This eliminates a troublesome operation and also difficulties in the preparation of uniform plates due to premature hardening of the agar. The remaining steps are as described previously,* except that incubation is at 30°, which incidentally reduces temperature instability of penicillin. The lag in growth due to spore germination permits better diffusion of the penicillin before growth limits the zone. Larger zones reduce the percentage deviation due to errors in measuring their diameters. The zone edges with Bacillus subtilis invariably are knife-sharp, and the growth stands in clear contrast to the zone of inhibition.

Those who wish to employ this modification of the Oxford cup method will do well to consult the detailed description of the modification published subsequently by Foster and Woodruff.[10]

Turbidimetric Method.—The turbidimetric method was described by Foster.[3] While it was said to be fairly accurate (10 to 15 per cent), the technic is rather difficult and a great deal of experience is required to carry it out satisfactorily. As described originally by Foster, the procedure is as follows:

Growth in various dilutions of unknown penicillin samples is compared with a standard curve of inhibition run daily side by side with the unknowns. Computation of the potency of the unknown with respect to the standard reference sample of established potency then is an easy matter. Accuracy is that common to microbiological work; namely, ± 10 to 15 per cent.

Fig. 1† shows the growth response as a function of penicillin concentration. The theoretical basis for the inhibition curve of penicillin and the assay method based on this principle seem established by the logarithmic nature of the inhibition.

Use of a stable reference standard is, of course, imperative. Activities usually are expressed in terms of Florey units, following the lead of the Oxford group. Penicillin preparations of proved stability should be standardized either directly or indirectly against penicillin preparations of known Florey unitage. Use of a standard eliminates variations due to the culture, media, personal factor, etc. In this work the Oxford strain of Staphylococcus aureus has been used.

To tubes containing 5 ml. of various dilutions of penicillin samples are added 5 ml. of sterile, double strength nutrient broth, inoculated just prior to apportionment. For inoculum, 0.4 ml. of a 20 hour nutrient broth culture of the test organism is added to 100 ml. of the double strength broth. Dilutions are made as follows: The original samples of penicillin are diluted with ice-cold sterile 0.02 M phosphate buffer at pH 7.2 so as to contain approximately 0.02 unit per ml. These, together with the standard, are kept in an ice bath until all the samples have been treated similarly. Different amounts, namely 0.5, 1.0, 2.0, 3.0, and 5.0 ml., are then added aseptically to tubes previously sterilized with 4.5, 4.0, 3.0, 2.0, and 0 ml. of buffer, respectively.

Aseptic precautions should be observed throughout. In assaying dry preparations of penicillin, contaminants are not a serious factor owing to the ultimate high dilution and short incubation. With Penicillium filtrates or penicillin solutions contaminations may, however, be serious. Such liquids, when possible, should be obtained aseptically and maintained sterile. Otherwise they should be kept cold (0–5°), or saturated with ether or chloroform to minimize contamination. These solvents are without effect on the test organism under these conditions.

* See Oxford method above. W. E. H.
† Not reproduced here. W. E. H.

After 16 hours (overnight) incubation at 37°, the tubes are shaken, the contents poured into calibrated Evelyn tubes, and the turbidimetric readings obtained. Galvanometer differences (per cent transmissible light) are plotted against penicillin concentration. Three to five levels are run on each unknown, depending on how many can be predicted to fall on the central (three-fourths) region of the curve. A short time (4 hour) assay employing this principle has been developed.

In practice the log curve may be used as reference; only 3 or 4 points are required to define the log curve.

Various modifications of this method have been suggested by Foster and Wilker,[11] by Joslyn,[12] and by Lee and associates.[13] Likewise, other turbidimetric methods have been described by McMahan[14] and by Holmes and Lockwood.[15]

Tissue Culture Method of Heilman.—This method was found by Dorothy Heilman[4] to be satisfactory for determination of the amount of penicillin present in given samples. The tissue culture preparation is an adaptation of one described by King, Henschel and Green[16, 17] in their studies on sulfonamides. The pneumococcus was used as the test organism since it grew exceedingly well in the tissue culture medium. Since the end point for complete inhibition was practically always the same, when this method was used, it was not necessary to use a standard in performance of the test. The procedure, as described by Heilman, is as follows:

Tissue Culture Medium.—Healthy adult male rabbits were used exclusively as a source of blood for the preparation of medium. Rabbits were not fed during the 24 hour period before they were used. Blood was obtained under sterile conditions by cardiac puncture or by carotid cannulation with the animal under light ether anesthesia. Serum was prepared and heparin was added to a portion of the blood for the preparation of plasma. The solution of heparin used contained 0.04 per cent of purified heparin (Connaught Laboratories) and 0.8 per cent of sodium chloride. This solution was sterilized by Berkefeld f.ltration and 0.25 c.c. was used for 15 c.c. of blood. Tubes containing blood to which heparin had been added were thoroughly chilled before being placed in the centrifuge. After the blood had been centrifuged the plasma was transferred to a sterile tube and packed in ice. Serum and plasma showing abnormal cloudiness or opalescence, or a considerable degree of hemolysis, were discarded. A slight degree of hemolysis did not appear to affect the results. A serum-chick embryo extract was prepared by extracting chick embryos of 8 days of incubation with rabbit's serum in the proportion of 1 embryo to 5 c.c. of serum.

Bacterial Cultures.—A strain of Diplococcus pneumoniae Type 7 originally isolated from exudate from an empyema cavity was used as the test organism. Cultures were grown in Hartley broth containing approximately 10 per cent of horse serum. When a culture had attained maximal growth, suitable dilutions were made in Hartley broth and added to the serum-chick embryo extract in the proportion of 1 part of the bacterial suspension to 40 parts of serum extract. The final concentration of the original bacterial culture in the tissue culture clot was approximately 1:10,000,000. This inoculum usually resulted in the appearance of 20 or more bacterial colonies in each preparation. It was found that a more uniform bacterial count could be obtained on different days by using a suspension of pneumococci stored in divided amounts in solid carbon dioxide than when freshly grown cultures were used. Tubes containing tissue extract to which pneumococic

TABLE 13

Assay of Penicillin

Source of penicillin	Sample No.	Test No.	Colonies per culture (controls)	Concentration of penicillin		Assay at source (Oxford units per mg.)	Assay, present method (Oxford units per mg.)	Reassay at source (Oxford units per mg.)
				Causing total inhibition (μg. per cc.)	Not causing total inhibition (μg. per cc.)			
A	1	1	60	1.00	0.50	98	84	
		2	100	1.00	0.90			
B	1	1	20	0.50	0.25	357	168	125
		2	36	0.50	0.40			
		3	15	0.50	0.40			
	2	1	20	0.50	0.25	138	210	
		2	12	0.40	0.30			
		3	36	0.40	0.30			
		4	22	0.40	0.30			
	3	1	21	1.00	0.50	182	140	
		2	24	1.00	0.50			
		3	15	0.60	0.50			
	4	1	60	0.32	0.16	200	262	
		2	16	0.32	0.16			
	5	1	26	0.41	0.40	215	205	
		2	25	0.43	0.41			
		3	32	0.41	0.40			
		4	20	0.40	0.36			
C	1	1	24	0.66	0.50	250	142	146
		2	28	0.62	0.59*			
		3	26	0.59	0.56			
		4	32	0.59	0.56			
		5	150	0.59	0.56			

* One colony only in all 4 cultures at this dilution.

TABLE 14

Assay of Penicillin in Terms of Oxford Units per Ampule

Source of penicillin	Sample No.	Test No.	Colonies per culture (controls)	Concentration of penicillin		Assay at source (Oxford units per ampule)	Assay, present method (Oxford units per ampule)	Reassay at source (Oxford units per ampule)
				Causing total inhibition (Oxford units per c.c.*)	Not causing total inhibition (Oxford units per c.c.)			
B	6	1	42	0.080	0.060	10,000	10,500	
	7	1	150	0.080	0.060	10,000	10,500	
		2	42	0.080	0.060			
C	2	1	22	0.107	0.094	30,000	23,550	21,000
		2	24	0.107	0.094			
		3	28	0.107	0.094			
D	1	1	25	0.106	0.084	10,000	8,400	
		2	32	0.100	0.084			
E	1	1	32	0.250	0.166	25,000	8,400	
		2	20	0.250	0.166			

* Values are expressed in terms of original assay at the source. The end-point in this method is 0.084 Oxford units per c.c.

had been added, as well as tubes containing plasma, were kept chilled throughout the experiment. It was found to be important to use freshly prepared extract for each day's determinations. Some variation resulted when plasma and extract that had been prepared the day before were used.

Penicillin.—The penicillin used to standardize the method was a preparation of the sodium salt of penicillin obtained from the Northern Regional Research Laboratories of the United States Department of Agriculture through the courtesy of Dr. Robert Coghill. By recent comparison with other standards by means of the Oxford method its potency had been determined as 28 Oxford units per mg. Additional tests were carried out with a standardized preparation of the calcium salt of penicillin obtained through the courtesy of Dr. Coghill. The potency of this preparation was 135 Oxford units per mg. Twelve other preparations from 5 different sources were tested [tables 13 and 14].* As soon as they were received, individual samples were weighed under sterile conditions and added to 0.8 per cent solution of sodium chloride to make a concentration of 1:500. These stock solutions were stored in divided amounts in solid carbon dioxide until they were needed for the preparation of suitable dilutions in 0.8 per cent solution of sodium chloride at the time the tests were made. Experiments with 1 sample of penicillin were usually carried out within a period of a few weeks, as prolonged storage of the stock solutions in solid carbon dioxide sometimes resulted in a loss of potency.

In instances in which the potency of penicillin received was expressed as the number of Oxford units per ampule and the total weight of the sample was not known, the results of tests were expressed in terms of Oxford units per ampule instead of Oxford units per mg. [table 14].† The results of the individual tests were expressed in terms of the potency as determined at the source, and the final estimation of the value of the product was arrived at by multiplying the number of Oxford units per ampule as determined at the source by the fraction $\dfrac{0.084}{\text{Oxford units necessary to inhibit}}$.‡

Plasma Clot Cultures.—Portions of each dilution of penicillin to be tested were added to both plasma and serum-chick embryo extract at the time the cultures were made in order to insure a uniform concentration of penicillin throughout each culture. Since the amount of medium necessary for each group of cultures was small, 0.1 c.c. portions of solution of penicillin were added to 0.9 c.c. of plasma and serum extract respectively. Control cultures received a tenth by volume of 0.8 per cent solution of sodium chloride instead of penicillin. The same mixing tubes and standardized pipets could be used for testing various concentrations of the same sample of penicillin by preparing cultures containing the least amount of penicillin first. Serum and plasma were removed carefully from the mixing tubes after one group of cultures had been made and before medium was prepared containing a greater amount of penicillin.

The preparation used in making the culture was a modified Maximow type of preparation in which the culture was planted on a 22 mm. round coverslip attached by a small drop of saline solution to a heavier glass slide. With a standardized pipet 1 drop (approximately 0.05 c.c.) of plasma containing penicillin was placed on the coverslip and evenly distributed by means of a sterile wire. Three drops of serum extract containing the test organism and penicillin were added to the drop of plasma on the coverslip and well mixed. Four cultures were prepared for each experimental condition. Each culture was covered with a sterile, hollow ground slide rimmed with petrolatum (Fig. 1).§ At the conclusion

---

* Tables 1 and 2 of Heilman's article. W. E. H.

† Table 2 of Heilman's article. W. E. H.

‡ When the U. S. Government penicillin standard became available the end point was revised to 0.07. W. E. H.

§ Not reproduced here. W. E. H.

of the experiment cultures were sealed with a mixture of paraffin and petrolatum and were incubated at 37° C. in a specially constructed down-draft incubator. Final observations were made after approximately 36 hours of incubation. At that time the number of bacterial colonies in each culture was determined with the aid of a dissection microscope at a magnification of 7X. An estimate was made of the average number of colonies present in control cultures not containing penicillin. An end-point was chosen arbitrarily as the lowest concentration of penicillin that would completely prevent the appearance of bacterial colonies in all 4 cultures. This end-point was determined several times for each preparation if the size of the sample would permit. The initial test in each instance was usually done with concentrations of penicillin spaced more widely apart than in subsequent tests in order to determine the range of activity of the sample. Several different preparations were tested on the same day.

Results.—It was found that the growth of the test organism was prevented by 3 μg. per c.c. of the standard sodium salt of penicillin but not by 2.86 μg. per c.c. Since the potency of this standard was 28 Oxford units per mg. the amount of penicillin necessary to prevent bacterial growth was presumably 0.084 Oxford units per c.c. in the final tissue culture clot. Using this value the potency of each of the other preparations was determined by dividing 84 by the number of micrograms of each sample necessary to cause total inhibition. In tests done with a second standard, a calcium salt of penicillin, 0.59 μg. per c.c. caused total inhibition of bacterial growth; thus the potency as determined by this method was 142 Oxford units per mg. This result showed an agreement of within 5 per cent with the original assay of potency of 135 Oxford units per mg.

The results of individual tests with preparations of penicillin from different sources appear in tables [13] and [14].* Similar results were usually obtained on different days with the same sample of penicillin, particularly when widely spaced concentrations of the drug were used as in earlier tests. When there were smaller differences between concentrations used, as in the case of sample B5, varied results were obtained; however, the variation in this instance was within a range of 10 per cent.

The difference between the results of assay of a product at the source and the value determined by this method was sometimes very great. All samples showing a greater potency by the present method than that claimed by the manufacturer were obtained from one source. In the case of 2 samples from source C the material was tested again at the source by the Oxford method and the results showed good agreement with the results obtained in this laboratory. Results of tests on preparations A and D did not differ more than 16 per cent from the results obtained at the source. Sample E was apparently less than half as potent as the estimate at the source would indicate.

Heilman pointed out that the disadvantages of the method are those which are common to tissue culture technic in general. The method was recommended not only for assay of penicillin but also for quantitative studies of other antibacterial agents. It was further pointed out by Heilman that the tissue culture medium appears to be more uniform than other bacteriologic media commonly used. Moreover, the same concentration of penicillin tested at different times regularly caused the same degree of inhibition of bacterial growth. Another advantage of the test lies in the fact that small amounts of penicillin are sufficient to perform a large number of tests. This method was not recommended for determining the amount of penicillin in the blood or other tissues of patients

* Tables 1 and 2 of Heilman's article. W. E. H.

who were receiving penicillin. It is strictly a method for standardizing the agent.

METHODS SUITABLE FOR DETERMINING THE PRESENCE OF PENICILLIN IN BODY FLUIDS

What was said of one of the methods of assay of penicillin, namely, that it is not suitable for determination of the amount of penicillin in the blood or body fluids, is true of most of them. To meet the problem of determining, as accurately as possible, levels of penicillin in the blood or body fluids, various methods have been devised. While these methods are satisfactory for clinical studies, their accuracy is not sufficiently high to be used in studies of a chemical nature. The test of the amount of active penicillin in the blood is measured by the power of the serum which contains penicillin to effect bacteriostasis. This is the test which lies behind use of the terms "penicillin activity," "bacteriostatic activity," "concentration of penicillin" in the blood or in the tissue fluids, "blood level of penicillin," "penicillin content" and so on.

The two methods which have been most extensively used are those described respectively by Rammelkamp[18] and by Fleming;[19] the latter is an adaptation of the Wright slide-cell technic. This latter method has been the most satisfactory in my experience for determination of the amounts of penicillin present in various body fluids of patients who are receiving penicillin.

The Method of Rammelkamp.[18]—This method has been used satisfactorily by a number of investigators to determine the amount of penicillin present in whole blood, erythrocytes, urine, spinal fluid, various exudates from infected cavities, including empyema cavities, and joint fluid. The method, as described by Rammelkamp, is as follows:

Methods.—The unknown samples of penicillin are stored at 5° C. until the time of testing. If the samples are known to be contaminated, sterlization is effected by passing them through a Seitz filter.

To the first 2 tubes of a series of small culture tubes, 0.2 c.c. of the unknown sample is added. The tubes, with the exception of the first one in the series, contain 0.2 c.c. of veal infusion broth. From the second tube, then, 0.2 c.c. of the broth-penicillin sample is removed and serial dilutions are made. In addition, if the solution to be tested is known to contain a very small quantity of penicillin, a further tube containing 0.5 c.c. of the unknown is added to the test.

A control run with each determination is made up from a standard of penicillin which is stored at 5° C. in a solution of 0.85 per cent sodium chloride in a concentration of 20 Florey units per c.c. This standard is then treated in a manner similar to the unknown samples.

The test organism is a Group A strain of hemolytic streptococcus obtained from the blood stream of a patient with erysipelas. The appropriate dilution of a 12-hr. broth culture is made in veal infusion broth containing 1 per cent erythrocytes so that the final number of organisms varies between 1,000 and 10,000 per c.c. The inoculum consists of 0.5 c.c. of this dilution and is added to each tube as well as to the control series containing dilutions of a known amount of penicillin. The final volume in each instance is 0.7 c.c. The cultures are then incubated for 18 hr. following which the tubes are examined for hemolysis. A 3 mm. loop of the cultures near the endpoint is streaked on blood agar plates as a check of sterility.

According to Rammelkamp, this test has proved satisfactory in his hands. The test is said to be sensitive to concentrations as low as 0.0039 unit of penicillin per 0.2 cc. of the solution. The amount of unknown fluid required is small (0.2 to 0.9 c.c.) and therefore the method is readily adaptable to clinical studies.

One disadvantage of the test lies in the fact that sterile precautions are necessary and it is recommended that some of the contents of the tubes near the end point be cultured on blood agar to insure sterility, which requires an additional period of twenty-four hours in order to complete the determination. Furthermore, it is necessary to filter the material to be tested if the samples are known to be contaminated.

Fleming's Modification of the Wright Slide-cell Technic for Determining Penicillin in Body Fluids.—At the Mayo Clinic this procedure, with one or two minor variations, has been found the most reliable method for this work. The details of the procedure, as it is used in the laboratories at the Mayo Clinic, have been described by Dorothy Heilman and me.[20] It is carried out as follows:

Materials.—Special materials needed for the test are (1) sterile whole human blood defibrinated by shaking with glass beads, (2) a twenty-four hour broth culture of Streptococcus pyogenes and (3) penicillin of known strength.

Preparation of Slide Cells.—1. Sterilize microscope slides by passing them through a Bunsen flame and allow them to cool. 2. Cut small pieces of paper of uniform thickness to the size of 25 by 2 mm. Paper with a dull finish from an old journal is satisfactory. 3. Dip the slips of paper in hot petrolatum; drain off the excess petrolatum and place the slips along each end of a microscope slide and across the slide at regular intervals to divide it into six compartments of equal size. 4. Place a second slide, flamed side down, on top of the first slide and press down (fig. [11]).* 5. Leave a weight on the preparation for a few minutes; then store slide cells in a covered dish in the refrigerator until they are used.

Method for Dilution of Test Material.—1. Use small test tubes 7.5 cm. long and 1 cm. in diameter, plugged with cotton and sterilized. For each sample of serum, spinal fluid and so forth to be tested, place a row of twelve tubes in a rack. For samples of urine fourteen tubes are used. 2. With a sterile 1 c.c. pipet place 0.2 c.c. of sterile 0.85 per cent solution of sodium chloride in all tubes except the first tube in each row. 3. With a sterile 0.2 c.c. pipet place 0.2 c.c. of the substance to be tested (blood serum and so forth) in the first tube. 4. Add 0.2 c.c. of the undiluted blood serum or other test material to the saline solution present in the second tube and mix well. 5. Transfer 0.2 c.c. of the mixture in the second tube to the third tube and mix. Transfer 0.2 c.c. of the contents of the third tube to the next tube and so on to the end of the row. Discard 0.2 c.c. of the mixture from the last tube.

* Figure 4 of Heilman and Herrell's article. W. E. H.

Method of Diluting the Solution of Standard Penicillin.—1. Make a solution of the standard penicillin in 0.85 per cent solution of sodium chloride so that 1 c.c. of solution will contain 1 unit of penicillin. 2. Place two rows of six test tubes each, one behind the other, in a rack. With a sterile 5 c.c. pipet place 1.5 c.c. of 0.85 per cent solution of sodium chloride in the first tube in the first row and 1 c.c. in each of the other tubes in the first row. 3. Place 0.5 c.c. of solution of standard penicillin (1 unit per cubic centimeter) in the first tube. Mix well. 4. Transfer 1 c.c. of the mixture in the first tube to the second tube. Mix well. 5. Transfer 1 c.c. of the mixture in the second tube to the third tube and so on. 6. With a 1 c.c. pipet transfer 0.2 c.c. of the solution of penicillin in the sixth tube to the empty tube behind it in the second row. Blow out the contents of the pipet before using it to measure the next dilution. 7. With the same pipet place 0.2 c.c. of the contents of the fifth tube in the first row to the tube behind it. Proceed in the same way until each of the tubes in the second row contains 0.2 c.c. of different concentrations of penicillin. 8. Remove the first row of tubes to another rack and save them for use in other tests to be done on the same day. Fresh dilutions of standard penicillin are prepared for each day's work.

Preparation of Slide-cell Cultures.—1. Heat the defibrinated human blood in a water bath at 50° C. for thirty minutes or store the blood in the ice-box for two days

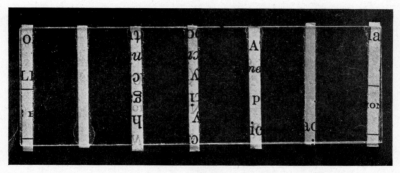

Fig. 11.—Plain slide cell as it appears before being filled with test material. (From article by Heilman and Herrell, American Journal of Clinical Pathology, January, 1945.)

in order to kill the leukocytes. 2. With a sterile 0.2 c.c. pipet add a twenty-four hour culture of Streptococcus pyogenes to the blood in the proportion of 0.005 c.c. of culture to each cubic centimeter of blood. Mix well. 3. With a 1 c.c. pipet add 0.2 c.c. of blood inoculated with Streptococcus pyogenes to each of the small tubes containing 0.2 c.c. of saline dilutions of the test material and penicillin standard. Shake the tubes to mix the contents. 4. With a capillary glass pipet take up some of the mixture of inoculated blood and penicillin solution from the sixth tube, the one containing the least amount of penicillin. 5. Allow the mixture to run from the capillary pipet into the sixth compartment of a slide cell, filling the compartment completely. Blow out the contents of the capillary pipet. 6. With the same pipet take up some of the contents of the fifth tube containing penicillin solution and fill the fifth compartment of the same slide cell. 7. Proceed in the same manner until the slide cell is filled with mixtures of each concentration of the penicillin standard and inoculated blood. 8. Place the slide cell on a glass plate (an old photographic plate is suitable). With a medicine dropper, run a hot mixture of equal parts of paraffin and petrolatum around the slide cell to seal it completely and attach it to the glass plate. 9. Fill slide cells with mixtures of the test substances and inoculated blood in the manner described for the penicillin standard. By transferring the suspensions containing the least amount of test substance first, the same capillary pipet may be used for all solutions containing the same test substance. Use a separate capillary pipet for tests involving different specimens. 10. As soon as slide cells are filled, place them close together on a glass plate and run the hot paraffin-petrolatum mixture between them and around the edges of each slide cell. Record data pertaining to individual slide cells on the glass plate with a wax pencil (fig. [12]).* 11. Incubate slide cell preparations in the horizontal position at 37° C. for eighteen hours. Figure [13]* shows a preparation after incubation.

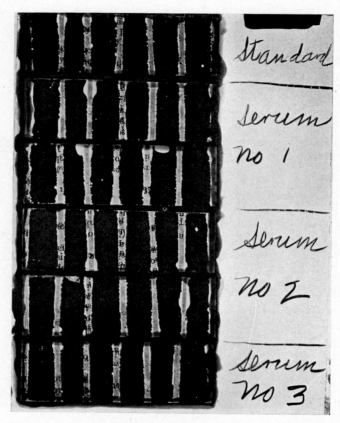

Fig. 12.—Slide-cell cultures on glass plate before incubation. (From article by Heilman and Herrell, American Journal of Clinical Pathology, January, 1945.)

Reading the Test.—1. Examine the slide cell containing the penicillin standard for the presence of hemolysis. Choose as an end point the concentration of penicillin that completely prevents hemolysis due to Streptococcus pyogenes. In our experience 0.03 unit per cubic centimeter (1/32 unit) usually causes inhibition (fig. [14])* but occasionally 0.06 unit per cubic centimeter (1/16 unit) is necessary to inhibit. 2. Determine the dilution of each test substance (serum, spinal fluid and so forth) that completely prevents hemolysis. Multiply the dilution factor by 0.03 or 0.06, depending on the results with

* Respectively figures 2, 3 and 4 of Heilman and Herrell's article. W. E. H.

the standard in the same test. For example, if a 1:4 dilution of the test substance causes complete inhibition and the end point with the standard is 0.03 unit, then the test material contains 0.12 unit per cubic centimeter of penicillin.

It is convenient to store samples of a stock solution of the penicillin standard in small tubes in solid carbon dioxide. If the penicillin is fairly pure, it will keep its potency for

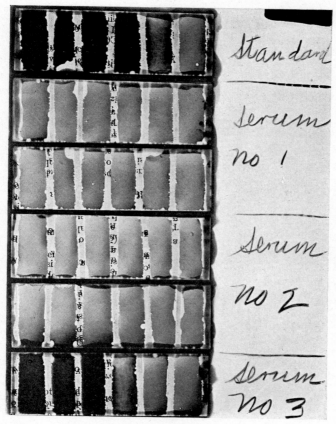

Fig. 13.—Same preparation as that shown in figure 12 after incubation at 37° C. for eighteen hours. The slide cell at the top contains the penicillin standard dilutions from 1:4 to 1:128 inclusive. The end point with the standard is 0.03 unit (see fig. 14). Serum sample 1 (second and third slide cells from the top) and serum sample 2 (fourth and fifth slide cells) do not give evidence of any penicillin activity. Hemolysis is complete in all dilutions. Serum sample 3 (in sixth slide cell) contains 0.12 unit of penicillin per cubic centimeter. (From article by Heilman and Herrell, American Journal of Clinical Pathology, January, 1945.)

several months when stored in this manner, provided it is not subjected to repeated freezing and thawing. When some of the contents of a tube have been used for making the standard solutions, the rest is discarded. The culture of Streptococcus pyogenes may be preserved in solid carbon dioxide in the same way. It is advisable to add an equal amount of horse serum to the culture before placing portions in small tubes prior to freezing.

It is not necessary to use sterile technic in the test, as ordinary contaminants do not grow readily in this medium and, when growth occurs, it rarely interferes with the results. We use sterile glassware and sterile blood and saline solutions but do not observe sterile precautions beyond this. Bacteriologic filtration of specimens to be tested is not necessary. Material to be tested does not have to be sterile if it is tested soon after it is received, so as to guard against loss of penicillin activity previous to the test.

Comparison of the Rammelkamp and Slide-cell Methods.—In order to determine which of the two methods previously described is the more reliable, certain comparative tests of the two methods were made.[21] Varying amounts of penicillin were added to human serum and were

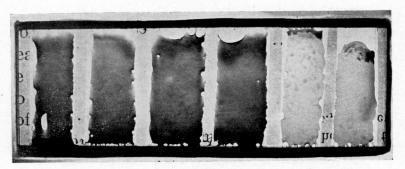

Fig. 14.—Slide cell containing test with standard penicillin after eighteen hours of incubation. The first four compartments from left to right contain the standard penicillin solution (1 unit per cubic centimeter) diluted 1:4 to 1:32. All four show complete inhibition of bacterial growth. The fifth compartment from left to right contains a 1:64 dilution of the penicillin standard. Here there is almost complete hemolysis due to growth of Streptococcus pyogenes. The next dilution shows complete hemolysis. The end point in this test is therefore 1/32 of 1 unit per cubic centimeter, or 0.03 unit per cubic centimeter. (From article by Heilman and Herrell, American Journal of Clinical Pathology, January, 1945.)

tested as unknowns by Heilman. The results of these experiments are shown in table 15. The Fleming method was found to be reliable for determining the actual concentration of penicillin in the serum. The percentage variation between the results obtained with the slide-cell technic and the actual concentration of penicillin was no greater than 50 per cent This variation is to be expected in any test wherein serial dilution methods are employed. Furthermore, the presence of large amounts of serum did not decrease the sensitivity of the test in detecting small amounts of penicillin. Small amounts (0.06 unit per cubic centimeter) were regularly detected when the Fleming method was used whereas these amounts were not detectable when the Rammelkamp method was used. It is possible, however, that others, more accustomed to the latter technic, could

TABLE 15

COMPARISON OF FLEMING AND RAMMELKAMP METHODS
FOR DETERMINING PENICILLIN CONTENT OF SERUM*

Sample number	Units per c.c. of serum†	Fleming method, units per c.c.	Error, per cent	Rammelkamp method, units per c.c.	Error, per cent
1	4.00	3.84	4.0	3.84	4.0
2	0.06	0.06	0	0	....
3	0.06	0.06	0	0	....
4	4.00	3.84	4.0	3.84	4.0
5	1.30	0.96	26.2	0.96	26.2
6	1.30	0.96	26.2	0.96	26.2
7	0.06	0.06	0	0	....
8	1.30	0.96	26.2	0.96	26.2
9	1.30	0.96	26.2	0.96	26.2
10	0.25	0.24	4.0	0.12	52.0
11	0.25	0.24	4.0	0.12	52.0
12	0.06	0.06	0	0	....
13	0.06	0.06	0	0	....
14	4.00	3.84	4.0	7.68	92.0
15	4.00	3.84	4.0	7.68	92.0
16	0.25	0.24	4.0	0.24	4.0
17	0.25	0.24	4.0	0.24	4.0
18	0	0	0	0	0
19	0	0	0	0	0
20	0	0	0	0	0
21	0.25	0.24	4.0	0.24	4.0
22	1.30	1.92	47.7	1.92	47.7
23	4.00	3.84	4.0	7.68	92.0

* From article by Herrell, Nichols and Heilman, Journal of the American Medical Association, August 12, 1944.
† Samples were run as unknowns.

detect these amounts. I already have mentioned the other advantages of the slide-cell method.

REFERENCES

1. Abraham, E. P., Chain, E., Fletcher, C. M., Gardner, A. D., Heatley, N. G., Jennings, M. A. and Florey, H. W.: Further observations on penicillin. Lancet. 2:177–188; 189 (Aug. 16) 1941.

2. Fleming, Alexander: On the antibacterial action of cultures of a penicillium, with special reference to their use in the isolation of B. influenzae. Brit. J. Exper. Path. 10:226–236 (June) 1929.

3. Foster, J. W.: Quantitative estimation of penicillin. J. Biol. Chem. 144:285–286 (June) 1942.

4. Heilman, Dorothy H.: A method for standardizing penicillin. Am. J. M. Sc. 207: 477–483 (Apr.) 1944.

5. Foster, J. W. and Woodruff, H. B.: Microbiological aspects of penicillin. I. Methods of assay. J. Bact. 46:187–202 (Aug.) 1943.

6. Rake, Geoffrey and Jones, Helen: A rapid method for estimation of penicillin. Proc. Soc. Exper. Biol. & Med. 54:189–190 (Nov.) 1943.

7. Heatley, N. G.: A method for the assay of penicillin. Biochem. J. 38:61–65 (No. 1) 1944.

8. Vincent, J. G. and Vincent, Helen W.: Filter paper disc modification of the Oxford cup penicillin determination. Proc. Soc. Exper. Biol. & Med. 55:162–164 (Mar.) 1944.

9. Foster, J. W. and Woodruff, H. B.: Improvements in the cup assay for penicillin. J. Biol. Chem. 148:723 (June) 1943.

10. Foster, J. W. and Woodruff, H. B.: Microbiological aspects of penicillin. VI. Procedure for the cup assay for penicillin. J. Bact. 47:43–58 (Jan.) 1944.

11. Foster, J. W. and Wilker, B. L.: Microbiological aspects of penicillin. II. Turbidimetric studies on penicillin inhibition. J. Bact. 46:377–389 (Oct.) 1943.

12. Joslyn, D. A.: Penicillin assay; outline of four-hour turbidimetric method. Science. n.s. 99:21–22 (Jan. 7) 1944.

13. Lee, S. W., Foley, E. J., Epstein, Jeanne A. and Wallace, J. H., Jr.: Improvements in the turbidimetric assay for penicillin. J. Biol. Chem. 152:485–486 (Feb.) 1944.

14. McMahan, J. R.: An improved short time turbidimetric assay for penicillin. J. Biol. Chem. 153:249–258 (Apr.) 1944.

15. Holmes, Lida F. and Lockwood, J. S.: Studies on bioassay of penicillin. Am. J. M. Sc. 207:267–268 (Feb.) 1944.

16. King, J. T., Henschel, A. F. and Green, B. S.: Influence of prontosil-soluble on beta hemolytic streptococci growing in tissue culture media. Proc. Soc. Exper. Biol. & Med. 38:810–812 (June) 1938.

17. King, J. T., Henschel, A. F. and Green, B. S.: The bacteriostatic and antitoxic actions of sulfanilamide; tissue culture studies. J. A. M. A. 113:1704–1709 (Nov. 4) 1939.

18. Rammelkamp, C. H.: A method for determining the concentration of penicillin in body fluids and exudates. Proc. Soc. Exper. Biol. & Med. 51:95–97 (Oct.) 1942.

19. Fleming, Alexander: Streptococcal meningitis treated with penicillin; measurement of bacteriostatic power of blood and cerebrospinal fluid. Lancet. 2:434–438 (Oct. 9) 1943.

20. Heilman, Dorothy H. and Herrell, W. E.: The use of Fleming's modification of the Wright slide cell technic for determining penicillin in body fluids. Am. J. Clin. Path. (Jan.) 1945.

21. Herrell, W. E., Nichols, D. R. and Heilman, Dorothy H.: Penicillin; its usefu'ness, limitations, diffusion and detection, with analysis of 150 cases in which it was employed. J. A. M. A. 125:1003–1010 (Aug. 12) 1944.

PART II

CLINICAL USE OF PENICILLIN: PREPARATIONS, SYNERGISM, ADMINISTRATION AND EFFECTIVENESS AGAINST DISEASES OF CERTAIN SYSTEMS

CHAPTER VIII

PREPARATIONS AND SYNERGISM OF PENICILLIN IN CLINICAL USE

CRUDE BROTH FILTRATES

Methods for preparing crude broth filtrates containing penicillin have been described in the first section of this book (p. 17). Fleming[1] as early as 1929, for example, used crude broth filtrates containing penicillin for local application to wounds and other infected surfaces. These broth filtrates are stable for at least one week when maintained at refrigerator temperature (5° C.). With the increasing supplies of penicillin that have become available, this form of treatment is being used less and less. Under conditions wherein the more purified preparations are not available, however, crude broth filtrates have proved a practical source of penicillin for use in the treatment of certain infected surfaces. It should be emphasized, nevertheless, that the potential danger of sensitizing patients to the mold protein is present when crude filtrates are employed, a fact which was pointed out by Raper and Coghill.[2]

To be mentioned in this connection, also, is the method of obtaining crude penicillin which was devised by Robinson and Wallace.[3] These investigators inoculated gauze dressings with Penicillium notatum. The dressings had been soaked in a medium that would favor growth of the mold. The dressings then were applied to infected surfaces. In some instances local lesions were treated by injecting crude liquid penicillin into the wound and then the inoculated gauze dressing was placed over the wound. The investigators reported that satisfactory results were obtained with a small number of patients so treated. The danger of sensitizing patients to mold products, however, must be remembered in connection with this form of treatment.

Fisher[4] also has described a crude penicillin filtrate which Crowe and his associates used rather extensively for external application in the field of otolaryngology. Hoyt, Levine and Pratt[5], moreover, have written of methods which facilitate the production of solutions of penicillin that are suitable for local use. Another form of crude penicillin which has been recommended for local use was described by Roberts and Murphy.[6] Penicillin agar was produced by growing Penicillium notatum on the surface of nutrient agar dishes. This agar, which contained varying amounts of penicillin, was then used for local application to superficial infected lesions. This method is claimed to be fairly simple and practical. However, the same difficulties may arise following its use as those mentioned in connection with other preparations which contain the crude substance.

SODIUM SALT OF PENICILLIN

For clinical purposes the sodium salt of penicillin has been most generally employed. This material usually is dispensed in sealed ampules which contain 100,000 units each. It is desirable that the material be dispensed in as near the dry state as possible. The sodium salt of penicillin is known to be very hygroscopic. It is also destroyed easily by alterations of the hydrogen ion concentration of the surrounding medium and it is very sensitive to oxidizing agents. Heat, primary alcohols and contact with heavy metals also alter the material. Because of these and other properties, the sodium salt of penicillin must be stored in the refrigerator at temperatures no higher than 5° C.

When the sodium salt is dissolved in physiologic saline or glucose solution, to be used for systemic therapy, it will retain its potency for at least forty-eight hours at room temperature. That this is true is further evident from the studies on the stability of penicillin at room temperature reported by Kirby.[7] If penicillin has been dissolved in glucose or physiologic saline solution and sealed in bottles, it can be kept in the refrigerator at 5° C. for as long as several weeks without loss of potency.

CALCIUM SALT OF PENICILLIN

The Oxford investigators, in 1942[8] and again in 1943,[9] reported their observations on the calcium salt of penicillin. They found the calcium salt nonhygroscopic and further pointed out that it could be handled more conveniently than the sodium salt. They, therefore, recommended it for local therapy. From the report of Clark and his associates[10] on the preparation of certain creams for local application in the treatment of burns, it also was evident that the calcium salt was easier to handle than the sodium salt. It was the impression, however, that the calcium salt was unsafe for intramuscular and intravenous use because of certain toxic reactions which had been found to follow its injection into experimental animals.

Nevertheless, it seemed evident from the studies[11-13] carried out at the Mayo Clinic that the calcium salt of penicillin was satisfactory not only for local use but also for various forms of systemic therapy. Using the tissue culture method for the study of cytotoxicity of bactericidal agents which had been previously described,[14] Dorothy Heilman and I found that the calcium salt was somewhat less toxic for cellular elements than the sodium salt of penicillin which, up to that time, had been most commonly used. The decrease of the radius of migration of lymphocytes from lymph node explants as compared with the controls was found to be 13 per cent when the calcium salt was used in concentrations of 1:1,000, whereas the decrease of the radius of migration in the presence of the same concentration of the sodium salt was found to be 27 per cent. Further, the calcium salt appeared to be relatively stable. In our lab-

TABLE 16

STUDIES OF TOXICITY OF SODIUM AND CALCIUM SALTS OF PENICILLIN
(TISSUE CULTURE)

Salt of penicillin	Source	Concentration in tissue culture clot	Migration of lymphocytes, % inhibition
Sodium	A	1:500	51
Calcium	B	1:500	37
Sodium	C	1:500	no inhibition
Sodium	C	1:200	66
Calcium	C	1:500	no inhibition
Calcium	C	1:200	25

oratory we were unable to detect any loss of activity of the calcium salt stored in the dry state, in sealed ampules, at room temperature for as long as six months. The material was kept away from the light. Because of these and other observations, my colleagues and I concluded that the calcium salt should prove safe for intravenous and intramuscular therapy. Subsequent experience has justified this conclusion, and it is now evident that the toxicity noted in the early work with the calcium salt was not due to the calcium in the preparation but, as pointed out later by Florey and Jennings,[15] "was almost certainly due to impurities." A more detailed comparison of the calcium and the sodium salts from three commercial sources, based on the tissue culture studies carried out by Dorothy Heilman, is shown in table 16.

Our studies on the calcium salt of penicillin appear to have received confirmation in the reports of György and Elmes.[16] It was evident from their experiments that the fairly well-purified calcium salt of penicillin is not more toxic for mice and man than is the sodium salt. With this, the reports of Welch and his colleagues[17, 18] are somewhat at variance. They were led to conclude, under the conditions of their experiment, that the calcium salt of penicillin was more toxic than the sodium salt. This is rather surprising in view of the results obtained by my colleagues and me and the results published by György and Elmes. It is my opinion that the data obtained from the studies reported by Welch and his associates do not warrant such unfavorable conclusions. I have found the calcium salt entirely satisfactory for local, intravenous, intramuscular and intrathecal administration. In preparing oil suspensions of penicillin, the calcium salt is much more desirable and satisfactory than the sodium salt.

OTHER SALTS OF PENICILLIN

Barium and ammonium salts of penicillin have been prepared by a number of investigators. While these preparations have been used for local and systemic treatment, at present definite statements cannot be made concerning their systemic use.

The magnesium salt of penicillin also has been prepared; however, according to Welch and his colleagues, the magnesium salt is extremely toxic in comparison with the sodium and calcium salts. From the results of their studies, they were inclinded seriously to question the clinical use of the magnesium salt, particularly for intrathecal injection. While strontium and potassium salts of penicillin also have been prepared, sufficient data are not available at present to warrant any general statement concerning their possible value for clinical use.

THE SYNERGISTIC ACTION OF PENICILLIN AND SULFONAMIDES

As I have mentioned in a previous chapter (p. 37), Ungar[19] reported that one of the sulfonamides, sulfapyridine, and penicillin appeared to be definitely synergistic in action. Likewise, the report of T'ung[20] suggested that antibacterial action was greater when penicillin was combined with sulfonamides than when penicillin was allowed to act alone on some pathogens. He pointed out, however, that this action was more noticeable on certain strains of organisms than on others. On the other hand, Hobby and Dawson[21] recently have reported that, under the conditions of their experiments, sulfadiazine or sulfapyridine and penicillin gave no evidence of true synergistic action. The organisms studied by them were Staphylococcus aureus and Streptococcus pyogenes. On the other hand, in connection with studies on these same organisms, Bigger[22] concluded that sulfathiazole was more effective than sulfanilamide or sulfapyridine in combination with penicillin. Whether or not penicillin and some of the sulfonamides exert true synergistic action, therefore, is still open to some question.

This much can be said, however, from a clinical standpoint. There is no contraindication to the simultaneous use of penicillin with any of the sulfonamides, at least this has been my experience. In fact, there is good evidence that at times a combination of sulfonamides with penicillin may be desirable. This is particularly true in the case of polyvalent infections wherein the physician is dealing with organisms which are sensitive to penicillin and organisms which are not sensitive to penicillin but which, at the same time, can be inhibited by one of the sulfonamides.

REFERENCES

1. Fleming, Alexander: On the antibacterial action of cultures of a penicillium with special reference to their use in the isolation of B. influenzae. Brit. J. Exper. Path. *10:* 226–236 (June) 1929.

2. Raper, K. B. and Coghill, R. D.: "Home made" penicillin. J. A. M. A. *123:*1135 (Dec. 25) 1943.

3. Robinson, G. H. and Wallace, J. E.: An inoculated penicillin dressing. Science. n.s. *98:*329–330 (Oct. 8) 1943.

4. Fisher, A. M.: The antibacterial properties of crude penicillin. Bull. Johns Hopkins Hosp. *73:*343–378 (Nov.) 1943.

5. Hoyt, R. E., Levine, M. G. and Pratt, O. B.: Preparation of crude penicillin for local application. Am. J. Clin. Path. (Tech. Suppl.) *8:*65–67 (July) 1944.

6. Roberts, Oliver and Murphy, Diarmuid: Penicillin agar. Irish J. M. Sc. s. 6, No. *223:*225–230 (July) 1944.

7. Kirby, W. M. M.: Stability of penicillin solutions at room and incubator temperatures. J. A. M. A. *125:*628–629 (July 1) 1944.

8. Florey, H. W. and Jennings, M. A.: Some biological properties of highly purified penicillin. Brit. J. Exper. Path. *23:*120–123 (June) 1942.

9. Florey, M. E. and Florey, H. W.: General and local administration of penicillin. Lancet. *1:*387–397 (Mar. 27) 1943.

10. Clark, A. M., Colebrook, Leonard, Gibson, Thomas and Thomson, M. L.: Penicillin and propamidine in burns; elimination of hemolytic streptococci and staphylococci. Lancet. *1:*605–609 (May 15) 1943.

11. Herrell, W. E. and Nichols, D. R.: The calcium salt of penicillin. Proc. Staff Meet., Mayo Clin. *18:*313–319 (Sept. 8) 1943.

12. Herrell, W. E.: The clinical use of penicillin; an antibacterial agent of biologic origin. J. A. M. A. *124:*622–627 (Mar. 4) 1944.

13. Herrell, W. E., Nichols, D. R. and Heilman, Dorothy H.: Penicillin; its usefulness, limitations, diffusion and detection, with analysis of 150 cases in which it was employed. J. A. M. A. *125:*1003–1010 (Aug. 12) 1944.

14. Herrell, W. E. and Heilman, Dorothy H.: Tissue culture studies on cytotoxicity of bactericidal agents. I. Effects of gramicidin, tyrocidine and penicillin on cultures of mammalian lymph node. Am. J. M. Sc. *205:*157–162 (Feb.) 1943.

15. Florey, H. W. and Jennings, M. A.: The principles of penicillin treatment. Brit. J. Surg. *32:*112–116 (July Suppl.) 1944.

16. György, Paul and Elmes, P. C.: Experiments on the toxicity of the calcium salt of penicillin. Proc. Soc. Exper. Biol. & Med. *55:*76–77 (Jan.) 1944.

17. Welch, Henry, Price, C. W., Nielsen, Jean K. and Hunter, A. C.: The acute toxicity of commercial penicillin. J. Lab. & Clin. Med. *29*:809–814 (Aug.) 1944.

18. Welch, Henry, Grove, D. C., Davis, Ruth P. and Hunter, A. C.: The relative toxicity of six salts of penicillin. Proc. Soc. Exper. Biol. & Med. *55*:246–248 (Apr.) 1944.

19. Ungar, J.: Synergistic effect of para-aminobenzoic acid and sulphapyridine on penicillin. Nature. *152*:245–246 (Aug. 28) 1943.

20. T'ung, Tsun: In vitro action of penicillin alone, and in combination with sulfathiazole, on Brucella organisms. Proc. Soc. Exper. Biol. & Med. *56*:8–11 (May) 1944.

21. Hobby, Gladys L. and Dawson, M. H.: Relationship of penicillin to sulfonamide action. Proc. Soc. Exper. Biol. & Med. *56*:184–187 (June) 1944.

22. Bigger, J. W.: Synergic action of penicillin and sulfonamides. Lancet. *2*:142–145 (July 29) 1944.

CHAPTER IX

METHODS OF ADMINISTRATION AND DOSAGE

LOCAL APPLICATION

In the treatment of infected superficial lesions, crude broth filtrates of cultures of Penicillium notatum, which contain penicillin, can be applied locally. Gauze dressings can be saturated with the material and kept in constant contact with the infected tissues. I have mentioned that this form of local treatment is of greatest value to those individuals who do not have available the more purified preparations of penicillin. Broth filtrates have been applied every few hours in many instances without difficulty.

One of the more purified preparations, either the sodium or the calcium salt, can be used for local treatment. However, the calcium salt is more satisfactory for this purpose, particularly if the preparation is used dry and is applied to raw surfaces. At times, under these conditions, the sodium salt may cause local irritation and pain. Solutions of either the sodium or the calcium salt can be employed for local treatment of wounds which involve soft tissue and bone. Physiologic saline or aqueous solutions containing 250 units of penicillin per cubic centimeter are suitable for this form of application. These solutions also can be instilled through small rubber tubes surgically placed in deeper wounds. Repeated injections of solution of penicillin through these tubes can be carried out several times a day. It is important to emphasize that solution of penicillin is not to be used for irrigation but rather for instillation. If solution of penicillin is used for irrigation, the material does not stay in contact with the infected surface long enough to permit bacteriostatic activity.

The British investigators[1] have used penicillin for local treatment in two other forms: 1. If a dry substance is desired, weighed amounts of penicillin are ground with sulfanilamide in a mortar until a homogeneous powder results. On occasions the final mixture contains as much as 5,000 Oxford units of penicillin per gram of powder. 2. Another preparation which the British have applied locally is a cream, of which the base is lanette wax and which contains 100 to 250 units of penicillin per gram. In general, in the treatment of severe and extensive inflammatory lesions, uniformly satisfactory results are more likely to be obtained by the use of systemic penicillin therapy alone or in combination with local therapy.

The local use of penicillin will be discussed in further detail in connection with its value in various infections, including wounds and other infected lesions.

INTRAMUSCULAR ADMINISTRATION

Intermittent Method.—The intermittent intramuscular administration of penicillin is simple and practical. Ten thousand to 20,000 Oxford units in 1 to 2 c.c. of isotonic solution of sodium chloride are injected intramuscularly every three hours day and night. A standard 22 gage intramuscular needle $2\frac{1}{2}$ inches (about 6 cm.) long is suitable. Local irritation occasionally may occur following these injections but serious difficulties are not encountered as a rule. One disadvantage lies in the fact that at least eight injections are required in every twenty-four hours. Furthermore, the concentration of penicillin in the blood rises rather sharply during the first hour following intramuscular administration and then falls to a low value during the hour before the next injection is made. Such sharp rises and falls in the concentration in the blood of any antibacterial agent are not, as a rule, desirable in treatment of bacterial infections. This is particularly true in the presence of severe, overwhelming septicemia.

Continuous Method.—Morgan and his colleagues[2] described a continuous intramuscular drip method for administration of penicillin. Sixty thousand to 90,000 Oxford units of the sodium salt of penicillin have been administered every twenty-four hours by this method. The entire quantity to be used is dissolved in a liter of physiologic saline solution and the rate of flow is adjusted to permit intramuscular administration of this amount in twenty-four hours. According to Morgan and his colleagues, this method maintains a more constant level of penicillin in the blood and, according to them, the administration can be accomplished with comparative freedom from pain or discomfort on the part of the patient. The disadvantages of this method include the danger of local infection and abscess. Concerning the possibility of some inactivation of penicillin by certain synthetic rubber tubing, see page 113.

McAdam, Duguid and Challinor[3] also have reported on this same method of administration. However, they use 100,000 Oxford units a day in 100 c.c. of solution and the rate of administration is regulated so as to deliver this amount in twenty-four hours. It was suggested by these observers, furthermore, that the material might be administered in this fashion directly into the site of local infection.

Harris[4] has described a continuous intramuscular infusion method of administering penicillin which is essentially the same as that previously described by Morgan and his colleagues. Under certain conditions I am sure that this method has a place in penicillin therapy.

Beeswax-oil Suspensions.—Since beeswax has proved useful in prolongation of the action of certain substances, such as histamine,[5] desoxy-corticosterone acetate[6] and heparin,[7] Romansky and Rittman[8] examined the possible use of mixtures of beeswax and peanut oil as a vehicle for prolonging the action of penicillin. Mixtures containing as much as 6 per cent beeswax in peanut oil were prepared. To these mixtures were added varying amounts of penicillin and, by shaking the assembled ingredients in bottles containing glass beads, the investigators were able to effect dispersion of the particles of penicillin. It was found that following intramuscular injection of this material, made to contain 5,000 to 10,000 Oxford units of penicillin per cubic centimeter, fairly adequate concentrations of penicillin in the blood of experimental animals were sustained for six to twelve hours. Furthermore, following intramuscular administration of 2 to 2.4 c.c. of the beeswax-peanut oil mixtures, to which had been added 41,500 to 66,400 Oxford units of penicillin, absorption was delayed and fairly adequate concentrations were maintained in the blood of human subjects for six to seven hours. Penicillin was present in the urine for twenty to thirty-two hours following this method of administration.

This is an exceedingly important addition to the methods of administering penicillin. In the treatment of certain conditions wherein long periods of administration of penicillin are not necessary (gonorrhea, p. 203), it may be possible to administer a complete course of treatment by means of a single intramuscular injection of the beeswax-peanut oil preparation. It may also prove of value in the treatment of certain chronic infections wherein delayed absorption and prolonged action are desirable.

Another significant finding in connection with studies on beeswax-peanut oil mixtures to which penicillin has been added is that various batches which are kept at room temperature for as long as sixty-two days do not lose potency.

The nonhygroscopic calcium salt of penicillin is the preparation of choice for addition to such mixtures. If available, I am inclined to believe that beeswax-sesame oil mixtures are equally as good as, if not better than, beeswax-peanut oil mixtures. Beeswax should not be mixed with animal oils as a vehicle for penicillin. If animal oils are employed, oil tumors are very likely to develop after multiple injections. Furthermore, while the beeswax-peanut oil preparation may prove useful under certain conditions, it probably will not replace the standard methods of administering penicillin for treatment of conditions such as severe, overwhelming septicemia, wherein high concentrations of penicillin in the blood are desirable and attainable immediately by intramuscular or intravenous administration of penicillin in physiologic solution of sodium chloride or glucose.

Effect of Chilling.—Further studies on efforts to prolong the action of penicillin following its intramuscular administration have been reported by Trumper and Hutter.[9] The principle they employed is that chilling slows circulation in and around the site of an intramuscular injection. Therefore, one or two hours before a single, large dose of penicillin in physiologic saline solution was to be administered intramuscularly, an ice bag was applied at the site of injection and it was left in place for five to twelve hours after the injection. By use of this method, effective concentrations in the blood were maintained for at least five hours, as compared with two and a half hours when single doses were administered without chilling. The investigators obtained satisfactory results in treatment of patients suffering with gonorrhea when using single injections of 50,000 units of penicillin. They concluded that, if chilling was employed, bacteriostatic concentrations of penicillin could be maintained by giving two or three, instead of eight to twelve, intramuscular injections over a period of twenty-four hours. They also pointed out that application of the ice bag in advance of the injections rendered the injections painless. Further, they concluded that chilling such as has been described resulted in a 50 per cent saving in the amount of penicillin required for each patient.

INTRAVENOUS ADMINISTRATION

Intermittent Method.—Penicillin disappears from the blood stream even faster after a single intravenous injection than after a single intramuscular injection. Furthermore, if penicillin is administered by single intravenous injection every three hours, eight separate venipunctures must be made each day. This method has been used, however, in some instances with satisfactory results. It is not a method of choice.

Continuous Method.—Since I am about to describe in some detail the continuous intravenous drip method of administering penicillin which is used at the Mayo Clinic, and since I have not particularly associated the name of the clinic with any of the intramuscular methods just described, perhaps I should make clear that intramuscular methods are used there also.

Half of the twenty-four hour dose of penicillin is dissolved in 1 liter of isotonic solution of sodium chloride. If the use of sodium chloride is undesirable, the material can be dissolved in a 5 per cent solution of dextrose made up in distilled water. However, the continuous administration of dextrose may of itself at times produce venous irritation. At the clinic, therefore, we dissolve the material in dextrose only in those cases in which the use of sodium chloride is undesirable. Next, an 18 gage Lewisohn transfusion needle is inserted deeply into the vein, usually a vein of the arm, and is anchored with adhesive plaster. Use of veins

on the dorsal surface of the hand or on the lateral aspect of the forearm allows the hand to be kept in pronation and renders this method
of administration much less uncomfortable than when the material is
administered with the arm in supination. A simple arm splint or
bandage is applied to keep the arm in position. This method is tolerated well by the patient and renders the administration of penicillin fairly

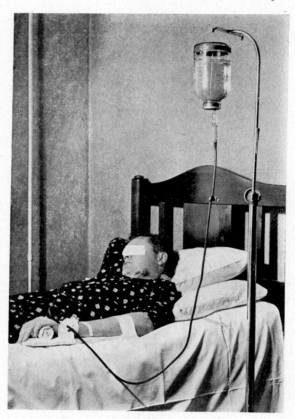

Fig. 15.—Administration of penicillin by the continuous intravenous drip method with
patient recumbent. The patient represented received penicillin in this manner for eight
days without withdrawal of the needle. He could move about with the needle in place.
(From article by Herrell, Journal of the American Medical Association, March 4, 1944.)

comfortable. It avoids eight separate intramuscular or intravenous injections in twenty-four hours. Some patients who receive penicillin in
this fashion may sit up at times during the course of the injection (figs.
15 and 16). It has been possible to administer penicillin without changing
the needle or disturbing the apparatus in some instances for as long as
eight days. Veins in the feet or legs can be used for this method of ad-

ministration but the veins of the arm are preferred because complications following occasional venous irritation or thrombosis are considerably less severe if the veins affected are in the upper rather than in the lower extremity.

From what has just been written, it is evident that local venous irritation at the site of injection may attend the use of the continuous intravenous drip method and, parenthetically, it may be said here that such

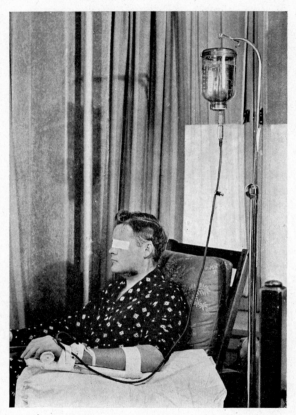

Fig. 16.—Administration with patient sitting. (From article by Herrell, Journal of the American Medical Association, March 4, 1944.)

irritation seems especially likely to occur with certain batches of penicillin which may contain impurities. Careful inspection of the intravenous apparatus and changing the site of injection at the first sign of irritation usually are sufficient to cope with this difficulty. Although we have administered penicillin for as long as eight days through the same vein and into the same site of injection, it is often necessary to change the apparatus every few days. In my experience, venous irritation does not occur in more than 5 to 10 per cent of cases. In this connection should be mentioned the possible inclusion of heparin in intravenous infusions as a means of preventing the thrombosis or venous irritation which may occur when the intravenous drip method is used. This use of heparin was suggested by Martin,[10] who found that 3 units of heparin per cubic centimeter of solution of penicillin made it possible to give the required amounts of penicillin without incident. He further pointed out that when infusions are given at the rate of 35 drops per minute, it would not seem possible to administer enough heparin materially to affect clotting time.

Now, to return to the technic of administration: Initially, 100 c.c. of the material is allowed to run into the vein at a fairly rapid rate. Following this, the rate of injection is regulated to 20 to 30 drops a minute. The second liter is attached to the continuous intravenous system eight to ten hours later, or whenever the material in the original bottle has been used. Cowan[10½] has reported that certain synthetic rubber tubing may inactivate penicillin. For intravenous drip therapy only natural rubber tubing, especially prepared, should be used.

We have used, as a rule, no more than 80,000 to 100,000 Oxford units per day and, in many instances, 40,000 units per day for intravenous therapy. Obviously, when increased supplies of penicillin are available, the problem of dosage may become of less and less significance. In our early work with penicillin low doses were employed in order to spread a small supply of penicillin as far as possible. If subsequent experience indicates that the hazard of delayed recurrence of the condition being treated is increased by using low dosage, obviously the amounts used must be increased. I consider, however, that 100,000 units per day is probably the maximal amount of penicillin necessary for treatment of those infections most commonly encountered. Delayed recurrences in the presence of metastatic lesions may occur at times regardless of the amount of penicillin used. Those infections which require a total daily dose larger than 80,000 to 100,000 Oxford units will be mentioned in connection with the treatment of certain specific infections.

The continuous intravenous drip method is the one of choice in the treatment of severe, overwhelming infections such as bacteriemia. Penicillin should be given by this route at least for the first few days of treatment. Under certain circumstances, the intermittent intramuscular method is entirely satisfactory. On the other hand, it is my impression that nearly twice as much penicillin is required for satisfactory intramuscular treatment as is required when the intravenous drip method is employed. That this is the case seems evident also from the report by White and others.[11] They declared that in their opinion 100,000 units of penicillin, given by the intravenous drip method, are as effective as 200,000 units administered by the intramuscular method.

5

SUBCUTANEOUS ADMINISTRATION

Penicillin can be administered intermittently or continuously by the subcutaneous route. However, absorption of material administered subcutaneously is erratic. Moreover, concentrated solutions of penicillin may at times prove irritating when given subcutaneously. It appears, therefore, that the intravenous or intramuscular method of administration is preferable to the subcutaneous method.

INTRATHORACIC ADMINISTRATION

In the treatment of suppurative intrathoracic disease such as empyema, it often is desirable to supplement systemic therapy with instillations of penicillin into the pleural space. In some instances, empyema can thus be satisfactorily treated without resorting to surgical drainage. For intrathoracic treatment, 40,000 to 50,000 units of penicillin is administered daily. The amount to be used should be dissolved in 40 to 50 c.c. of physiologic saline solution and instilled directly into the pleural space following thoracentesis. It is recommended that this procedure be carried out once every twenty-four to forty-eight hours (see p. 158).

INTRA-ARTICULAR ADMINISTRATION

In the discussion of diffusion of penicillin (p. 77) I mentioned the results of studies carried out by my colleagues and me which indicate that adequately antibacterial amounts of penicillin may reach the joint fluid following intramuscular or intravenous administration, whether the patients are suffering from acute suppurative disease of joints or whether they do not present evidence of inflammation of joints. It is often desirable, however, to supplement systemic therapy by means of instillation of penicillin into affected joints. This can be accomplished without any serious effects. Ten thousand to 20,000 Oxford units of penicillin dissolved in 10 c.c. of isotonic saline solution can be instilled into infected joints after aspiration has been performed. Since penicillin remains in the structure for at least twenty-four hours, it is not necessary to repeat the injection oftener. The material can be administered every day or every other day for several times.

INTRATHECAL ADMINISTRATION

In a previous chapter (p. 75) it was pointed out that penicillin does not readily diffuse into the cerebrospinal structures following its systemic administration. This appears certainly true of the patient who, after being subjected on therapeutic indications to administration of penicillin and spinal puncture, yet is found to be normal. It seems true, also, of subjects suffering with certain diseases, such as syphilis, involving the cerebrospinal structures. Although small amounts of penicillin may reach the cerebrospinal fluid in certain types of infections (acute meningitis for instance) it seems essential to supplement systemic therapy by daily instillations of 10,000 to 20,000 Oxford units of penicillin directly into the spinal canal. At least this should be done during the early period of treatment of severe diseases involving the spinal cord and meninges. This procedure, as a matter of fact, can be carried out for a considerable period without producing any important reactions. The amount of penicillin administered should be dissolved in 10 c.c. of isotonic solution of sodium chloride. Either the sodium or the calcium salt of penicillin has proved satisfactory for this form of treatment.

Five thousand to 10,000 units of penicillin can be instilled also once or twice daily into the ventricular system of the brain if small tubes have been left in place for this purpose at the time some surgical procedure is carried out.

INFUSION OF PENICILLIN BY WAY OF THE BONE MARROW

A satisfactory method for administration of various therapeutic agents by way of the bone marrow has been described by Tocantins and O'Neill.[12] The sternum or clavicle can be used and, in children, the tibia or femur has been employed. It has been found possible to administer as much as 1 liter of solution by this route when the infusion needle was left in place for as long as sixteen hours. The average rate of infusion recommended by Tocantins and O'Neill was between 0.4 and 9 c.c. per minute. Likewise Turkel and Bethell[13] also have described a satisfactory instrument and technic for administration of fluids through the bone marrow.

Since either glucose or salt solution can be administered by way of the bone marrow, Morgan and his colleagues[2] used this method for administration of penicillin in these solutions. It appeared, from the report of Morgan and his colleagues, that as much as 46,000 units of penicillin could be administered in nine hours by this route. This method, however, is not recommended except under very unusual circumstances; for instance, when suitable veins are not available or when, for any reason, as in the presence of extensive burns, the intramuscular or intravenous method is not considered practicable.

ORAL AND INTRACOLONIC ADMINISTRATION

At present, administration of penicillin orally is not satisfactory and is not generally recommended. The hydrochloric acid in the stomach will destroy penicillin. Enteric coating to protect penicillin against gastric acidity does not satisfactorily solve the problem since, when enteric coating is employed, penicillin may find its way into the large intestine, where it is inactivated by certain bacterial enzymes present there. If a patient presents complete achlorhydria, penicillin can be administered by mouth and absorbed into the general circulation in amounts sufficient to justify this method of administration. The method may be of value in the treatment of patients with achlorhydria, then, if other acceptable methods are not practicable. Whether penicillin can be administered successfully by the oral route[14, 15, 16, 17] to human beings, alone, combined with antacids or in various vehicles (see pages 73 and 332), will depend on further clinical trials. Intracolonic administration of penicillin is of no value for reasons which I have already mentioned.

PENICILLIN SNUFF

Snuff containing 5 parts of penicillin by weight, 5 parts of menthol and 90 parts of lycopodium has been recommended by some investigators.[18] The material is administered by this route as often as every four hours. Except in the most superficial types of infections in the nose, however, this method is not likely to be followed by satisfactory results unless, perhaps, systemic therapy also is employed.

PENICILLIN AS AN INHALANT

It was evident from the report of Bryson and his colleagues[19] that penicillin could be used as an inhalant. It is so employed by having the patient breathe nebulized penicillin according to the standard procedure recommended for this purpose. When this form of treatment is used (see bronchitis and bronchiectasis, p. 153) patients may inhale at regular intervals throughout the day varying amounts of penicillin. One cubic centimeter of physiologic saline solution, containing 2,500 Oxford units of penicillin, can be nebulized and inhaled by a patient over a period of ten minutes. This procedure can be carried out as often as three times an hour throughout the day, excluding time out for eating and sleeping. As much as 75,000 to 80,000 Oxford units can be administered by this method. This procedure must not be confused with vaporization methods, wherein the heat that is employed is likely to inactivate penicillin.

REFERENCES

1. Florey, H. W. and Cairns, Hugh: Penicillin in war wounds; a report from the Mediterranean. Lancet. *2:*742–745 (Dec. 11) 1943.

2. Morgan, H. V., Christie, R. V. and Roxburgh, I. A.: Experiences in the systemic administration of penicillin. Brit. M. J. *1:*515–516 (Apr. 15) 1944.

3. McAdam, I. W. J., Duguid, J. P. and Challinor, S. W.: Systemic administration of penicillin. Lancet. *2:*336–338 (Sept. 9) 1944.

4. Harris, F. I.: Continuous intramuscular infusion of penicillin. J. A. M. A. *126:*232 (Sept. 23) 1944.

5. Code, C. F. and Varco, R. L.: Prolonged action of histamine. Am. J. Physiol. *137:*225–233 (Aug.) 1942.

6. Code, C. F., Gregory, R. A., Lewis, R. E. and Kottke, F. J.: Prolonged action of desoxycorticosterone acetate. Am. J. Physiol. *133*:240–241 (June) 1941.

7. Bryson, J. C. and Code, C. F.: Prolonged anticoagulant action of heparin in a beeswax mixture. Proc. Staff Meet., Mayo Clin. *19*:100–107 (Feb. 23) 1944.

8. Romansky, M. J. and Rittman, G. E.: A method of prolonging the action of penicillin. Science. n.s. *100*:196–198 (Sept. 1) 1944.

9. Trumper, Max and Hutter, A. M.: Prolonging effective penicillin action. Science. n.s. *100*:432–434 (Nov. 10) 1944.

10. Martin, Peter: Heparin in intravenous infusions, including penicillin therapy. Brit. M. J. *2*:308 (Sept. 2) 1944.

10½ Cowan, S. T.: Effect of rubber tubing on solutions of penicillin. Lancet. *1*:178–179 (Feb. 10) 1945.

11. White, W. L., Flippin, H. F., Lockwood, J. S. and Murphy, F. D.: The indications for penicillin; its dosage and administration. Clinics. *3*:309–323 (Aug.) 1944.

12. Tocantins, L. M. and O'Neill, J. F.: Infusion of blood and other fluids into the circulation via the bone marrow. Proc. Soc. Exper. Biol. & Med. *45*:782–783 (Dec.) 1940.

13. Turkel, Henry and Bethell, F. H.: A new and simple instrument for administration of fluids through bone marrow. War Med. *5*:222–225 (Apr.) 1944.

14. Libby, R. L.: Oral administration of penicillin in oil. Science. n.s. *101*:178–180 (Feb. 16) 1945.

15. Little, C. J. H. and Lumb, George: Penicillin by mouth. Lancet. *1*:203–206 (Feb. 17) 1945.

16. McDermott, Walsh, Bunn, P. A., Benoit, Maria, DuBois, Rebeckah and Haynes, Willetta: Oral penicillin. Science. n.s. *101*.228–229 (Mar. 2) 1945.

17. Charney, Jesse, Alburn, H. E. and Bernhart, F. W.: Urinary excretion of penicillin in man after oral administration with gastric antacids. Science. n.s. *101*:251–253 (Mar. 9) 1945.

18. Delafield, M. E., Straker, Edith and Topley, W. W. C.: Antiseptic snuffs. Brit. M. J. *1*:145–150 (Feb. 1) 1941.

19. Bryson, Vernon, Sansome, Eva and Laskin, Sidney: Aerosolization of penicillin solutions. Science. n.s. *100*:33–35 (July 14) 1944.

CHAPTER X

INFECTIONS INVOLVING THE BLOOD STREAM AND HEART

In the present chapter I propose to deal with those infections of the blood stream and heart, exclusive of sinus thrombosis, in which penicillin has been used. The use of penicillin in the treatment of sinus thrombosis is discussed in the chapter on infections of the skin and soft tissues, such as severe orbital and nasal cellulitis (p. 182).

BACTERIEMIA NOT ACCOMPANIED BY SUBACUTE BACTERIAL ENDOCARDITIS

Bacteriemia, or septicemia, constitutes one of the most serious problems in the treatment of bacterial infections. Available statistical data indicate that the prognosis in cases of bacteriemia was exceedingly grave until the introduction of modern chemotherapy, beginning with the sulfonamides. For example, before the introduction of sulfonamides, patients fifty years of age or older who became victims of staphylococcal or streptococcal bacteriemia had only one chance in ten to recover—in other words, the recovery rate was 10 per cent. Subsequent to the introduction of sulfonamides, under intensive and adequate treatment, recovery rates in this age group as high as 60 per cent were experienced by some investigators. Nevertheless, the problems involved in the successful use of sulfonamides have been rather formidable. Even in the most experienced hands it is evident, therefore, that at least four of ten patients failed to survive for one reason or another. The development of resistance to sulfonamides on the part of the micro-organism, the feeble bactericidal action of these compounds, as well as their toxicity, are responsible for some of the failures which occurred when sulfonamides were used in treatment.

With the introduction of penicillin as a chemotherapeutic agent by the group of investigators at Oxford,[1] it was evident even in their early experience that a new and far more effective agent had become available for treatment of bacteriemia. Two of the ten cases included in the now famous report by Abraham and others were examples of severe bacteriemia against which penicillin was successfully used in treatment. Probably no therapeutic agent has been more rigidly tested than has penicillin. When only limited supplies were available, for example, only the most critically ill, including bacteriemic patients, received the benefit of the agent. Likewise, the first four cases reported in the American literature[2] in which penicillin had been used were examples of over-whelming infection due to Staphylococcus aureus, including bacteri-emia.

Subsequent to the first British and American reports on the effec-tiveness of penicillin in bacteriemia, reports of a fairly large number of cases of a similar type appeared. The order of appearance of the sub-sequent reports on bacteriemia not accompanied by subacute bacterial endocarditis, of which I have knowledge, was as follows: Guerra Perez Carral,[3] Herrell,[4] Florey and Florey,[5] Keefer and others,[6] Blumberg,[7] Flannery,[8] Hageman and others,[9] Likely and Swirsky,[10] Lyons,[11] Silver-thorne,[12] von Gutfeld,[13] Hellman and Guilfoil,[14] Mitchell and Kam-inester,[15] Dawson and Hobby,[16] Herrell,[17] Bloomfield and others,[18] Tillett and others,[19] Watson,[20] Deeds,[21] De Gowin,[22] Erickson,[23] Christie and Garrod,[24] Anderson and Hill,[25] MacLeod,[26] Wickstrom and Heb-ble,[27] Boller,[28] Leopold,[29] MacNeal and Pease,[30] Ayala Gonzalez and Vejar,[31] Herrell and others,[32] Rosenberg and Arling,[33] Evans[34] and Wollgast.[35]

This series of reports represents a total of 244 cases of bacteriemia in which penicillin has been used. As has just been said, cases of bac-teriemia associated with subacute bacterial endocarditis are not in-cluded in this figure. In the 244 cases of bacteriemia, 186 patients recov-ered following the use of penicillin, a recovery rate of 76 per cent. The above percentage represents a cross section of results obtained by a large number of investigators. It also includes cases which represent experience obtained very early in the studies on penicillin. Many pa-tients were treated very late in the course of their disease and under adverse conditions. It may be possible, in some series of cases, to obtain even better results, particularly if the patients are seen early in the course of the disease and more especially if treatment with penicillin is possible before sulfonamide therapy is first employed. In one series of cases of bacteriemia in which treatment was given at the Mayo Clinic,[32] for example, twenty-five of twenty-eight consecutive patients recovered, a recovery rate of 89 per cent. The group of cases of bacter-iemia from which these data are drawn are summarized in table 17. It now appears that under conditions which permit early, adequate treat-ment with penicillin, the recovery rate in this disease has increased from 10 per cent before the days of modern chemotherapy, to nearly 60 per cent following the use of sulfonamides and now, with penicillin, to 75 per cent or more. In few conditions can such remarkable progress in such a short period be reported.

Staphylococcal Bacteriemia.—Of the 244 cases of bacteriemia without subacute bacterial endocarditis, listed above, the majority were examples of staphylococcal bacteriemia and most of the patients concerned had been found to resist adequate treatment with sulfonamides. The recovery rate in this group of cases of staphylococcal bacteriemia was 135 out of 185, or approximately 73 per cent. It would appear that this figure is fairly representative of the early experience in the treatment of staphylococcal bacteriemia with penicillin. The recovery rate quoted by Anderson,[36] who mentioned 550 cases of staphylococcal bacteriemia (which undoubtedly included a number of cases previously reported) was 71 per cent. Since time is such an exceedingly important factor in

TABLE 17

RESULTS OF TREATMENT WITH PENICILLIN IN 244 CASES OF BACTERIEMIA

Organism	Cases	Results	
		Recovery	Failure
Staphylococcus aureus	183	133	50
Staphylococcus albus	2	2	0
Streptococcus pyogenes	16	15	1
Diplococcus pneumoniae	21	17	4
Anaerobic streptococci	2	2	0
Neisseria intracellularis	14	13	1
Micrococcus tetragenous	1	1	0
Proteus bacillus	1	0	1
Nonhemolytic streptococci	3	2	1
Salmonella*	1	1	0
Total	244	186	58

* Recovery in this case not likely to have been attributable to penicillin. W. E. H.

the outcome of staphylococcal septicemia, it is evident that a higher recovery rate would have been experienced had enough penicillin been available to treat all of the patients concerned, without waiting for sulfonamide resistance or failure under treatment with sulfonamides to occur. Suffice to say, however, that the results in many of the cases have been almost dramatic.

Shown in figure 17 is an example of overwhelming staphylococcal septicemia in which penicillin was used effectively. The condition almost certainly would have been fatal had not penicillin been available. Sulfonamide therapy had been tried and had failed.

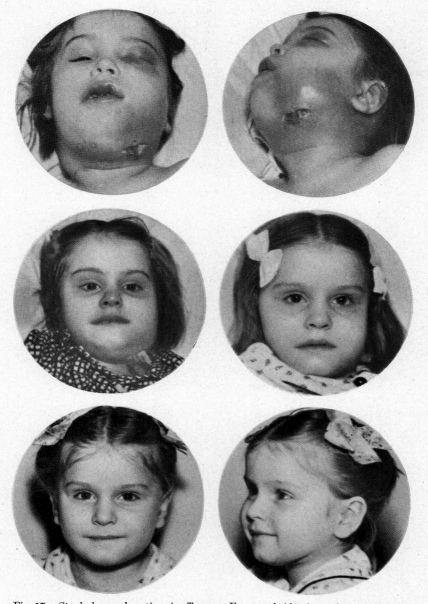

Fig. 17.—Staphylococcal septicemia. *Top row*. Front and side views of patient at onset of penicillin therapy. Extensive facial cellulitis and edema of both eyes. Patient moribund. *Middle row*. Appearance of child, *left*, ninety-six hours and, *right*, nine days after onset of treatment. *Bottom row*. Front and side views of patient before dismissal. Complete recovery.

Streptococcal Bacteriemia.—Results to date have been fairly satisfactory in the treatment of streptococcal infections with sulfonamides. For that reason, the group of cases of this type in which penicillin has been employed is not as large as the group representing staphylococcal bacteriemia. Of the 244 cases previously referred to, sixteen were examples of streptococcal bacteriemia. Fifteen of the sixteen patients recovered satisfactorily.

Figure 18 represents a patient suffering with streptococcal bacteriemia which followed dental extraction and in treatment of whom sulfonamides had failed completely. The patient was treated with the calcium salt of penicillin and satisfactory recovery resulted.

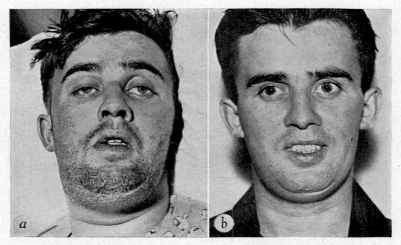

Fig. 18.—Streptococcal bacteriemia. Appearance of patient; *a*, on admission, *b*, on dismissal.

Bacteriemia Due to Miscellaneous Micro-organisms.—In the group of 244 cases of bacteriemia referred to above there occurred examples of bacteriemia owing to Diplococcus pneumoniae, Neisseria intracellularis, anaerobic streptococci, micrococci, micro-organisms of the genus Proteus, nonhemolytic streptococci, and micro-organisms of the genus Salmonella. The number of cases in this miscellaneous group was forty-three, in thirty-six of which recovery resulted.

Clinical Response.—One of the interesting features of patients under treatment with penicillin for bacteriemia not associated with subacute bacterial endocarditis is the temperature curve. As a rule, the temperature subsides gradually and very seldom by crisis such as frequently is seen following successful sulfonamide therapy. In many instances the temperature chart does not give an accurate index of the improvement of the patient (fig. 19). Furthermore, in cases in which treatment for bacteriemia is successful, the blood cultures usually will become negative within twenty-four to seventy-two hours following onset of treatment.

Why Patients with Bacteriemia, not Associated with Subacute Bacterial Endocarditis, Fail to Recover Following Penicillin Therapy.—For the most part, failures in these cases have occurred because the patients were not treated early enough in the course of their infection. In my experience, as will appear a few paragraphs further on, if a patient has evidence of acute vegetative endocarditis before, or at the time of institution of, penicillin therapy, the outlook is poor. Three patients who

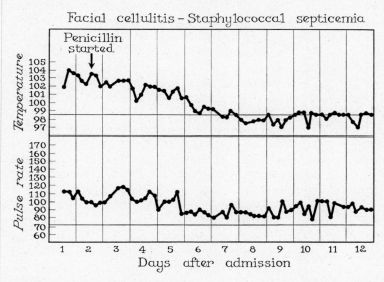

Fig. 19.—Record of temperature and pulse rate in a case of facial cellulitis complicated by staphylococcal septicemia.

failed to recover in a series of twenty-eight whose cases were reported by my colleagues and me,[32] all gave clinical evidence suggestive of the presence of acute endocarditis when treatment with penicillin was begun. All were found to have vegetative endocarditis at the time of necropsy. Much less frequently can unsatisfactory results be attributed to development of resistance on the part of the micro-organism to the action of penicillin. Failure to maintain a constant level of penicillin in the blood is most likely to result in the development of such resistance.

Contraindications.—There are practically no contraindications to the use of penicillin in the treatment of bacteriemia. Severely and critically ill patients, even those with cardiac or renal failure, have been satisfactorily treated with the drug. Penicillin also can be used intensively in treatment of the parturient patient. I have had patients who have been delivered of normal children during the course of penicillin therapy successfully administered for bacteriemia. That penicillin reaches the fetal blood stream was evident from the studies mentioned in the chapter on absorption, diffusion and excretion of penicillin (p. 77).

Plan of Treatment.—In practically no other condition is it more essential to maintain a constant level of penicillin in the blood, particularly for the first few days, than in the treatment of bacteriemia. Whenever suitable veins are available and contraindications do not exist to the administration of 2 liters of physiologic saline or glucose solution per day, penicillin should be administered to patients with bacteriemia, at least for the first few days, by the continuous intravenous drip method. In most instances uncomplicated bacteriemia will respond satisfactorily to the intravenous administration of 40,000 to 50,000 Oxford units of penicillin in 1 liter of physiologic saline or 5 per cent glucose solution given morning and evening. If the rate of flow is adjusted to 20 to 30 drops per minute, usually it will not be necessary to give additional fluids through the continuous intravenous system. (See description of this method in the chapter on methods of administration, p. 110.)

If intravenous infusions are contraindicated, or if it is impracticable to give them, 15,000 to 20,000 Oxford units of penicillin dissolved in 3 or 4 c.c. of physiologic saline solution should be injected every three hours day and night into the muscles of the buttocks or into other muscles. To prevent the local irritation at the site of injection which may result from eight separate punctures a day, it is desirable to alternate from one area to another when using the intramuscular method.

Adequate intake of fluid is essential and the patient should be encouraged to eat an adequate amount of food, preferably a diet high in vitamins and in calories. Unless anemia is present, it is not necessary to give transfusions of whole blood.

If the offending micro-organism is not highly sensitive to penicillin, it may be desirable at times to combine sulfonamides with penicillin in the treatment of bacteriemia. This is especially true in the presence of blood stream infections wherein, as occasionally may occur, two organisms are present, one sensitive to penicillin and the other not sensitive to penicillin (mixed infection with gram-positive and gram-negative pathogens). Under such conditions, penicillin and sulfonamides can be given simultaneously without difficulty. The sulfonamide is administered in solution intravenously or the substance is given by mouth in sufficient quantity to cause the concentration of the sulfonamide in the blood to rise to 12 to 16 mg. per 100 c.c. The solution of sulfonamide can be introduced directly into the tubing of the intravenous apparatus that contains the penicillin.

SUBACUTE BACTERIAL ENDOCARDITIS

Intensive investigations on the effectiveness of penicillin against subacute bacterial endocarditis were not undertaken in the beginning of studies on the use of penicillin because limited supplies of penicillin were available. It was evident, however, from the report by Florey and Florey[5] and from the report from the Mayo Clinic,[4] that when penicillin was used in the treatment of subacute bacterial endocarditis due to a sensitive strain of streptococcus, the blood stream of the patient could be sterilized and fever would subside. However, when penicillin was withdrawn, the infection recurred, blood cultures again became positive and clinical relapse supervened.

Seventeen such cases were included in the report by Keefer and others.[6] In only three was temporary improvement recorded. These investigators were aware of the fact that better results might have been obtained in these cases, when due to susceptible strains of the causative organism, if treatment could have been started very early and carried out over a longer period with massive doses of penicillin. Likewise, ten cases of subacute bacterial endocarditis were reported by Dawson and Hobby.[16] They considered that five of the patients received quantities of penicillin which were totally inadequate to give satisfactory results. Of the other five patients, one was reported to be in good health nine months after penicillin had been administered. The condition of two temporarily improved and two died.

The results obtained by Loewe and his colleagues[37] were somewhat more encouraging. These investigators combined penicillin with heparin and administration was by the continuous intravenous drip method. Some of their patients received as much as 200,000 Oxford units of penicillin per day and some patients each received a total dose of as much as 7,890,340 Oxford units. The heparin was administered either subcutaneously or with the penicillin. Heparin was included with the idea of reducing the incidence of thrombosis, and possibly with the idea of controlling the formation of heavy endocardial vegetations made up of fibrin; such vegetations decrease the chance that the antibacterial agent will come into adequate contact with the infecting micro-organism. The coagulation time of the blood of the patients who received heparin and penicillin was held at somewhere between thirty and sixty minutes. Seven cases of subacute bacterial endocarditis in which treatment was with penicillin and heparin were reported by Loewe and his colleagues. They were successful in sterilizing the circulating blood and relieving the clinical manifestations of the disease in all of the seven cases. In a subsequent report,[38] this same group of investigators reported equally promising results in the treatment of twenty-two additional patients suffering with subacute bacterial endocarditis. Likewise, MacNeal and others,[39] and Collins,[40] have reported on clinical arrest of the course of subacute bacterial endocarditis by the use of penicillin.

It will be necessary, of course, to follow this group of cases for a considerable time before final statements can be made concerning the effectiveness of penicillin in this disease.

My colleagues and I have administered penicillin in a small group of cases of subacute bacterial endocarditis in which the micro-organisms present in the blood were found to be sensitive to penicillin. In this study, much larger doses of penicillin were used than were employed in the earlier investigations at the Mayo Clinic. In a few cases, the condition has remained clinically arrested for several months. In most of them, however, it has recurred. If patients with subacute bacterial endocarditis are to be treated, it is exceedingly important to test the micro-organism that is recovered from the blood for sensitivity to penicillin. It is well established that different strains of streptococci in the so-called viridans group vary considerably in sensitivity. In the chapter on studies made in vitro it was pointed out that considerable variation exists between the sensitivity of Streptococcus salivarius (sensitive) and Streptococcus faecalis (rather resistant). Even with the use of large doses of penicillin I have been unsuccessful in the treatment of patients whose bacterial endocarditis was attributable to the rather resistant Streptococcus faecalis. Streptococcus salivarius and other sensitive strains of streptococci have responded occasionally in a satisfactory manner. It should be emphasized, however, that although the infection may be removed from the blood stream and the heart, the heart is still the site of endocarditis with valvular disease. The patients are faced, therefore, with two possible sequelae, one of which is spontaneous recurrence or reinfection, which may follow some minor surgical procedure such as dental extraction. It is recommended, therefore, that these patients be given penicillin before and after any operations performed subsequent to their endocarditis, even if apparent cure has been obtained. The other sequela which confronts these patients is the usual complication of heart disease. For example, a patient may be freed completely of the bacterial phase of the disease only to die subsequently of congestive heart failure associated with the intrinsic cardiac lesion.

It is my conviction that probably the greatest usefulness of penicillin to patients suffering with intrinsic cardiac lesions may be in its prophylactic employment before and after surgical procedures which are known to be followed frequently by transient bacteriemia and subsequent subacute bacterial endocarditis. If adequate supplies of penicillin are available, this preoperative and postoperative use of the material is to be highly recommended for patients who are victims of endocarditis or who are likely to develop this disease.

Plan of Treatment.—*Penicillin Alone.*—When positive blood cultures are obtained in suspected cases of bacterial endocarditis, the micro-organism should be tested for sensitivity against various concentrations of penicillin. If the organism is sensitive in the range of 0.1 to 0.01 Oxford units per cubic centimeter, satisfactory results are more likely to be obtained than if it is less sensitive. With one or two possible exceptions, treatment of this infection requires the largest dose of penicillin that usually is recommended. For children, as much as 150,000 Oxford units of penicillin per day is recommended; to adults, between 200,000 and 300,000 Oxford units per day should be administered. Constant concentrations of penicillin in the blood are best maintained by administering the material by the intravenous drip method. Blood cultures are obtained every two or three days and administration of penicillin is continued for fifteen to twenty days, or even longer in some instances. Administration of penicillin should not be discontinued until three successive negative blood cultures have been obtained and the patient is free of fever. Some investigators[41] have recommended that penicillin therapy be continued in these cases for a period of months.

Penicillin with Heparin.—The hazards of the successful use of heparin are well known to students of chemotherapy. Its universal use is not recommended. If successful response can be obtained by the use of penicillin alone, it is our practice at the clinic not to use heparin. It can be administered, however, without difficulty by combining it with penicillin in physiologic saline or glucose solution. It also can be given in amounts of 300 mg. every other day subcutaneously. When incorporated in the intravenous drip system in which penicillin is present, 200 mg. of heparin per day is considered a satisfactory amount.

Penicillin with Sulfonamides.—In some instances wherein the infecting micro-organism is slightly resistant to, but is inhibited to some degree by, penicillin, it may be desirable to combine penicillin with sulfonamides. If sulfonamides are used, it is desirable to maintain a concentration of this material in the blood of 14 to 18 mg. per 100 c.c. The sulfonamide can be administered orally or it can be incorporated in the solution of penicillin used for the intravenous drip therapy. Further investigations of this plan of treatment are necessary before its usefulness can be finally evaluated.

Comment.—While continued investigation of the use of penicillin in treatment of subacute bacterial endocarditis is amply justified, I am inclined to adopt a very cautious attitude in interpretation of results. If sufficient supplies of penicillin are available, however, certainly patients who have this disease in an early form should have the benefit of this form of treatment. If the blood streams of these individuals can be kept sterile for a long period, it seems likely that spontaneous healing could occur in some cases.

SUPPURATIVE PERICARDITIS

Acute suppurative pericarditis owing to pyogenic coccal infections will respond satisfactorily to the use of penicillin in certain instances. It is exceedingly desirable to treat the patients intensively either by the intravenous drip or by the intramuscular route of administration. In addition to systemic administration of penicillin, the substance should be instilled locally into the pericardial sac. It is recommended that pus be aspirated frequently from the pericardial sac—at least once a day in the early stages of the disease. Following aspiration, 10,000 to 20,000 Oxford units of penicillin should be instilled in 5 or 10 c.c. of physiologic saline solution. The amount of the solution will depend on the amount of pus withdrawn from the pericardium and also will depend on the size of the cardiac silhouette as measured by roentgenoscopy or roentgenography, as recommended by White.[42]

INFECTIONS OF THE BLOOD STREAM AND HEART IN WHICH PENICILLIN IS OF DOUBTFUL OR NO VALUE

Acute Rheumatic Fever.—Many students of acute rheumatic fever have presented evidence that the disease can be caused by, or can be associated with, infection owing to certain strains of Streptococcus pyogenes. This organism is highly sensitive to the action of penicillin. It was natural, therefore, for investigators to attempt to evaluate the possible use of penicillin in treatment of this disease. Denny and his colleagues[43] reported four cases in which penicillin had been used in treatment of acute rheumatic fever. Penicillin did not appear favorably to affect the course of the disease of two rather acutely ill patients. In two of these cases the disease was mild and was reported to respond satisfactorily. In general, however, the experience of most investigators would tend to indicate that penicillin is of doubtful value, or of no value, in the treatment of rheumatic fever.

A very careful study of the treatment of rheumatic fever with penicillin was conducted by Foster and others.[44] Thirty-eight patients with acute rheumatic fever received penicillin. The investigators concluded that there was no evidence of benefit following its use. They further concluded that in some cases it appeared clinically that the course of the disease was actually aggravated. They also observed two patients in whom characteristic manifestations of acute rheumatic fever developed while the patients were receiving penicillin for severe infections due to group A Streptococcus pyogenes. Simultaneously with the report by Foster and others, there appeared another report by Watson and others[45] who had treated with penicillin eight young adults who had acute rheumatic fever. The course of treatment was given over a period of two weeks and total doses as high as 3,470,000 Oxford units were administered to some patients. Of considerable interest is the fact that Streptococcus pyogenes was isolated in cultures from the nasopharynx in six of these eight cases at the time of admission of the patients. Growth of this organism was completely inhibited by 0.015 Oxford unit. It was further evident that concentrations far in excess of inhibitory amounts were maintained in the blood of these patients during most of the period of treatment. On the other hand, treatment with penicillin failed to alter the course of the disease.

While these negative results which were obtained following the use of penicillin in these cases do not completely eliminate the possibility of the hemolytic streptococcal origin of acute rheumatic fever, they are indeed suggestive. It can be stated with reasonable certainty, however, that the acute clinical phase of the disease, be its origin streptococcal or not, is not favorably affected by administration of amounts of penicillin which can be assumed to be adequate. Penicillin may have some place in the prevention of acute streptococcal infection of the throat, which is of common occurrence among patients who have rheumatic fever, and thereby penicillin may be of value in the prevention of recurrent episodes of rheumatic fever. If so, the effect of penicillin would be similar to the now well-established prophylactic effect of sulfonamides in cases of rheumatic fever. It will be recalled that sulfonamides, while of no value against acute rheumatic fever, have definitely been established as valuable agents in the prophylaxis against recurrences. If it becomes feasible to administer penicillin in some form to these ambulatory patients, the use of this relatively nontoxic chemotherapeutic agent should be investigated further.

Bacteriemia Due to Insensitive Micro-organisms.—To date penicillin has proved of doubtful or no value in the treatment of bacteriemia due to gram-negative organisms belonging to the colon-typhoid-dysentery group. Penicillin is likewise ineffective in the treatment of tularemia and brucellosis. It is ineffective against bacteriemia due to microorganisms of the genus Proteus, Pseudomonas aeruginosa or Klebsiella pneumoniae.

Blood Dyscrasias.—Penicillin is of no value in the treatment of such conditions as mononucleosis or leukemia, either acute or chronic.

Malaria.—Lyons[11] and my colleagues and I[32] have reported complete lack of success in attempts to treat with penicillin patients who have malaria due to Plasmodium vivax.

REFERENCES

1. Abraham, E. P., Chain, E., Fletcher, C. M., Gardner, A. D., Heatley, N. G., Jennings, M. A. and Florey, H. W.: Further observations on penicillin. Lancet. 2:177–188; 189 (Aug. 16) 1941.

2. Herrell, W. E., Heilman, Dorothy H. and Williams, H. L.: The clinical use of penicillin. Proc. Staff Meet., Mayo Clin. 17:609–616 (Dec. 30) 1942.

3. Guerra Perez Carral, F.: La quimioterapia por microorganismos. La penicilina en el tratamiento de las endocarditis. Arch. latino am. de cardiol. y hemat. 13: 25–42 (Jan.-Feb.) 1943.

4. Herrell, W. E.: Further observations on the clinical use of penicillin. Proc. Staff Meet., Mayo Clin. 18:65–76 (Mar. 10) 1943.

5. Florey, M. E. and Florey, H. W.: General and local administration of penicillin. Lancet. 1:387–397 (Mar. 27) 1943.

6. Keefer, C. S., Blake, F. G., Marshall, E. K., Jr., Lockwood, J. S. and Wood, W. B., Jr.: Penicillin in the treatment of infections; a report of 500 cases. J. A. M. A. 122:1217–1224 (Aug. 28) 1943.

7. Blumberg, M. L.: Staphylococcus aureus septicemia. Arch. Pediat. 60:580–582 (Oct.) 1943.

8. Flannery, W. E.: A case of hemolytic streptococcus septicemia successfully treated with penicillin. Lawrence Co. M. Soc. Bull. No. 2, (Oct.) 1943; Nat. Eclectic M. A. Quart. 35:13 (Dec.) 1943.

9. Hageman, P. O., Martin, S. P. and Wood, W. B., Jr.: Penicillin, a clinical study of its effectiveness. Proc. Central Soc. Clin. Research. 16:18–19 (Nov. 5) 1943.

10. Likely, D. S. and Swirsky, M. Y.: Staphylococcus aureus septicemia treated with penicillin, with report of drug side effects. J. A. M. A. 123:956–958 (Dec. 11) 1943.

11. Lyons, Champ: Penicillin therapy of surgical infections in the U. S. Army; a report. J. A. M. A. 123:1007–1018 (Dec. 18) 1943.

12. Silverthorne, N.: Penicillin in treatment of hemolytic staphylococcal septicemia. Canad. M. A. J. 49:516–517 (Dec.) 1943.

13. von Gutfeld, F. J.: The use of penicillin in statu nascendi. Virginia M. Monthly. 71:39 (Jan.) 1944.

14. Hellman, A. M. and Guilfoil, E. F.: Treatment with penicillin after the failure of sulfa drugs in a case of vaginal plastic followed by blood stream infection. Am. J. Obst. & Gynec. 47:125–126 (Jan.) 1944.

15. Mitchell, R. M. and Kaminester, Sanford: Penicillin; case report of a patient who recovered from puerperal sepsis hemolytic streptococcus septicemia. Am. J. Surg. n.s. 63:136–140 (Jan.) 1944.

16. Dawson, M. H. and Hobby, Gladys L.: The clinical use of penicillin; observations in one hundred cases. J. A. M. A. 124:611–622 (Mar. 4) 1944.

17. Herrell, W. E.: The clinical use of penicillin; an antibacterial agent of biologic origin. J. A. M. A. 124:622–627 (Mar. 4) 1944.

18. Bloomfield, A. L., Rantz, L. A. and Kirby, W. M. M.: The clinical use of penicillin. J. A. M. A. 124:627–633 (Mar. 4) 1944.

19. Tillett, W. S., Cambier, Margaret J. and McCormack, J. E.: The treatment of lobar pneumonia and pneumococcal empyema with penicillin. Bull. New York Acad. Med. 20:142–178 (Mar.) 1944.

20. Watson, C. J.: Discussion. J. A. M. A. 124:798 (Mar. 18) 1944.

21. Deeds, Douglas: Discussion. J. A. M. A. 124:798–799 (Mar. 18) 1944.

22. De Gowin, E. L.: Discussion. J. A. M. A. 124:799 (Mar. 18) 1944.

23. Erickson, O. C.: Staphylococcus albus osteomyelitis and septicemia treated with penicillin. J. A. M. A. 124:1053–1054 (Apr. 8) 1944.

24. Christie, R. V. and Garrod, L. P.: A review of the work of a penicillin therapeutic research unit. Brit. M. J. *1*:513–514 (Apr. 15) 1944.

25. Anderson, J. D. and Hill, L. F.: Penicillin in the treatment of severe staphylococcic bacteriemia with complications; report of a case. J. Iowa State M. Soc. *34*:191–198 (May) 1944.

26. MacLeod, K. J.: Report of a case of septicaemia: cure by penicillin. M. J. Australia. *1*:585 (June 24) 1944.

27. Wickstrom, O. W. and Hebble, H. M.: Acute suppurative ethmoiditis with orbital abscess and septicemia treated with penicillin. U. S. Nav. M. Bull. *42*:1379–1380 (June) 1944.

28. Boller, R. J.: Case of staphylococcic septicemia treated with penicillin. J. A. M. A. *125*:629–631 (July 1) 1944.

29. Leopold, J. S.: Staphylococcus albus septicemia in an infant aged six weeks; recovery with penicillin. Arch. Pediat. *61*:347–351 (July) 1944.

30. MacNeal, W. J. and Pease, M. C.: Fulminant meningococcemia treated with penicillin calcium. Am. J. Dis. Child. *63*:30–31 (July) 1944.

31. Ayala Gonzalez, Abraham and Vejar, C. L.: Pyogenous hepatitis with staphylococci bacteremia treated with penicillin. Gastroenterology. *3*:33–38 (July) 1944.

32. Herrell, W. E., Nichols, D. R. and Heilman, Dorothy H.: Penicillin; its usefulness, limitations, diffusion and detection, with analysis of 150 cases in which it was employed. J. A. M. A. *125*:1003–1010 (Aug. 12) 1944.

33. Rosenberg, D. H. and Arling, P. A.: Penicillin in the treatment of meningitis. J. A. M. A. *125*:1011–1016 (Aug. 12) 1944.

34. Evans, A. L.: Penicillin in acute and chronic infections. J. M. A. Georgia. *33*:249–251 (Aug.) 1944.

35. Wollgast, C. F.: The clinical use of penicillin; a report of 115 cases treated in an army hospital. Texas State J. Med. *40*:225–230 (Aug.) 1944.

36. Anderson, D. G.: Clinical experience with penicillin. New York State J. Med. *44*:1651–1654 (Aug. 1) 1944.

37. Loewe, Leo, Rosenblatt, Philip, Greene, H. J. and Russell, Mortimer: Combined penicillin and heparin therapy of subacute bacterial endocarditis; report of seven consecutive successfully treated patients. J. A. M. A. *124*:144–149 (Jan. 15) 1944.

38. Loewe, Leo, Rosenblatt, Philip, Greene, H. J. and Russell, Mortimer: Combined penicillin and heparin treatment of subacute bacterial endocarditis. Bull. New York Acad. Med. *20*:416 (July) 1944.

39. MacNeal, W. J., Blevins, Anne and Poindexter, C. A.: Clinical arrest of bacterial endocarditis by bacteriostatic agents, particularly penicillin. Bull. New York Acad. Med. *20*:415–416 (July) 1944.

40. Collins, B. C.: Subacute bacterial endocarditis treated with penicillin. J. A. M. A. *126*:233 (Sept. 23) 1944.

41. Poindexter, C. A.: The use of penicillin in the treatment of subacute bacterial endocarditis due to Streptococcus viridans. Mod. Concepts Cardiovascular Dis. *13*:1–2 (Nov.) 1944.

42. White, W. L.: The use of penicillin in surgical infections. Am. J. M. Sc. *208*:248–255 (Aug.) 1944.

43. Denny, E. R., Shallenberger, P. L. and Pyle, H. D.: Clinical observations in the use of penicillin. J. Oklahoma M. A. *37*:193–205 (May) 1944.

44. Foster, F. P., McEachern, G. C., Miller, J. H., Ball, F. E., Higley, C. S. and Warren, H. A.: The treatment of acute rheumatic fever with penicillin. J. A. M. A. *126*:281–282 (Sept. 30) 1944.

45. Watson, R. F., Rothbard, Sidney and Swift, H. F.: The use of penicillin in rheumatic fever. J. A. M. A. *126*:274–280 (Sept. 30) 1944.

CHAPTER XI

INFECTIONS OF THE CENTRAL NERVOUS SYSTEM, INCLUDING THE EYE

MENINGITIS

It was evident from studies in vitro and in vivo that penicillin is effective against the organisms most commonly responsible for meningitis; namely, Neisseria intracellularis, Diplococcus pneumoniae, staphylococci and, finally, streptococci including certain sensitive strains of green-producing streptococci as well as anaerobic streptococci. It is not surprising, therefore, that investigators have attempted to evaluate the possible effectiveness of penicillin in the treatment of meningitis owing to a variety of pathogenic organisms.

Meningococcal Meningitis (Meningitis Caused by Neisseria Intracellularis).—It is well established that certain sulfonamides, such as sulfapyridine, sulfadiazine and sulfamerazine, have proved of considerable value in the treatment of meningococcal meningitis. For that reason, the effectiveness of penicillin in the treatment of meningococcal meningitis was not intensively studied during the early investigations on penicillin, when supplies of the material were exceedingly limited. Keefer and others[1] reported on the results obtained in treatment with penicillin of five patients suffering with meningococcal meningitis. Of these five patients, four recovered. Of especial significance is the fact that the one failure occurred in a case in which penicillin was not administered intrathecally. On the other hand, one patient recovered without intrathecal injection of penicillin. Similarly, Dawson and Hobby[2] reported on the treatment with penicillin of two patients suffering with meningococcal meningitis. One of these patients had become anuretic following treatment with sulfonamides. Penicillin then was administered and the patient recovered. The other patient was an infant to whom penicillin was administered intramuscularly; none was given intrathecally. As in the experience of Keefer and others just mentioned, this patient failed to recover. Lyons[3] used penicillin in the treatment of one patient whose meningococcal meningitis appeared to have been arrested by use of sulfadiazine and meningococcal antiserum; however, multiple metastatic abscesses developed as a complication of the disease. The use of penicillin, according to Lyons, prevented recurrence of the meningitis and the patient recovered.

My colleagues and I[4] reported on the use of penicillin in treatment of two patients who had meningococcal meningitis. Both patients received penicillin by the combined intrathecal and intravenous routes. One of the patients was suffering with meningococcal bacteriemia as well as meningitis. This patient recovered. The patient who did not have bacteriemia failed to recover. Both of these patients were seen late in the course of their infection and both had been treated intensively with sulfonamides, without benefit. It seems likely that more satisfactory results will be obtained now that patients can be treated immediately with penicillin, without waiting to determine, first, whether treatment with sulfonamides will be successful.

One of the most exhaustive studies on the value of penicillin in treatment of meningococcal meningitis was made by Rosenberg and Arling.[5] They reported results obtained with penicillin in treatment of a series of seventy-six patients who had meningococcal meningitis. When the few isolated cases previously reported are combined with those reported by Rosenberg and Arling, it appears that, of the eighty-six cases of meningococcal meningitis, satisfactory results were obtained in eighty-two, a recovery rate of 95 per cent. In their report, Rosenberg and Arling agreed that to obtain the most satisfactory results penicillin should be administered intrathecally as well as systemically. It should be pointed out, however, that Rosenberg and Sylvester's[6] subsequent studies tended to indicate that small amounts of penicillin may pass into the cerebrospinal fluid of patients suffering with acute meningococcal meningitis following intravenous and intramuscular administration. They stated, however, that the quantities of penicillin which reached the spinal fluid following intravenous and intramuscular administration of the preparation to patients with meningitis varied considerably with different individuals. It should be mentioned here that Dawson and Hobby[2] already had suggested that penicillin might traverse the blood brain barrier in cases in which inflammation was present in the meninges. Likewise Cairns and others[7] were able to detect penicillin in the cerebrospinal fluid in a case of meningitis two hours after the intravenous injection of 100,000 units of penicillin. In some instances, then, satisfactory results might be obtained in meningitis from systemic therapy with penicillin, without the aid of its intrathecal administration. The decision as to whether systemic penicillin therapy alone is justified in these cases must await further studies. At all events, at the moment there seems insufficient reason to alter the recommendation that penicillin be administered intrathecally and systemically.

Although small amounts of penicillin may reach the general circulation following its intrathecal administration, it is my conviction that the material should be given also intramuscularly or intravenously in treatment of meningitis. This procedure, as compared with intrathecal administration only, unquestionably will result in more satisfactory management of the bacteriemic phase of the disease and will be followed by more satisfactory results in treatment of other complications of meningitis, such as metastatic lesions, epididymitis, arthritis and so forth.

To be mentioned in connection with what already has been said about the use of penicillin in treatment of meningococcal meningitis is the report by Meads and others.[8] The report was based on clinical and laboratory findings in a series of nine cases of meningococcal meningitis. These investigators found five consecutive cases in which the strains of meningococci were relatively resistant to penicillin. They were inclined to the opinion that their results with penicillin, when viewed in the light of accumulated results with sulfonamide therapy, favored the sulfonamides as the drugs of choice in treatment of meningitis caused by meningococci of group I. Doubtless the difference in susceptibility of different strains of Neisseria intracellularis to the action of penicillin should be investigated further.

The *plan of treatment* is as follows: As soon as the diagnosis has been established, 10,000 to 20,000 Oxford units of penicillin, dissolved in 10 c.c. of physiologic saline solution, should be administered immediately by the intrathecal route. This injection should be repeated every twenty-four hours until two negative cultures of the cerebrospinal fluid have been obtained. In addition, 80,000 to 100,000 Oxford units of penicillin in 2 liters, either of physiologic saline solution or of 5 per cent solution of glucose, should be administered by the intravenous drip method every twenty-four hours. If the intravenous method is not considered desirable, 10,000 Oxford units of penicillin in 2 c.c. of physiologic saline solution should be administered intramuscularly every three hours. Systemic therapy should be continued until satisfactory clinical response has been obtained. The average daily intake of fluid should approximate 3,000 c.c. and, when the intravenous drip method is employed, 2,000 c.c. of the daily intake of fluid will be accounted for by the material given in this fashion.

Pneumococcal Meningitis.—From the reports available, there seems to be general agreement that pneumococcal meningitis has not responded as dramatically to penicillin therapy as has meningococcal meningitis. The difficulty in the treatment of pneumococcal meningitis probably is accounted for by the fact that strains of pneumococci vary considerably in their sensitivity to penicillin. Also, the nature of the pathologic process in pneumococcal meningitis differs from that in meningococcal meningitis. The formation of heavy exudates, with possible walling off of regions which consequently are not penetrated by penicillin, has to be considered in the presence of meningitis due to Diplococcus pneumoniae.

The report of Keefer and others[1] emphasizes the rather poor response of pneumococcal meningitis to penicillin therapy. Recovery or improvement was recorded in only seven of twenty-one cases of pneumococcal meningitis in the series they reported. Many of the patients, however, probably were seen late in the course of the disease and after failure with other standard methods of treatment, including administration of sulfonamides, had occurred. Single cases of pneumococcal meningitis, in which treatment was with penicillin, were reported by Barker;[9] McNulty;[10] Evans;[11] Hageman, Martin and Wood;[12] Meola;[13] Rosenberg and Arling;[5] Litvak, Appelbaum and Greene,[14] and Vickery and Dey.[15]

Cairns and others[7] reported on the intrathecal treatment with penicillin of eight patients who had pneumococcal meningitis. In only three cases was intramuscular therapy combined with intrathecal therapy. In six of the eight cases reported by them, the patients recovered. In an addition to this report, the investigators mentioned that they had treated with penicillin another group of eight patients suffering with pneumococcal meningitis. Six of these eight patients recovered, making a total of twelve recoveries in sixteen cases. Dawson and Hobby[2] likewise reported four cases of pneumococcal meningitis in which all four patients recovered following administration of penicillin. In two of these cases, sulfonamides and pneumococcal antiserum had been used in combination with penicillin. In two, sulfonamides alone had been employed but were ineffective.

Examination of the reports just cited disclosed that of forty-nine cases of meningitis owing to Diplococcus pneumoniae, improvement or recovery occurred in only thirty-one, a recovery rate of 63 per cent. The recovery rate in 200 cases of pneumococcal meningitis, which probably included some cases previously reported, was said by Anderson[16] to be somewhere near 45 per cent. This figure is rather surprisingly low; however, it does emphasize the fact that even with penicillin therapy this infection continues to carry a high mortality rate. It is safe to state that penicillin, however, is probably as effective as any other single therapeutic agent in the treatment of pneumococcal meningitis. In the present state of knowledge, it seems that penicillin probably should be combined with sulfonamides in the treatment of pneumococcal meningitis. It would appear from the report of Waring and Smith[17] that, using this combination of sulfonamides and penicillin, they treated twelve consecutive patients who had pneumococcal meningitis, with only one failure.

The *plan of treatment* is as follows: The quantity of penicillin used, and the method of administration in the treatment of pneumococcal meningitis are essentially the same as those outlined for the treatment of meningococcal meningitis. However, it is recommended that sulfonamides (sulfadiazine or sulfamerazine) be combined with systemic and intrathecal administration of penicillin. The sulfonamide may be administered orally or intravenously and enough of the sulfonamide should be administered to establish concentrations in the blood of 14 to 18 mg. per 100 c.c. Unless some toxic reaction occurs, administration of the sulfonamide should be continued for as long as penicillin is given. The course of treatment for pneumococcal meningitis will be longer than it is for meningococcal meningitis. In fact, it may be necessary to give penicillin intrathecally every day for many days in order to obtain satisfactory results. In addition to intrathecal administration, intensive systemic administration is necessary. Ample experimental evidence to support this recommendation is found in the studies of Pilcher and Meacham[18] on the beneficial effects of the addition of intravenous therapy to intrathecal therapy.

It may be feasible at times to administer penicillin intracisternally in these cases, a procedure which Ayer[19] reported as being without apparent harm.

Staphylococcal Meningitis.—Fortunately, meningitis due to Staphylococcus aureus is not a common occurrence. Certainly its frequency is considerably less than that of meningococcal or pneumococcal meningitis. On the other hand, when staphylococcal meningitis has developed in the past, the problem of successful treatment has been rather formidable. Intensive treatment with sulfonamides has been followed by occasional recoveries. At the time of preparation of this report, a few patients had been treated with penicillin. In the report on 500 miscellaneous infections, made by Keefer and others,[1] staphylococcal meningitis was recorded as having been encountered in only five cases. In two of these, the meningitis was associated with bacteriemia. Of these five patients, two recovered; one of the two had bacteriemia and one did not. The other three patients failed to recover. Likewise, in a series of 209 cases of acute infection in which penicillin was used, Lyons[3] encountered staphylococcal meningitis in two. Both of the patients recovered following administration of penicillin. Evans[11] used penicillin in two cases of staphylococcal meningitis, one of which occurred as a complication of a brain abscess; in the other case, staphylococcal meningitis followed cervical laminectomy for a tumor. Both patients recovered following intrathecal administration of penicillin. Dawson and Hobby[2] also used penicillin in one case in which staphylococcal meningitis followed removal of a brain tumor. The result was considered satisfactory although the patient died of ventricular block without evidence of infection. My colleagues and I[4] were unsuccessful in the treatment of one case of overwhelming staphylococcal meningitis. This patient received daily intrathecal injections of penicillin combined with penicillin administered by the intravenous drip method.

In this small group of eleven cases of staphylococcal meningitis, improvement or recovery occurred in seven, a satisfactory record for the use of penicillin.

The *plan of treatment* recommended is as follows: At least 20,000 Oxford units of penicillin should be administered daily in 10 c.c. of physiologic saline solution by the intrathecal route. Also, 80,000 to 100,000 Oxford units should be administered daily by either the intramuscular or the intravenous route. This is exceedingly important in the presence of bacteriemia or severe infection. Intervals of time and volumes of solution to use in intramuscular and intravenous administration can be found in, or calculated from, the exposition of the plan of treatment for meningococcal meningitis, given earlier in this chapter.

If the clinical response reaches a standstill under intrathecal administration combined with systemic therapy, it may be feasible to administer 5,000 to 10,000 units of penicillin directly into the ventricles, a procedure which was recommended by McCune and Evans.[20] On the other hand, introduction of a needle into the ventricles in the acute stages of meningitis should be performed with great caution and not until penicillin has been thoroughly tried for several days by the methods of administration already outlined.

Streptococcal Meningitis.—One of the first cases in which penicillin proved effective in the treatment of streptococcal meningitis was included in a report by Florey and Florey[21] and later was reported in somewhat more detail by Fleming.[22] The organism present was a non-hemolytic streptococcus which was found to be sensitive to penicillin. All medications had failed and the patient's condition appeared to be hopeless. Recovery followed penicillin therapy. According to Florey and Florey, this was the first patient to have received penicillin by the intrathecal route and there appeared to be no ill effects from this method of administering the material. The patient received a total of 1,305,000 Oxford units of penicillin intramuscularly in fourteen days. The total amount received by the intrathecal route was 22,500 Oxford units. For single intrathecal injections 2,500 to 5,000 Oxford units were used.

Likewise, Wollgast[23] reported the recovery of a patient suffering with meningitis in which the micro-organism of infection was reported to be Streptococcus viridans. The patient had failed to respond to sulfonamide therapy and to penicillin administered intrathecally. Forty cubic centimeters of air was injected following introduction of penicillin into the subarachnoid space. Within twenty-four hours thereafter, improvement was said to have been marked and the patient recovered.

Three cases of meningitis due to Streptococcus pyogenes were included in the report by Keefer and others.[1] One patient who had bacteriemia in addition to the meningitis recovered. The other two patients died.

While meningitis due to anaerobic streptococci is of uncommon occurrence, my colleagues and I[4] have treated one patient who harbored an anaerobic streptococcus. The organism isolated from this patient was found to be sensitive to penicillin. Sulfonamides and other agents had proved ineffective. The patient made a satisfactory initial response to penicillin administered by the combined intrathecal and intravenous routes. The spinal fluid became bacteriologically sterile and it appeared that the meningitis responded satisfactorily. On the other hand, the patient died following rupture of an abscess into the frontal lobe of the brain.

In view of the established high mortality of streptococcal meningitis, especially meningitis due to streptococci which are insensitive to, or resistant to, sulfonamides, it seems reasonable to hope that penicillin may prove of value in treatment of this disease.

The *plan of treatment* recommended is essentially the same as that outlined for the treatment of pneumococcal and staphylococcal meningitis.

WOUNDS INVOLVING THE BRAIN AND BRAIN ABSCESS

Wounds involving the brain, as well as brain abscesses, constitute important therapeutic problems under conditions of combat and in civilian practice alike. In the management of wounds of the brain sustained in the Battle of Sicily, certain investigators found penicillin to be of considerable value. Bacteriologic examinations of material aspirated from wounds of the brain revealed that gram-positive cocci often disappeared from these wounds within forty-eight hours after treatment with penicillin had been begun. It was evident that very early treatment of wounds of the brain was essential if satisfactory results were to be obtained. For example, if the wounds were three days old or older, they did not respond as satisfactorily as did wounds treated earlier. Of twenty-three patients suffering with wounds involving the brain, and who received penicillin, according to the report by Florey and Cairns,[24] twenty recovered. In spite of the fact that many of these wounds were purulent, healing was satisfactory following use of penicillin.

In a subsequent report on the general subject, Cairns[25] mentioned bacteriologic studies in thirty-six cases observed in the Sicilian campaign. The wounds were three to twelve days old. The predominating microorganism in twenty-three cases was Staphylococcus aureus. Streptococcus pyogenes and Staphylococcus aureus were present in four cases and Diplococcus pneumoniae was isolated in one case. Other organisms found included Staphylococcus albus, organisms of the genus Clostridium and coliform organisms. It was evident that, if these wounds continued to suppurate, they would be associated with the development of brain abscesses. This complication probably can be prevented by using penicillin early in the course of the infection and by combining the local use of penicillin with its systemic administration.

Penicillin has been used in a few cases in which brain abscess developed following trauma to the head. Pulvertaft[26] reported on the successful use of penicillin combined with sulfadiazine after surgical drainage had been instituted. The predominating organisms present in the cases studied by Pulvertaft were Staphylococcus aureus and Streptococcus pyogenes. In one case, two days after implantation of sulfadiazine and penicillin into the cavity through a catheter, the wound appeared healthy. Administration of penicillin was continued for several days. In this case, recovery from the brain abscess occurred yet the patient died of an intercurrent extradural abscess in the lumbar region. The brain, at necropsy, revealed no signs of the recent abscess which had been treated with penicillin. Brain abscesses complicating meningococcal and other infections have been mentioned. In a report on the general subject of penicillin therapy, Wollgast[23] was inclined to the opinion that results in the treatment of abscesses of the brain and of subdural abscesses have been rather discouraging.

A rather extensive study on the use of penicillin in treatment of brain abscess and of wounds involving the brain, was reported by Cairns.[27] In recent wounds of the brain (up to seventy-two hours old), calcium penicillin was applied as a powder in which 5,000 Oxford units of penicillin was combined with 1 gm. of one of the sulfonamides. Following the local use of penicillin, primary closure was performed. Of 129 cases in which treatment was as has just been described, fatal infections developed in only two. In older wounds of the brain, after excision and closure, sodium or calcium penicillin solution (250 to 1,000 Oxford units per cubic centimeter) was instilled through tubes left in at the time of operation. The penicillin was injected twice daily for three to five days. Of twenty-three cases in which old wounds of the brain were so treated by Cairns, in only three did major intracranial infection develop subsequently. Cairns further recommended that 4,000 to 8,000 Oxford units of penicillin be introduced into the lateral ventricle or intrathecally as prophylaxis against meningitis. It was recommended that the penicillin be administered immediately before operation for the following conditions: removal of a chronic brain abscess; closure of a cerebrospinal fistula, or repair of the dura after wounds involving the brain.

Plan of Treatment.—*Wounds.*—It is recommended that recent wounds of the brain (up to seventy-two hours old) receive an application of the powder containing 5,000 Oxford units of penicillin per gram of one of the sulfonamides such as was used by Cairns. Sulfathiazole is not recommended since it may cause irritation when applied directly to brain tissue. Local application of the penicillin-sulfonamide powder should then be followed by primary closure. If wounds involving the brain are more than three days old, they should be excised, cleansed and closed and small rubber tubes should be left in place, through which either the calcium or the sodium salt of penicillin can be instilled. Instillation of penicillin in physiologic saline solution through these tubes can be carried out two or three times a day for five to seven days. The solution recommended contains 500 to 1,000 Oxford units of penicillin per cubic centimeter. Since the infections frequently are of the mixed or polyvalent type, it may be advisable at times to combine 50 mg. of sulfadiazine, each time, with the penicillin that is instilled. In addition to the penicillin that is given locally, whenever possible it should be administered, for the same period, intramuscularly or intravenously in amounts of 80,000 to 100,000 Oxford units a day. This is exceedingly important, since delayed development of metastatic foci can be prevented by combining systemic penicillin therapy with local therapy. Intervals of time and volumes of solution to use in intramuscular and intravenous administration can be found in, or calculated from, the exposition of the plan of treatment for meningococcal meningitis, given earlier in this chapter.

Brain Abscess.—When feasible, the abscess should be opened and, using the same amounts for the same interval of time as has been recommended previously, penicillin should be instilled through a catheter. Administration of sulfadiazine in the amounts recommended previously also can be combined with administration of penicillin. The systemic administration of penicillin, moreover, is exceedingly important in these cases.

INFECTIONS OF THE EYE EXCLUSIVE OF GONORRHEA AND SYPHILIS

It appears, from most of the available reports, that following systemic administration of penicillin, concentrations of the material in the tissues of the eye and in the tears are not attainable in amounts thought to be therapeutically effective. Therefore, local use of penicillin in the form of corneal baths, or by employing the iontophoretic method of introducing the material, as suggested by von Sallmann and Meyer,[28] may be essential in the treatment of at least certain types of ocular infections. That little or no penicillin reached the tissues of the eye following systemic administration of quantities usually considered therapeutically effective, was further evident from the reports of Struble and Bellows.[29] However, when the quantities of penicillin given systemically are fairly large, the substance does reach the tissues of the eye in amounts which could be expected to prove therapeutically effective.

The first report on the local treatment of infections of the eye with penicillin was made by the Oxford investigators in 1941.[30] In four cases, conjunctivitis appeared to respond satisfactorily to the local use of penicillin. In a subsequent study, Florey and Florey[21] used penicillin in the treatment of eighty-nine infections of the eye. Forty-six were examples of blepharitis; eighteen were cases of acute conjunctivitis; nineteen were examples of chronic conjunctivitis and six were represented by dacryocystitis. Although a variety of micro-organisms were found present in these cases, the predominating one was Staphylococcus aureus. All of the patients received local treatment with an ointment made by dissolving penicillin in distilled water and incorporating the solution in petrolatum (vaseline). The final strength of the ointment was 600 to 800 Oxford units per gram. In the treatment of acute conjunctivitis, the material was applied locally every hour during the day and every two hours during the night. Treatment was continued until negative cultures were obtained. This form of treatment proved effective even in cases of acute conjunctivitis complicated by corneal ulceration. The corneal ulcerations were said to have healed in five to seven days. In cases of blepharitis and conjunctivitis, the treatment was continued in some instances for several weeks. The investigators recommended that if ointments proved irritating, penicillin in physiologic saline solution could be used as drops every one or two hours. The recommended concentration of penicillin in the saline solution was 1,000 Oxford units per cubic centimeter.

Lyons[3] also used penicillin in treatment of three patients who had conjunctivitis owing to Staphylococcus aureus. Satisfactory results were obtained in all three. Cashell,[31] furthermore, reported satisfactory results from treatment with penicillin of certain ocular infections. He found penicillin effective against a variety of organisms, including Staphylococcus aureus, Streptococcus pyogenes, Diplococcus pneumoniae and Neisseria gonorrhoeae. This observer recommended use of either drops or ointment and, in his experience, a concentration of 500 Oxford units per cubic centimeter or per gram appeared to be the most satisfactory one for local treatment. The types of infections listed by Cashell as suitable for treatment included: (1) acute conjunctivitis and blepharitis due to Staphylococcus aureus, streptococci or pneumococci, (2) chronic blepharitis, (3) infected corneal ulcers due to trauma or associated with the above named conditions, (4) perforating corneal injuries wherein there was risk of intra-ocular infection. Likewise, Crawford and King[32] have reported on the successful local use of penicillin in treatment of various infections of the eyes and margins of the lids. Milner[33] also reported satisfactory results in the treatment of certain acute infections involving the eyes, although he was of the opinion that penicillin was not of great value in the treatment of chronic conjunctivitis.

In spite of the evidence that penicillin does not diffuse readily into the tissues of the eye, my colleagues and I[34] at times have obtained satisfactory results in the treatment of extensive inflammatory lesions, including cellulitis involving the eye and orbit, by administration of penicillin systemically without resorting to local treatment. An example is a case in which the patient was suffering with extensive cellulitis which involved both orbits and the tissues of the face. The cellulitis followed an intranasal infection and was complicated by staphylococcal septicemia. Sulfonamide therapy had failed. At the time penicillin therapy was started, the patient was gravely ill and no vision was present in either eye. The extensive cellulitis responded dramatically to systemic administration of penicillin and the patient recovered vision in one eye but not in the other, probably due to damage to the nerve resulting from the great amount of retro-orbital edema that was associated with the severe infection. Photographs of this patient before, during and after treatment are shown in figure 20.

A similar case in which orbital cellulitis and septicemia were satisfactorily treated and, in fact, the course of the disease was changed from almost certain fatality to gradual recovery, was reported by Wickstrom and Hebble.[35] The course of this patient's illness also had been unaffected by fairly intensive sulfonamide therapy. Likewise, Sloane[36] has reported a case of severe orbital cellulitis complicating sinusitis in which recovery occurred, without the necessity of surgical drainage, following intravenous administration of penicillin for ten days. In this case, also, intensive sulfadiazine therapy had not affected the course of the disease.

My colleagues and I[4] have administered penicillin systemically for severe infection of the eye without resorting to local therapy. An example of such an infection was presented by a patient who was suffering with extensive blepharitis and conjunctivitis owing to Neisseria intracellularis (meningococci). Following systemic administration of penicillin, the patient recovered promptly (fig. 21). Harner and Smith[37] also reported satisfactory results in the treatment of severe iridocyclitis when penicillin was administered by the intramuscular route.

These results suggest that at least antibacterial amounts of penicillin reach the orbital tissues following adequate systemic administration of the material, although quantities of penicillin present cannot be detected by ordinary methods. Further, these results lend support to the studies on diffusion of penicillin into the eye reported by Struble and Bellows.[29] Further studies on the general subject of penicillin in the treatment of ocular infections have been reported by Bellows.[38] The results he obtained were in general agreement with the clinical observations reported earlier by Florey and Florey. In treatment of acute staphylococcal conjunctivitis, cures were achieved within forty-eight hours in ten of twelve cases. Even more remarkable was the efficacy of penicillin in treatment of chronic conjunctivitis. Bellows commented that penicillin might prove of equal value in prevention of intra-ocular infections following surgical operation. He pointed out that penicillin reaches the ocular tissues

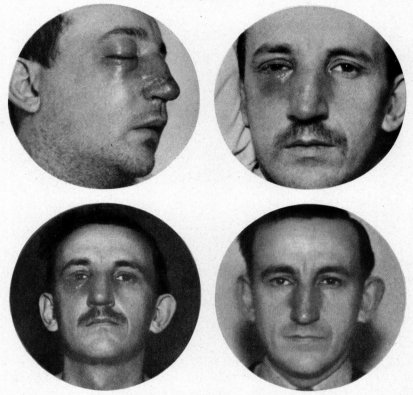

Fig. 20.—Severe orbital cellulitis. *Upper row, left*, before administration of penicillin; *right*, during penicillin therapy. *Lower row, left*, at completion of treatment with penicillin; *right*, several months after dismissal.

within a few minutes after intravenous injection of rather large amounts of the material. On the other hand, he asserted, local application of penicillin leads to high concentrations of the drug in the tissues of the anterior segment of the globe. Bellows recommended the following preparations for clinical use: (1) a simple ointment with a base of grease, (2) an oil-in-water emulsion type of preparation and (3) lubricating jelly. The desired amount of penicillin is then incorporated in one of these preparations for local application. A fourth preparation which the author recommended was an ointment containing penicillin made up in a stearate type of base. This preparation was not recommended except for use on the skin of the lids because, if placed in direct contact with the cornea it might damage the corneal epithelium.

Other important studies on the use of penicillin in treatment of ocular infections have been reported by Keyes.[39] This investigator concluded that penicillin was the drug of choice in treatment of ocular infections associated with Neisseria gonorrhoeae, streptococci and sensitive staphylococci. He further suggested that it should be used in treatment of diseases caused by Neisseria intracellularis, Neisseria catarrhalis or pneumococci. It was evident from his studies that the relief afforded by penic-

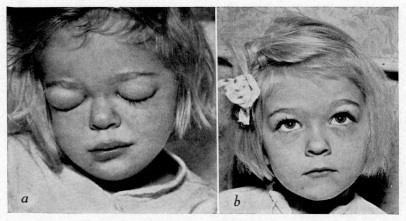

Fig. 21.—Severe meningococcal ophthalmitis. a, Before treatment with penicillin; b, after treatment.

illin, when it was effective, was usually prompt and, in some instances, was considerably better than that afforded by other methods of treatment. He further emphasized the importance of careful bacteriologic studies, together with sensitivity tests, to determine the possible effect of penicillin in vitro against the organism of infection. Also, he recommended the prophylactic use of penicillin in connection with intra-ocular operations and injuries.

The use of penicillin in treatment of infections of the eye associated with gonorrhea and syphilis will be discussed in the chapters on gonorrhea (p. 206) and on syphilis (p. 228).

Plan of Treatment.—For superficial ulcerations, conjunctivitis, acute and chronic blepharitis and dacryocystitis due to susceptible organisms, local instillations into the eye in the form of a cream containing as much as 5,000 Oxford units of penicillin per gram, or physiologic saline solution containing 1,000 to 5,000 Oxford units per cubic centimeter are recommended. The instillations should be made every one or two hours and continued until satisfactory clinical response is obtained. In severe infections, including cellulitis and deep-seated involvement, local treatment should be combined with intramuscular or intravenous methods of administration. At times satisfactory results can be obtained by using the latter methods alone. For the systemic treatment of ocular infections, it is recommended that 80,000 to 100,000 Oxford units of penicillin be given per day, either by the intermittent intramuscular method or by the continuous intravenous drip method (see methods of administration, chapter IX).

CONDITIONS OF THE CENTRAL NERVOUS SYSTEM AND EYE IN WHICH PENICILLIN IS OF DOUBTFUL OR NO VALUE

That the next sentence may have full significance, it must first be said that meningitis, brain abscesses and ocular infections, as well as infections of wounds of the brain, if they are owing to susceptible gram-positive organisms or to the gram-negative organisms Neisseria intracellularis and Neisseria gonorrhoeae, respond to penicillin. Up to the present time, however, penicillin has been found to be of doubtful or no value in the treatment of corresponding diseases and infections due to most other gram-negative organisms.

Penicillin is of no value in the treatment of infections of the central nervous system and eye due to Mycobacterium tuberculosis. If it is of no value in the treatment of infections due to certain resistant micro-organisms such as those of the group Torula, Blastomyces dermatitidis (one of the causes of blastomycosis), of the genus Coccidioides and so forth. Infections owing to organisms of the genus Sporotrichum, Klebsiella pneumoniae (Friedländer's bacillus) and Hemophilus influenzae will not be found to respond to treatment with penicillin. Penicillin is of no value in the treatment of virus infections such as poliomyelitis, encephalitis and so forth.

For the use of penicillin in the treatment of actinomycosis, syphilis and gonorrhea see chapters dealing with these general subjects.

REFERENCES

1. Keefer, C. S., Blake, F. G., Marshall, E. K., Jr., Lockwood, J. S. and Wood, W. B., Jr.: Penicillin in the treatment of infections; a report of 500 cases. J. A. M. A. *122*:1217–1224 (Aug. 28) 1943.

2. Dawson, M. H. and Hobby, Gladys L.: The clinical use of penicillin; observations in one hundred cases. J. A. M. A. *124*:611–622 (Mar. 4) 1944.

3. Lyons, Champ: Penicillin therapy of surgical infections in the U. S. Army; a report J. A. M. A. *123*:1007–1018 (Dec. 18) 1943.

4. Herrell, W. E., Nichols, D. R. and Heilman, Dorothy H.: Penicillin; its usefulness, limitations, diffusion and detection, with analysis of 150 cases in which it was employed. J. A. M. A. *125*:1003–1010 (Aug. 12) 1944.

5. Rosenberg, D. H. and Arling, P. A.: Penicillin in the treatment of meningitis. J. A. M. A. *125*:1011–1016 (Aug. 12) 1944.

6. Rosenberg, D. H. and Sylvester, J. C.: The excretion of penicillin in the spinal fluid in meningitis. Science. n.s. *100*:132–133 (Aug. 11) 1944.

7. Cairns, H., Duthie, E. S., Lewin, W. S. and Smith, H. V.: Pneumococcal meningitis treated with penicillin. Lancet. *1*:655–659 (May 20) 1944.

8. Meads, Manson, Harris, H. W., Samper, B. A., Finland, Maxwell, with the technical assistance of Clare Wilcox: Treatment of meningococcal meningitis with penicillin. New England J. Med. *231*:509–517 (Oct. 12) 1944.

9. Barker, L. F.: Gradenigo syndrome complicated by pneumococcic meningitis; recovery after intensive treatment with penicillin and sulfadiazine. Am. J. M. Sc. *206*:701–703 (Dec.) 1943.

10. McNulty, P. H.: Pneumococcal meningitis secondary to fractured skull treated with penicillin. Manitoba M. A. Rev. *24*:11–12 (Jan.) 1944.

11. Evans, A. L.: The treatment of intracranial infections with penicillin; report of three cases. J. A. M. A. *124*:641–643 (Mar. 4) 1944.

12. Hageman, P. O., Martin, S. P. and Wood, W. B., Jr.: Penicillin: clinical study of its therapeutic effectiveness. J. A. M. A. *124*:798 (Mar. 18) 1944.

13. Meola, Frank: Pneumococcus meningitis treated with penicillin: report of case. Ohio State M. J. *40*:327–328 (Apr.) 1944.

14. Litvak, A. M., Applebaum, Emanuel and Greene, Morton: Pneumococcic meningitis; complete recovery of a six month old infant treated with penicillin. Am. J. Dis. Child. *67*:485–486 (June) 1944.

15. Vickery, Donald and Dey, Lindsay: Pneumococcal meningitis treated with penicillin. M. J. Australia. *1*:537–538 (June 10) 1944.

16. Anderson, D. G.: Clinical experience with penicillin. New York State J. Med. *44*:1651–1654 (Aug. 1) 1944.

17. Waring, A. J., Jr. and Smith, Margaret H. D.: Combined penicillin and sulfonamide therapy; in the treatment of pneumococcic meningitis. J. A. M. A. *126*:418–424 (Oct. 14) 1944.

18. Pilcher, Cobb and Meacham, W. F.: The chemotherapy of intracranial infections. IV. The treatment of pneumococcal meningitis by intrathecal administration of penicillin. J. Neurosurg. *1*:76–81 (Jan.) 1944.

19. Ayer, J. B.: Medical progress. Neurology. New England J. Med. *228*:422–431 (Apr. 1) 1943.

20. McCune, W. S. and Evans, J. M.: Intraventricular penicillin in the treatment of staphylococcic meningitis. J. A. M. A. *125*:705–706 (July 8) 1944.

21. Florey, M. E. and Florey, H. W.: General and local administration of penicillin. Lancet. *1*:387–397 (Mar. 27) 1943.

22. Fleming, Alexander: Streptococcal meningitis treated with penicillin; measurement of bacteriostatic power of blood and cerebrospinal fluid. Lancet. *2*:434–438 (Oct. 9) 1943.

23. Wollgast, C. F.: The clinical use of penicillin; a report of 115 cases treated in an army hospital. Texas State J. Med. *40*:225–230 (Aug.) 1944.

24. Florey, H. W. and Cairns, Hugh: Penicillin in war wounds; a report from the Mediterranean. Lancet. *2*:742–745 (Dec. 11) 1943.

25. Cairns, Hugh: Gunshot wounds of the head in the acute stage. Brit. M. J. *1*:33–37 (Jan. 8) 1944.

26. Pulvertaft, R. J. V.: Local therapy of war wounds. I. With penicillin. Lancet. *2*:341–346 (Sept. 18) 1943.

27. Cairns, Hugh: Penicillin in head and spinal wounds. Brit. J. Surg. *32*:199–207 (July Suppl.) 1944.

28. von Sallmann, L. and Meyer, K.: Penetration of penicillin into the eye. Arch. Ophth. *31*:1–7 (Jan.) 1944.

29. Struble, G. C. and Bellows, J. G.: Studies on the distribution of penicillin in the eye; and its clinical application. J. A. M. A. *125*:685-690 (July 8) 1944.

30. Abraham, E. P., Chain, E., Fletcher, C. M., Gardner, A. D., Heatley, N. G., Jennings, M. A. and Florey, H. W.: Further observations on penicillin. Lancet. *2*:177–188; 189 (Aug. 16) 1941.

31. Cashell, G. T. W.: Treatment of ocular infections with penicillin. Brit. M. J. *1*:420–421 (Mar. 25) 1944.

32. Crawford, T. and King, E. F.: The value of penicillin in the treatment of superficial infections of the eyes and lid margins. Brit. J. Ophth. *28*:373–383 (Aug.) 1944.

33. Milner, J. G.: Penicillin in ophthalmology. Brit. M. J. *2*:175–178 (Aug. 5) 1944.

34. Herrell, W. E., Heilman, Dorothy H. and Williams, H. L.: The clinical use of penicillin. Proc. Staff Meet., Mayo Clin. *17*:609–616 (Dec. 30) 1942.

35. Wickstrom, O. W. and Hebble, H. M.: Acute suppurative ethmoiditis with orbital abscess and septicemia treated with penicillin. U. S. Nav. M. Bull. *42*:1379–1380 (June) 1944.

36. Sloane, H. O.: Orbital cellulitis treated successfully with penicillin. J. A. M. A. *126*:164–166 (Sept. 16) 1944.

37. Harner, C. E. and Smith, J. C.: Severe iridocyclitis treated with penicillin. U. S. Nav. M. Bull. *43*:546–548 (Sept.) 1944.

38. Bellows, J. C.: Penicillin therapy in ocular infections. Am. J. Ophth. s. 3., *27*:1206–1218 (Nov.) 1944.

39. Keyes, J. E. L.: Penicillin in ophthalmology. J. A. M. A. *126*:610–615 (Nov. 4) 1944.

CHAPTER XII

INFECTIONS OF THE RESPIRATORY SYSTEM

INFECTIONS OF THE PARANASAL SINUSES AND MIDDLE EAR

Since penicillin is effective against a variety of pathogenic organisms, including certain anaerobes frequently present in cultures obtained from infected sinuses as well as in cultures from the infected middle ear, it seemed that penicillin might prove an effective agent in treatment of infections involving these structures. Little or no irritation of these mucous membranes is evident following contact with penicillin.

Bordley and his colleagues,[1] at Johns Hopkins Hospital, were among the first to report on the effectiveness of penicillin in treatment of this type of infection. They used the crude broth filtrate containing penicillin which had been prepared by Fisher, of the medical department of their institution. According to their report, the filtrate from cultures of the mold was suitable for local application in infected wounds and for instillation into the middle ear and accessory nasal sinuses. The broth filtrate used by them was prepared in a manner described in the chapter dealing with preparations of penicillin (p. 101). The filtrate was kept sterile and was refrigerated. Varying amounts of the material were applied locally in treatment of infections of the paranasal sinuses. Its local use also was combined with various operative procedures performed on the paranasal sinuses and ears. According to the observers named, penicillin was more effective than either the sulfonamides or gramicidin in combating not only staphylococcal but also pneumococcal infections and infections with anaerobic streptococci.

Keefer and others,[2] and Lyons,[3] reported on one case each in which penicillin was administered systemically in treatment of acute pansinusitis due to Streptococcus pyogenes and Staphylococcus aureus. In the case reported by Lyons, the organism of infection was Streptococcus pyogenes and a satisfactory result was obtained. Death occurred in the case reported by Keefer and coauthors although this likely was due to a secondary complication.

Denny, Shallenberger and Pyle[4] likewise reported on the effectiveness of penicillin in the treatment of chronic pansinusitis owing to Streptococcus pyogenes. In the case reported by these authors previous treatment had been surgical but the infection persisted. Rapid clinical response was said to follow intramuscular administration of 15,000 Oxford units of penicillin every three hours for several days. Streptococcus pyogenes disappeared promptly from the lesion.

My colleagues and I[5] have used penicillin successfully in treatment of acute infections involving the paranasal sinuses and middle ear, due to susceptible organisms. My impression is that systemic use of penicillin is more suitable in this type of case than is local application in the form of sprays or nasal douches. Swanson and Baker[6] have reported on the successful local and systemic use of penicillin in treatment of acute and chronic otitis media and acute labyrinthitis.

Since penicillin requires several hours to act on susceptible pathogenic organisms, it does not seem likely that local instillations would be sufficient to rid the region of all bacteria present. Certainly, deep-seated infections involving these structures will scarcely be reached by local application of penicillin. While acute and subacute infections may respond to penicillin therapy only, I am inclined to the opinion that in chronic cases of long standing, the greatest usefulness of penicillin lies in a combination of penicillin plus necessary surgical drainage. The reports by Hauser and Work,[7] and by Putney,[8] on treatment of sinusitis with penicillin appear to be in general agreement with this viewpoint concerning the possible role of penicillin in treatment of these infections.

Osteomyelitis of the facial and cranial bones secondary to (1) infections of sinuses, (2) intranasal surgical operation and (3) mastoiditis, is discussed in connection with the treatment of osteomyelitis in the chapter dealing with diseases of the skeletal system (p. 164).

INFECTIONS OF THE THROAT

Septic sore throat and acute tonsillitis owing to Streptococcus pyogenes are, as a rule, satisfactorily treated with one of the sulfonamides. Under certain conditions, however, wherein sulfonamides are not well tolerated by the patient, or in those conditions in which sulfonamides have proved ineffective, penicillin therapy may be followed by satisfactory results. Delafield, Straker and Topley[9] used penicillin snuff in treatment of carriers whose nasal discharges were heavily infected with staphylococci. The preparation used by them contained 1 part by weight of penicillin, 5 parts of menthol and 94 parts of lycopodium. The treatment was administered six times per day. Although the penicillin they used was of relatively low potency, the number of staphylococci in the nasal secretions of the patients was greatly decreased during the period of treatment. At the time when Delafield and his colleagues did the reported work, supplies of penicillin did not permit systemic use of the material for prophylaxis. It was their impression, however, that penicillin was of considerable value in eliminating carrier infections and they further suggested that mixtures of penicillin and sulfathiazole might be used.

6

Fisher[10] used broth filtrates containing penicillin to spray the throats and nasal passages of a group of persons who were carriers of group A streptococci. While the results were encouraging in some instances, failures occurred in others. It seemed evident from Fisher's studies that local treatment was not effective against deep-seated infections, including chronic infection of tonsils. This lends support to the statement which I have made in connection with these deep-seated infections; namely, that penicillin, if it is to be used locally, also should be administered systemically.

The successful use of penicillin in treatment of severe pharyngitis and other infectious conditions of the throat, due to Staphylococcus aureus, has been reported by Dunayer, Buxbaum and Knobloch.[11] They applied penicillin by means of a swab directly to the tonsils and to the pharynx every three hours for three days and four times a day thereafter for three days. They also reported on the successful local use of penicillin in treatment of hemolytic streptococcal infections, including so-called surgical scarlet fever. Likewise, Denny, Shallenberger and Pyle[4] reported excellent results in treatment of acute suppurative tonsillitis owing to beta hemolytic streptococci; previously the condition had been unsuccessfully treated with sulfonamides. For treatment in this type of case, Denny and his colleagues used 10,000 to 15,000 Oxford units of penicillin intramuscularly every three or four hours until clinical response was obtained.

Petersen, Northrup and I[12] examined the effectiveness of penicillin in treatment of diphtheria carriers. Large amounts of penicillin were administered intramuscularly for one to two weeks. In a few cases negative cultures were obtained during the time penicillin was being administered or shortly after the course of penicillin had been completed. However, there were recurrences. This is rather surprising in view of the high degree of sensitivity of Corynebacterium diphtheriae to the action of penicillin in vitro. The result is not surprising, however, in view of the finding of F. R. Heilman[13] that guinea pigs and hamsters could not be protected against experimental infections with diphtheria. If some carriers cannot be freed of the organism by means of penicillin therapy, the doubt seems reasonable that penicillin would be of much value in treatment of acute diphtheria. If penicillin is used against this infection, I would without exception insist that its administration be combined with standard procedures such as the use of antitoxin. In striking contrast to the experience of my colleagues and me is the report by Turner[14] on the successful local use of penicillin in treatment of patients who harbored Corynebacterium diphtheriae in the upper part of the respiratory tract. More work remains to be done on this general subject.

PNEUMONIA

All are aware that sulfonamides have proved exceedingly effective in the treatment of pneumonia due to Diplococcus pneumoniae. On the other hand, sulfonamides have not been entirely satisfactory for treatment in certain cases of pneumonia owing to streptococci and staphylococci. In view of the sensitivity of these organisms to penicillin, it appeared that the substance might prove an effective adjunct to sulfonamides for treatment in cases in which the named organisms were causative. Penicillin also has been used satisfactorily for treatment in certain cases of pneumococcal pneumonia in which the causative microorganisms had become sulfonamide resistant.

Reports from the Mayo Clinic,[15, 16] as well as reports by Keefer and associates[2] and by Lyons,[3] have indicated that penicillin is effective for treatment in certain cases of pneumonia, including those complicating severe, overwhelming septicemia. This was particularly true in connection with treatment of patients suffering from pneumonia complicating bacteriemia owing to Staphylococcus aureus. It was true also when pneumonia was associated with overwhelming infections due to Streptococcus pyogenes.

Pneumococcal Pneumonia.—Tillett, Cambier and McCormack[17] reported that penicillin has been found effective in treatment of pneumococcal pneumonia. Of forty-six patients treated, only three died. Pneumococcic bacteriemia was present in fourteen cases and in every instance disappeared following administration of penicillin. The experience indicated that penicillin was at least equally as effective as sulfadiazine for treatment in these cases. The investigators were led to conclude further that under certain circumstances penicillin was particularly advantageous as compared with sulfadiazine. The advantages of penicillin include the almost complete freedom from serious toxic manifestations that attends its use as well as the fact that penicillin usually is effective against sulfonamide-fast strains of pneumococci. Furthermore, it was evident from the studies of Tillett and his colleagues that penicillin rather rapidly sterilizes the blood stream in cases of bacteriemia and at a more rapid rate than does sulfadiazine. Rapidity of action is important in preventing complications incident to bacteriemia; it is generally agreed that many of the failures with sulfadiazine are due to secondary complications probably associated with uncontrolled bacteriemia. Examples of such complications are metastatic abscesses, endocarditis and so on.

Dawson and Hobby[18] also obtained satisfactory results in treatment of pneumococcal pneumonia. In ten cases of pneumococcal pneumonia reported by them, nine patients responded satisfactorily. In the one failure, the patient was parturient and overwhelming septicemia was present. In spite of the fact that this patient died, the blood stream and pleural fluid were sterile twelve hours after treatment with penicillin had been started. Dawson and Hobby administered 10,000 Oxford units of penicillin intramuscularly every four hours for one and a half to two days. Wollgast[19] also has reported satisfactory results in treatment of a small number of patients who had pneumococcal pneumonia.

Since sulfonamides generally have been effective in treatment of infections owing to Diplococcus pneumoniae, it is understandable that as long as supplies of penicillin were limited, only a limited number of patients were treated with this agent. It is essential that a large group of patients be treated with penicillin before comparative effectiveness of this form of treatment and of treatment with sulfonamides can be finally evaluated.

Staphylococcal Pneumonia.—Bennett and Parkes[20] studied the effectiveness of penicillin in a small group of cases of pneumonia owing to Staphylococcus aureus which had proved resistant to sulfonamide therapy. All of the patients treated with penicillin recovered completely. Included in the report was one case of pneumonia complicated by empyema owing to Staphylococcus aureus. The investigators also found penicillin exceedingly effective in treatment of severe bronchopneumonia. Other cases in which severe staphylococcal pneumonia has been successfully treated with penicillin have been reported by Bloomfield and others[21] and by the surgical staff at a United States Naval Hospital.[22] I already have mentioned that pneumonia secondary to, or complicating, staphylococcal bacteriemia has responded satisfactorily to intensive penicillin therapy.

Streptococcal Pneumonia.—Denny, Shallenberger and Pyle[4] reported dramatic results following treatment of pneumonia due to both alpha and beta types of streptococci. In treatment of this condition, penicillin was administered both intramuscularly and by the intravenous drip method. The cases of streptococcal pneumonia reported by Denny and coauthors had failed to respond clinically to adequate sulfonamide therapy. Wollgast[19] also reported on the effectiveness of penicillin in treatment of pneumonia owing to Streptococcus pyogenes. Christie and Garrod,[23] furthermore, have reported on the successful use of penicillin in treatment of severe, sulfonamide resistant, streptococcal pneumonia of six weeks' duration. The patient recovered after receiving a total of 750,000 Oxford units of penicillin by the intravenous route.

Atypical Pneumonia.—Experience with penicillin in treatment of primary atypical pneumonia has been somewhat limited. Preliminary evidence, however, suggests that penicillin has little effect on the course of this disease which probably is due to an insusceptible virus. In a previous chapter (p. 61), however, it was pointed out that there was good evidence from the experiments reported by F. R. Heilman and me[24, 25] that penicillin should prove effective in the treatment of patients with pneumonia due to either the virus of ornithosis or the virus of psittacosis (p. 243).

Plan of Treatment.—For treatment of pneumonia in general, penicillin should be administered either by the intramuscular route or by the intravenous drip method. In most instances the intramuscular route is preferable and 10,000 to 15,000 Oxford units of penicillin should be given every three hours in 2 or 3 c.c. of physiologic saline solution. Duration of treatment will depend on clinical response. It appears that uncomplicated pneumococcal pneumonia will not require more than three to four days' treatment. Slightly longer periods of treatment may be necessary in treatment of staphylococcal pneumonia, pneumonia owing to streptococci and, possibly, pneumonia owing to the susceptible viruses. Intramuscular administration is preferred particularly if marked congestion is present or if cardiac complications are evident, for then intravenous administration of large amounts of fluid is undesirable. In the presence of bacteriemia due to susceptible organisms, it may be advisable to administer penicillin by the intravenous drip method for at least the first one or two days. While the intravenous drip method is in use, a total daily dose of 80,000 Oxford units, as a rule, will prove sufficient.

Since the duration of treatment in some cases of pneumonia is short, administration of penicillin in beeswax-oil mixtures, which was described in the chapter on methods of administration (p. 108), may prove satisfactory.

BRONCHITIS AND BRONCHIECTASIS

At present it is difficult to evaluate the possible role of penicillin in the treatment of bronchitis and bronchiectasis in cases in which susceptible organisms are present. However, a suitable method of treating these infections has been described by Bryson, Sansome and Laskin.[26] The penicillin is introduced directly into the bronchial tree by allowing the patient to inhale the material after nebulization. Obviously, although penicillin may prove effective against the bacterial phase of the disease, it will not bring about restoration of normal physiologic processes in a bronchial tree which already is the site of marked pathologic changes owing to long-standing infection.

Sims[27] used penicillin for treatment in a few cases of acute laryngo-tracheo-bronchitis (nondiphtheritic croup). The nature of the illness in each case was so severe that tracheotomy had been necessary. The penicillin was administered by the systemic route. According to Sims, the response left little or no doubt that penicillin favorably altered the grave prognosis. It was further evident from his report that penicillin was superior to sulfonamides for treatment.

Plan of Treatment.—By use of a standard glass nebulizer which is operated by compressed air, varying amounts of penicillin in solution can be nebulized. It is possible for a patient to inhale, in ten minutes, 1 c.c. of nebulized saline solution containing from 2,500 to 5,000 Oxford units of penicillin. This can be done as often as three times an hour throughout the day. By this method, patients can inhale without difficulty as much as 75,000 to 80,000 Oxford units in one day. (See chapter on methods of administration.) For systemic treatment, 80,000 Oxford units a day should be administered by either the intermittent intramuscular or the continuous intravenous drip method.

EMPYEMA AND LUNG ABSCESS

All evidence available tends to support the idea that penicillin is of considerable value in treatment of pulmonary suppurative disease such as empyema and lung abscess, particularly if the lesion is due to susceptible organisms. Such organisms include Diplococcus pneumoniae, Staphylococcus aureus, Streptococcus pyogenes, anaerobic streptococci and probably certain spirilla. Although systemic penicillin therapy usually is indicated for treatment in these cases, it was evident from the report of Keefer and others[2] that it may not be possible to sterilize the exudate of empyema cavities without combining intrapleural treatment with systemic treatment. Daily intrapleural injection of varying amounts of penicillin in a high percentage of cases will result in sterilization of the exudate although thoracotomy and surgical drainage will be necessary occasionally.

Pneumococcal Empyema.—Tillett, Cambier and McCormack[17] reported on the intrapleural injection of penicillin in treatment of eight patients suffering with pneumococcal empyema. In seven of the eight cases the infection was eliminated following local treatment and surgical drainage was not required. Six of these seven patients recovered and the only permanent residuum was a small area of pleural thickening. One case was an example of pyopneumothorax and, following penicillin therapy, the pyothorax cleared up satisfactorily. The pneumothorax was associated with a bronchopleural fistula which had been present before treatment was started and both pneumothorax and fistula persisted. The patients who recovered completely were followed for four to six months and all remained free of symptoms. The strains of Diplococcus pneumoniae obtained from empyema cavities of patients who had been treated previously with sulfadiazine were found to possess varying degrees of sulfonamide resistance.

Likewise, Christie and Garrod[23] reported on the use of penicillin in treatment of sixteen patients who had empyema. Following one or two intrapleural injections of 15,000 to 30,000 Oxford units, the pus could be sterilized but subsequent surgical drainage was necessary. I am inclined to believe that the quantity of penicillin used by Christie and Garrod was not adequate and for that reason it is understandable that surgical drainage became necessary more often in this group of cases than in the group reported by Tillett and his colleagues.[17] Hageman, Martin and Wood[28] have successfully treated pneumococcal empyema with intrapleurally administered penicillin. Others who have successfully treated pneumococcal empyema with penicillin include Wollgast,[19] Jeffrey and Thomson,[29] Pilcher and others,[30] and Butler and coauthors.[31] While many of these investigators found it unnecessary to resort to surgical drainage following daily injections of adequate amounts of penicillin into these cavities, rib resection frequently will be necessary to remove fibrin as well as walled-off and encapsulated collections of pus. Some observers have considered that penicillin should be given systemically as well as intrapleurally.

Staphylococcal and Streptococcal Empyema.—Empyema of staphylococcal or streptococcal origin also has been satisfactorily treated with penicillin. As in the case of pneumococcal empyema, it has been recommended that intrapleural administration of the material should be combined with its systemic administration. Florey and Florey[32] were among the first to report on the successful treatment of streptococcal empyema by means of penicillin. Likewise, Blake and Craige[33] were successful in treatment of certain types of suppurative disease of the lung including empyema, using penicillin. Bennett and Parkes[20] also reported satisfactory results in treatment of empyema owing to staphylococci or streptococci. Two of their cases were examples of streptococcal empyema which had been unaffected by sulfonamide therapy and in which complete recovery followed use of penicillin.

Two cases of empyema owing to Streptococcus pyogenes were reported by Keefer and others;[2] both patients recovered. These investigators also reported recovery in seven of nine cases of staphylococcal empyema. Lyons[3] reported one case of empyema owing to Streptococcus pyogenes in which penicillin was used unsuccessfully; however, two patients with staphylococcal empyema improved after penicillin therapy. Likewise, Dawson and Hobby[18] successfully treated a patient with empyema due to Staphylococcus aureus by means of intrapleural instillation and intramuscular injection of penicillin. Denny, Shallenberger and Pyle,[4] furthermore, reported dramatic results in treatment of streptococcal empyema with penicillin when the infection had been found clinically resistant to sulfonamide therapy. One patient described by Denny and coauthors was critically ill with extensive empyema owing to the beta type of hemolytic streptococci. Following use of penicillin, this patient recovered completely without surgical intervention. The patient received between 10,000 and 12,500 Oxford units of penicillin intramuscularly every three hours. Butler, Perry and Valentine[31]

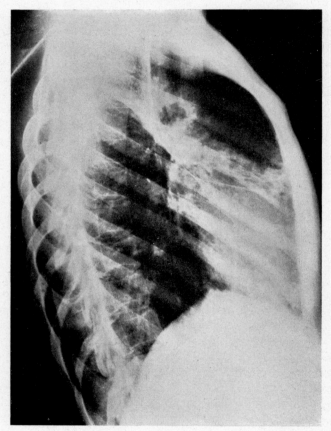

Fig. 22.—Pulmonary abscess in upper pulmonary field before treatment with penicillin

also found penicillin effective in treatment of empyema of streptococcal origin. They further pointed out, however, that frequent aspirations often leave a thickened pleura which occasionally results in reduced vital capacity and fibrosis. It seemed likely to these investigators that rib resection frequently would be necessary to remove masses of fibrin present in the cavities in spite of the fact that the pleural cavity had been sterilized.

Lung Abscess.—Striking clinical improvement has been observed in a few instances in which penicillin has been used in treatment of lung abscess. Some of the lesions have been reported to heal completely without the necessity of surgical intervention. Florey and Florey[32] reported one of the first cases of this type in which penicillin was used. In this report appeared roentgenograms showing multiple pulmonary cavities

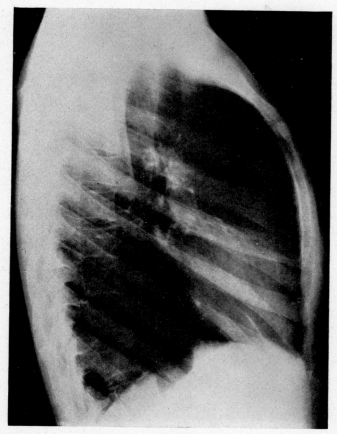

Fig. 23.—Same case as that represented in figure 22. Complete recovery after treatment with penicillin.

as well as pulmonary consolidation. The final roentgenograms, taken at the end of the course of treatment with penicillin, revealed that these lesions had practically healed. Likewise, Keefer and others,[2] Dawson and Hobby,[18] and also Lyons[3] have reported satisfactory results with penicillin in treatment of pyogenic lung abscesses.

My colleagues and I[5] have successfully treated pulmonary abscesses with penicillin. Roentgenograms in one of the cases in which a pulmonary abscess was successfully treated are shown in figures 22 and 23. This patient's pulmonary abscess was a complication of staphylococcal bacteriemia. The patient received penicillin by means of the intravenous drip method and surgical intervention was not necessary. Complete healing occurred.

Plan of Treatment.—*Empyema.*—In treatment of empyema, as I have already indicated, it is recommended that intrathoracic instillation of penicillin be combined with its systemic administration. In many instances, however, intrapleural administration of penicillin alone may be followed by satisfactory results. For intrathoracic instillations following thoracentesis, 40,000 to 50,000 Oxford units of penicillin dissolved in 40 to 50 c.c. of physiologic saline solution are instilled into, and left in, the pleural space. This procedure may be carried out once every twenty-four to forty-eight hours. When surgical drainage previously has been established for empyema and a closed system is being employed, the same quantities of penicillin may be introduced through drainage tubes and the tubes clamped for several hours in order to keep the penicillin from escaping from the pleural space. This is an effective adjunctive procedure for the postoperative use of penicillin.

When systemic therapy is combined with intrathoracic instillation of penicillin, it is recommended that patients receive 10,000 Oxford units of penicillin intramuscularly every three hours or that approximately 80,000 Oxford units of penicillin be administered by the intravenous drip method each twenty-four hours.

Lung Abscess.—Systemic administration of penicillin is recommended as a routine in treatment of lung abscess. Ten thousand to 15,000 Oxford units (5,000 units per cubic centimeter of solution) should be administered intramuscularly every three hours or 80,000 to 100,000 Oxford units should be administered each day by the intravenous drip method. The course of the disease should be followed by frequent roentgenograms and treatment continued until there is evidence of improvement or resolution of the process.

Local treatment is not used unless surgical intervention becomes necessary. If the abscess is drained surgically, small rubber tubes should be left in place at the time surgical drainage is established. Penicillin then should be instilled directly into these tubes two or three times a day. Solutions containing 500 to 1,000 Oxford units of penicillin per cubic centimeter are satisfactory for this purpose. As much of the solution as can be run in without spilling over should be used and should be left in place until absorbed.

TREATMENT BEFORE AND AFTER SURGICAL OPERATION ON THE THORAX

Evidence is accumulating that penicillin is effective in preoperative preparation and postoperative treatment of patients who must undergo, or who have undergone, surgical operation for inflammatory or malignant lesions of the lung. The hazard of postoperative empyema and mediastinitis is greatly reduced if penicillin is administered during the immediately preoperative and the postoperative periods. The temperature and pulse chart of a patient suffering from an extensive inflammatory lesion of the entire lung, and who was subjected to total pneumonectomy, is shown in figure 24. This patient received penicillin before and after operation and, in spite of the extensive suppurative disease

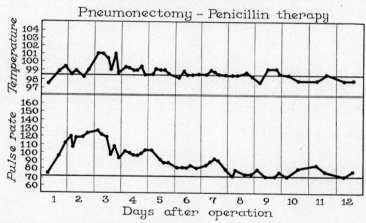

Fig. 24.—Absence of marked or sustained rise in temperature or pulse rate following pneumonectomy for extensive suppurative disease of lung. Penicillin was administered preoperatively and postoperatively.

present at the time of operation, convalescence was extraordinarily uneventful. Also, the temperature and pulse chart of a patient who did not receive penicillin preoperatively and in whom extensive mediastinitis developed following surgical operation is shown in figure 25. This patient was practically moribund when treatment with penicillin was begun but, following administration of penicillin, convalescence was uneventful.

Although introduction of penicillin into the pleural cavity failed to prevent empyema in cases of hemothorax with infection, according to Nicholson and Stevenson,[34] its local use was of considerable value in prevention of infection following operative procedures for removal of foreign bodies from the lung or pleural cavity. That use of penicillin was of value in conjunction with surgical procedures for removal of foreign bodies was further evident from the report of d'Abreu, Litch-field and Thomson[35] on the use of penicillin in treatment of war wounds of the thorax. Their report showed that as a prophylactic agent against infection penicillin is of great value. In a series of sixty-four cases in which penicillin was used in conjunction with surgical procedures for wounds of the chest, including hemothorax with infection and empyema, not a single death occurred, according to the report of these British investigators. In a contrast series of forty cases in which penicillin was not used, there were six deaths. The investigators concluded that pen-icillin reduced the mortality as well as the period of invalidism after wounds of the thorax.

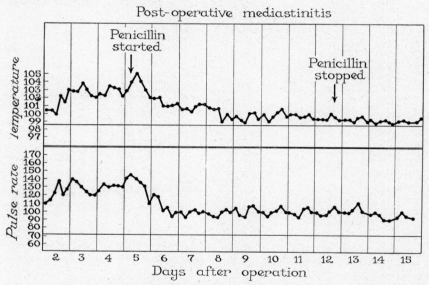

Fig. 25.—Severe postoperative mediastinitis. Patient was gravely ill when treatment with penicillin was started. Recovery was uneventful.

Plan of Treatment.—In the preparation of a patient with pulmonary suppurative disease or tumor, penicillin is administered for approxi-mately four or five days before operation. When there is evidence of cardiac embarrassment, or if for any other reason injection of large amounts of fluid is not desirable, 10,000 to 15,000 Oxford units of pen-icillin are given intramuscularly every three hours. If injection of 2,000 c.c. of fluid is not contraindicated, 80,000 to 100,000 Oxford units of penicillin can be administered each day by the intravenous drip method. Following operation, administration of the same quantity of penicillin is continued for seven to fourteen days, depending on the postoperative course.

Solutions containing penicillin also can be instilled through tubes left in place for this purpose at the time the wound is closed. The procedure for this method of administration is identical with that described under the treatment of empyema.

INFECTIONS OF THE RESPIRATORY SYSTEM IN WHICH PENICILLIN IS OF DOUBTFUL OR NO VALUE

Penicillin is of doubtful or no value in treatment of pulmonary tuberculosis. It is of value, however, in treatment of secondary infections complicating pulmonary tuberculosis.

Penicillin is of no value in treatment of pulmonary lesions owing to gram-negative organisms (Hemophilus influenzae and so forth).

Penicillin is of no value in treatment of infections due to Klebsiella pneumoniae (Friedländer's bacillus). It is of no value in treatment of yeast or fungus infections of the lung; it is useless against pulmonary blastomycosis, coccidiosis, torulosis or moniliasis.

Penicillin is of doubtful value in the treatment of extensive pulmonary actinomycosis in spite of the fact that the organism is susceptible to the action of penicillin (see actinomycosis, chapter XVIII, p. 240).

REFERENCES

1. Bordley, J. E., Crowe, S. J., Dolowitz, D. A. and Pickrell, K. L.: The local use of the sulfonamides, gramicidin (tyrothricin) and penicillin in otolaryngology. Ann. Otol., Rhin. & Laryng. *51*:936–944 (Dec.) 1942.

2. Keefer, C. S., Blake, F. G., Marshall, E. K., Jr., Lockwood, J. S. and Wood, W. B., Jr.: Penicillin in the treatment of infections; a report of 500 cases. J. A. M. A. *122*:1217–1224 (Aug. 28) 1943.

3. Lyons, Champ: Penicillin therapy of surgical infections in the U. S. Army; a report. J. A. M. A. *123*:1007–1018 (Dec. 18) 1943.

4. Denny, E. R., Shallenberger, P. L. and Pyle, H. D.: Clinical observations in the use of penicillin. J. Oklahoma M. A. *37*:193–205 (May) 1944.

5. Herrell, W. E., Nichols, D. R. and Heilman, Dorothy H.: Penicillin; its usefulness, limitations, diffusion and detection, with analysis of 150 cases in which it was employed. J. A. M. A. *125*:1003–1010 (Aug. 12) 1944.

6. Swanson, C. A. and Baker, D. C., Jr.: The use of penicillin in diseases of the ear. J. A. M. A. *126*:616–620 (Nov. 4) 1944.

7. Hauser, I. J. and Work, W. P.: The treatment of sinusitis by penicillin. Tr. Am. Acad. Ophth. (In press.)

8. Putney, F. J.: Uses of penicillin in diseases of the nose and throat. J. A. M. A. *126*:620–621 (Nov. 4) 1944.

9. Delafield, M. E., Straker, Edith and Topley, W. W. C.: Antiseptic snuffs. Brit. M. J. *1*:145–150 (Feb. 1) 1941.

10. Fisher, A. M.: The antibacterial properties of crude penicillin. Bull. Johns Hopkins Hosp. *73*:343–378 (Nov.) 1943.

11. Dunayer, Charlotte, Buxbaum, Lillian and Knobloch, Hilda: Crude penicillin: its preparation and clinical use externally. Ann. Surg. *119*:791–795 (May) 1944.

12. Petersen, M. C., Northrup, W. F. and Herrell, W. E.: Unpublished data.

13. Heilman, F. R.: Personal communication to the author.

14. Turner, Elizabeth K.: Penicillin in paediatrics: preliminary report of cases of varying diseases treated with penicillin at the Children's Hospital, Melbourne. M. J. Australia. 2:205–213 (Aug. 26) 1944.

15. Herrell, W. E.: Further observations on the clinical use of penicillin. Proc. Staff Meet., Mayo Clin. 18:65–76 (Mar. 10) 1943.

16. Nichols, D. R. and Herrell, W. E.: Penicillin in the treatment of staphylococcic sepsis. M. Clin. North America. (July) 1944, pp. 860–868.

17. Tillett, W. S., Cambier, Margaret J. and McCormack, J. E.: The treatment of lobar pneumonia and pneumococcal empyema with penicillin. Bull. New York Acad. Med. 20:142–178 (Mar.) 1944.

18. Dawson, M. H. and Hobby, Gladys L.: The clinical use of penicillin; observations in one hundred cases. J. A. M. A. 124:611–622 (Mar. 4) 1944.

19. Wollgast, C. F.: The clinical use of penicillin; a report of 115 cases treated in an army hospital. Texas State J. Med. 40:225–230 (Aug.) 1944.

20. Bennett, T. I. and Parkes, Trevor: Penicillin in sulphonamide-resistant pneumonias; with special reference to staphylococcal infection and empyema. Lancet. 1:305–308 (Mar. 4) 1944.

21. Bloomfield, A. L., Rantz, L. A. and Kirby, W. M. M.: The clinical use of penicillin. J. A. M. A. 124:627–633 (Mar. 4) 1944.

22. Staff Surgical Conference, U. S. Naval Hospital, San Diego, California: Summary of experience with penicillin on a surgical service. U. S. Nav. M. Bull. 42:85–86 (Jan.) 1944.

23. Christie, R. V. and Garrod, L. P.: A review of the work of a penicillin therapeutic research unit. Brit. M. J. 1:513–514 (Apr. 15) 1944.

24. Heilman, F. R. and Herrell, W. E.: Penicillin in the treatment of experimental ornithosis. Proc. Staff Meet., Mayo Clin. 19:57–65 (Feb. 9) 1944.

25. Heilman, F. R. and Herrell, W. E.: Penicillin in the treatment of experimental psittacosis. Proc. Staff Meet., Mayo Clin. 19:204–207 (Apr. 19) 1944.

26. Bryson, Vernon, Sansome, Eva and Laskin, Sidney: Aerosolization of penicillin solutions. Science. n.s. 100:33–35 (July 14) 1944.

27. Sims, E. B.: Acute laryngo-tracheo-bronchitis treated by penicillin and sulphonamides. M. J. Australia. 2:234–236 (Sept. 2) 1944.

28. Hageman, P. O., Martin, S. P., and Wood, W. B., Jr.: Penicillin: clinical study of its therapeutic effectiveness. J. A. M. A. 124:798 (Mar. 18) 1944.

29. Jeffrey, J. S. and Thomson, Scott: Penicillin in battle casualties. Brit. M. J. 2:1–4 (July 1) 1944.

30. Pilcher, R. S., and others: Discussion on cases treated by penicillin. Proc. Roy. Soc. Med. 37:499–506 (July) 1944.

31. Butler, E. C. B., Perry, K. M. A. and Valentine, F. C. O.: Treatment of acute empyema with penicillin. Brit. M. J. 2:171–175 (Aug. 5) 1944.

32. Florey, M. E. and Florey, H. W.: General and local administration of penicillin Lancet. 1:387–397 (Mar. 27) 1943.

33. Blake, F. G. and Craige, Branch, Jr.: Penicillin in suppurative disease of the lungs. Yale J. Biol. & Med. 15: 507–516 (Jan.) 1943.

34. Nicholson, W. F. and Stevenson, C. R.: Intrapleural penicillin in penetrating wounds of the chest. Brit. J. Surg. 32:176–179 (July Suppl.) 1944.

35. d'Abreu, A. L., Litchfield, J. W. and Thomson, Scott: Penicillin in the treatment of war wounds of the chest. Brit. J. Surg. 32:179–198 (July Suppl.) 1944.

CHAPTER XIII

INFECTIONS OF THE SKELETAL SYSTEM

ACUTE AND SUBACUTE OSTEOMYELITIS

In view of the rather marked antibacterial activity of penicillin against the micro-organisms most commonly encountered in osteomyelitis (Staphylococcus aureus, Streptococcus pyogenes and various anaerobes including micro-aerophilic streptococci), it is understandable that most investigators early in their studies on penicillin attempted to evaluate its use in treatment of osteomyelitis, both acute and chronic. It was evident from the original report by the Oxford investigators,[1] in 1941, that penicillin would be found effective in treatment of acute hematogenous osteomyelitis. In one of their original cases, penicillin was used in treatment of a fourteen year old boy suffering with staphylococcal bacteriemia and early osteomyelitis of the left femur. Sulfathiazole had been administered previously. A satisfactory result was obtained; the patient received a total of 17.2 grams of penicillin. In a subsequent report by Florey and Florey,[2] it was pointed out that rarefaction of bone increases with clinical improvement and that the roentgenologic appearance of bones in osteomyelitis should be interpreted in the light of this observation. Other investigators who subsequently reported satisfactory results in treatment of acute hematogenous osteomyelitis include Keefer and others,[3] Herrell and Nichols,[4] Lyons,[5] Dawson and Hobby,[6] Hageman and others,[7] Robertson[8] and Riddell.[9]

Still further reports on the general subject have been made by a number of investigators. Altemeier,[10] for example, reported on six cases of early acute osteomyelitis in which penicillin was administered. Surgical drainage was necessary in only two of them. As was pointed out by this investigator, there is evidence that if penicillin is administered in cases of acute osteomyelitis, before thrombosis of the nutrient vessels has occurred, open operation may be unnecessary in many cases. Likewise, Wollgast[11] reported on the use of penicillin for treatment in twenty cases of osteomyelitis, in sixteen of which it appeared that cures resulted.

Christie[12] reported on the use of penicillin for infections of bone with sinuses; in most of the cases, the infections had been present for four weeks or longer. Of thirty-four patients treated with penicillin, fourteen were reported as cured and the condition of thirteen as improved. The course of the disease remained unchanged in seven. Therefore, less than half of these patients could be considered cured. It was also evident from Christie's studies that, while the presence of sequestra was not a contraindication to penicillin therapy, results were not so good in the presence of sequestra as in cases in which sequestra were absent. Apparently surgical treatment should be combined with penicillin therapy if better results are to be obtained in cases of osteomyelitis in which sinuses or sequestra are present. That penicillin was responsible for the satisfactory results obtained when combined with surgical operation was evident from Christie's conclusions. For example, the good results obtained when operation was performed and penicillin therapy also was employed were not duplicated following identical operations if penicillin was not used. Evidence of the inability of penicillin to replace surgical measures in treatment of osteomyelitis which had endured for any considerable time was suggested by the studies reported by Dill.[13] It was evident from Dill's report, however, that storminess of the postoperative course of osteomyelitis was reduced when penicillin was given a week before operation and its administration was continued during the postoperative period.

Although it is generally agreed that acute osteomyelitis responds satisfactorily to intensive treatment with penicillin, two important considerations must be mentioned. 1. In the presence of suspected acute osteomyelitis, intensive penicillin therapy may result in complete control of the lesion and symptoms may disappear. At the same time, roentgenologic evidence of localized infection of bone may be absent or considerably delayed. It is important, therefore, to be aware of this effect and to treat the patients for some time after clinical cure is apparent. 2. If a definite lesion of bone is present without symptoms (masking effect), frequent roentgenograms are necessary to identify, and to follow, the course of the lesion which, in many instances, will require surgical drainage. In general, it can be stated that osteomyelitis of flat bones appears to respond more satisfactorily than osteomyelitis of long bones and that less frequently the infections of flat bones require surgical intervention.

Spreading Osteomyelitis of Cranial and Facial Bones.—One of the most difficult problems confronting the otolaryngologist is spreading osteomyelitis of cranial bones, which may complicate severe sinus infections or which may follow intranasal or intracranial surgical procedures for these infections. While the organism responsible for this infection may at times be Staphylococcus aureus, more frequently anaerobic organisms or partially anaerobic organisms, such as micro-aerophilic streptococci, are responsible. Not infrequently the infection may involve the bones of the face and continue to spread into the frontal bones.

Surgical intervention combined with sulfonamides, as a rule, has not given entirely satisfactory results.

Williams and Nichols[14] reported on the successful use of penicillin combined with surgical eradication of sequestra and infected bone in the treatment of severe and usually progressive spreading osteomyelitis of the type under consideration here. Likewise, Iglauer[15] has reported on the successful use of penicillin against this type of osteomyelitis, in

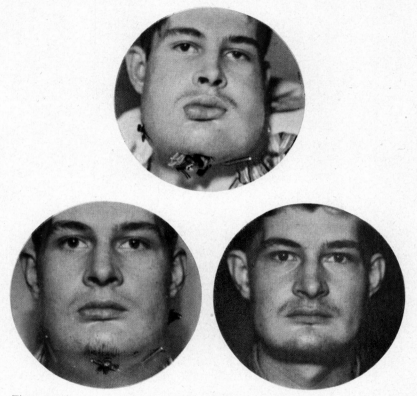

Fig. 26.—Extensive osteomyelitis of the mandible. Cultures revealed micro-aerophilic streptococci. *Top*, before treatment. *Lower left*, eleven days later, during penicillin therapy. *Lower right*, twelve weeks after dismissal.

cases in which sulfonamides had been found completely ineffective. In one report from the Mayo Clinic[16] were listed nine cases of spreading osteomyelitis of the maxillary or frontal bones in which penicillin was successfully used. Penicillin was administered during the preoperative, as well as the postoperative, period. It may be necessary to continue administration of penicillin for as long as two to three weeks after operation in some instances.

Kirby and Hepp[17] also have experienced satisfactory results in treatment of osteomyelitis of facial bones by combining administration of penicillin with surgical methods when the latter were indicated. They, too, emphasized the importance of giving penicillin for a considerable time following sequestrectomy or other surgical procedures. They recommended that surgical procedures be postponed until penicillin had been administered for at least three weeks and that all devitalized bone be removed at one time. According to reports by Putney[18] and by Colbert,[19] equally satisfactory results have been obtained in treatment of osteomyelitis of the cranial and facial bones by combining penicillin with adequate surgical drainage.

Osteomyelitis of the Mandible.—Penicillin has been used successfully in treatment of osteomyelitis of the mandible. In this instance, also, it is essential to combine administration of penicillin with adequate surgical removal of devitalized bone (fig. 26). It was evident from the report of Mowlem[20] that penicillin might prove of value in treatment of osteomyelitis of the mandible. Sixteen patients were treated by this investigator and healing and regeneration of bone took place satisfactorily. He concluded that what heretofore had been an extremely chronic lesion had become, with the use of penicillin, one in which convalescence could be markedly shortened.

Plan of Treatment.—In treatment of acute or subacute osteomyelitis, including spreading osteomyelitis of the cranial and facial bones, it is recommended that 80,000 to 160,000 Oxford units of penicillin be administered per day. The material can be given by either the intramuscular or the intravenous route, according to the technic described in the chapter on methods of administration and dosage.

When surgical procedures are carried out in combination with administration of penicillin for treatment of acute or subacute osteomyelitis, it may be desirable at times to combine local with systemic use of penicillin. The material can be administered locally in this condition in the form of a solution containing 250 to 500 units per cubic centimeter. Solutions of penicillin also can be instilled three or four times daily into the wounds through small rubber tubes left in place at the time of operation.

MASTOIDITIS AND PETROSITIS

The desirability of primary closure of mastoid wounds has been apparent to otologists for many years. On the other hand, most chemotherapeutic agents which preceded the introduction of penicillin were not sufficiently effective to permit primary closure as a routine. While the local and systemic use of sulfonamides has contributed materially toward making primary closure a rational procedure, the use of sulfonamides is not without certain dangers, which include lack of complete bacteriostasis and the possibility of certain toxic reactions.

As in the case of infections involving bone in general, it is naturally difficult to evaluate the effectiveness of any new chemotherapeutic agent in relation to mastoiditis. Reports on the use of penicillin combined with surgical measures in treatment of mastoid infections, however, have been encouraging. A few satisfactory results have been obtained in treatment of early, acute mastoiditis without resorting to surgical intervention. Twenty-two cases of mastoid infection were reported by Florey and Florey.[2] Sixteen of the patients had had the disease for from four days to four weeks. The remaining six patients presented chronic mastoid infection associated with periodic acute exacerbations. The organisms present were predominantly Streptococcus pyogenes, Diplococcus pneumoniae and Staphylococcus aureus. In this series of cases, mastoidectomy was performed and the wounds closed completely from below. A fine rubber tube was inserted through the upper end of the wound. Solutions of penicillin containing 250 to 500 units per cubic centimeter, dissolved in distilled water, were instilled every six hours through these surgically placed tubes. Primary healing occurred in fourteen of the sixteen cases of acute mastoiditis and in five of the six cases of chronic mastoiditis. The ears were found to be dry either at the first dressing (five days after operation) or within ten days after operation in the majority of cases.

A similar experience to that of Florey and Florey with the use of penicillin as an adjunct to surgical treatment of suppurative mastoiditis has been reported by Johnson and Weinstein.[21] Twenty-three patients who had suppurative mastoiditis following scarlet fever and measles were treated by simple mastoidectomy and local application of penicillin in the mastoid cavity. At the time of operation, a ureteral catheter was left in place, through which the penicillin could be introduced into the cavity. Ten thousand Oxford units of penicillin were instilled into the wound every eight hours for four days (a total dose of 120,000 units). In a few cases it was necessary to give a second course of treatment; however, in seventeen cure was complete following a single course. Healing of the wound occurred satisfactorily and a dry external auditory canal was present by the fifth postoperative day, a finding which is in complete agreement with the earlier report by Florey and Florey. Johnson and Weinstein emphasized the advantage of penicillin over the sulfonamides for this form of treatment, particularly since there was little risk of sensitization following use of penicillin and since the speed of healing was considerably increased.

In another report on the general subject, Swanson and Baker[22] stated that they had used penicillin satisfactorily in combination with surgical treatment for acute mastoiditis. The technic employed by them was essentially the same as that recommended by the Floreys. Primary healing occurred in nineteen of the twenty-two cases included in Swanson and Baker's report.

Keefer and others,[3] as well as Lyons,[5] Dawson and Hobby,[6] Hageman and others[7] and my colleagues and I,[16] have reported cases in which mastoiditis appeared to respond favorably to penicillin. The material was administered systemically alone in some instances; in others, both systemically and locally. In the group of cases reported by my colleagues and me, penicillin was used systemically in treatment of acute otitis media and early mastoiditis. In four out of five of the cases, recovery occurred without surgical intervention. It is necessary to bear in mind, however, the masking effect of penicillin in these cases and exceeding caution is required to avoid becoming too assured of good final results when the striking symptomatic response has been secured. Such premature assurance may permit an infection of low grade, but which requires surgical intervention, to develop into a dangerous infection. The masking effect of penicillin, just mentioned, is similar to, if not more pronounced than, that exerted by the sulfonamides. Frequent roentgenographic studies of the mastoid cells, therefore, are essential parts of the treatment of mastoiditis with penicillin.

Dawson and Hobby[6] successfully used penicillin in treatment of mastoiditis and petrositis complicating pneumococcal meningitis. They were unsuccessful in one instance wherein the organism of infection was a streptococcus; however, in this case, treatment with penicillin was begun in the terminal stages of the disease. It should be emphasized that, in treatment of this complication, penicillin should be given over a fairly long period of time. Crowe and his associates[23] also have reported satisfactory results in treatment of mastoiditis when penicillin was applied locally in combination with standard surgical procedures.

Plan of Treatment.—*Local.*—The method of treatment recommended by Florey and Florey[2] is a satisfactory one. Following primary closure after surgical treatment of mastoid infections, penicillin is instilled through small rubber tubes that have been left in place in the wound. Penicillin in amounts of 250 to 500 Oxford units per cubic centimeter, dissolved in distilled water or physiologic saline solution, is instilled into the tubes three or four times daily.

Systemic.—If reliance is placed on the systemic use of penicillin alone in treatment of mastoiditis, fairly large amounts of the substance should be administered. In treatment of infants and small children, it is recommended that at least 40,000 Oxford units of penicillin be given each day by the intramuscular route (5,000 units every three hours). In treatment of larger children, the same amount of the material can be administered by the intravenous drip method. For adults, a total daily dose of 80,000 to 100,000 Oxford units is recommended and can be administered by either the intermittent intramuscular route or the intravenous drip method.

CHRONIC OSTEOMYELITIS

In the beginning of studies on the clinical use of penicillin there was considerable enthusiasm for its use in treatment of chronic hematogenous osteomyelitis. Time has to some degree tempered this enthusiasm. It is well established that the presence of sequestra and walled-off foci of infection in bone presents the same problem in penicillin therapy as in any other form of chemotherapy previously available in treatment of chronic, recurring osteomyelitis. It was evident from the report of Keefer and others[3] that improvement or recovery was likely to follow administration of penicillin in many cases of chronic osteomyelitis. By improvement it was meant, of course, that wounds and sinuses frequently healed completely and under treatment exudates might become free of staphylococci. It was also evident, however, that recurrences would follow withdrawal of penicillin and that a considerable period of time would be necessary before results could be finally evaluated.

Subsequent experience has amply justified a cautious attitude in interpretation of results obtained in long-standing chronic osteomyelitis. It seems evident at present that successful use of penicillin in treatment of chronic staphylococcal osteomyelitis, especially of the long bones, depends on thorough eradication of foci and sequestra. Altemeier[10] also expressed the opinion that in treatment of chronic osteomyelitis, surgical drainage, including sequestrectomy and so forth, is essential even though penicillin is employed. It was evident from the studies of Lyons,[5] and of Anderson and his colleagues,[24] moreover, that surgical intervention, with incomplete or primary closure of wounds, was indicated in conjunction with the use of penicillin in treatment of many of the infections under consideration in these paragraphs. Lyons was further of the opinion that penicillin alone occasionally would bring about a satisfactory result in cases of osteomyelitis of flat bones provided no sequestrum was present. I am inclined to agree, on the basis of my experience, that this is true in some cases of chronic osteomyelitis involving flat bones.

It is my conviction that the greatest usefulness of penicillin in chronic osteomyelitis lies in the prevention, rather than in the treatment, of the chronic recurring osteomyelitis which may follow acute hematogenous osteomyelitis. If early and adequate penicillin therapy is possible in cases of acute osteomyelitis, it may be possible to eradicate the disease before foci become established. Once these foci have become established they constitute a continuous menace.

Plan of Treatment.—In treatment of chronic osteomyelitis, both systemic and local treatment frequently are used.

Systemic.—Approximately 80,000 Oxford units a day should be administered by either the intramuscular (10,000 units every three hours) or the intravenous route. Duration of treatment depends entirely on the response; this is evidenced by the amount of drainage and the progress of the disease as measured by roentgenologic and other indications of improvement. A course of treatment as long as two to three weeks frequently is indicated.

Local.—For local treatment, a solution of either the calcium or the sodium salt of penicillin, which contains 1,000 Oxford units per cubic centimeter, can be instilled directly into sinuses or into small rubber tubes extending well down into sinuses. The material should be instilled at least twice every twenty-four hours. In cases in which saucerization of bone has been employed, a mixture of powdered penicillin and a powdered sulfonamide, which contains 5,000 Oxford units of penicillin per gram, can be applied locally. In some instances, it may be desirable to use for this purpose a cream containing 250 to 500 units of penicillin per gram (see local therapy, p. 107).

COMPOUND FRACTURES WITH OR WITHOUT LOCALIZED OSTEOMYELITIS

Opinions are not uniform as to the value of penicillin in treatment of compound fractures, with or without localized osteomyelitis. Robertson[8] in his early studies was not particularly impressed with the results obtained from the use of penicillin administered locally and systemically in osteomyelitis following compound fractures. Robertson considered surgical removal of sequestra absolutely essential for successful use of penicillin, regardless of how the material was administered. On the other hand, Florey[25] reported that local and systemic use of penicillin permitted primary closure of many wounds, including compound fractures. Of 171 patients so treated, 104 obtained complete union; sixty obtained subtotal union. Failures were said to have occurred in only seven cases. In many cases of compound fractures studied by Florey, a solution of penicillin was instilled through small tubes leading into the wounds. A mixture of powdered penicillin and a powdered sulfonamide also was administered by insufflation.

Lyons[5] investigated the value of penicillin in treatment of badly infected gunshot fractures and felt that outstandingly successful results might be achieved by combining administration of penicillin with conservative surgical procedures. In addition, Lyons recommended extreme care to restore the patient's blood volume and to relieve his depleted nutritional state. These objects are accomplished by dietary measures and blood transfusion. Lyons concluded, however, that putrid wound infection is a contraindication to extensive surgical treatment or to primary closure of the wound. At variance with some reports on the use of penicillin in treatment of battle casualties, Jeffrey and Thomson[26] were inclined to the opinion that, in a group of patients with compound fractures of the femur, there was very little difference in incidence of localized infection among those who received penicillin as compared with those who did not receive it. The disappointing results, however, as they pointed out, may have been due to difficulty in obtaining adequate drainage. There was no doubt from their report, however, that major cellulitis was prevented by the use of penicillin. For example, in a group of 140 patients with open fracture of the femur, seventy received penicillin and seventy served as controls. Only one death occurred in the group of seventy patients who received penicillin (1.4 per cent). This death was due to a cerebral lesion and apparently not to septicemia. In the control group, six deaths occurred (8.6 per cent). Furthermore, amputations were necessary in six of the seventy cases in which penicillin was not employed. Amputations were necessary in only two of the cases in which penicillin was used and these two amputations were not performed because of cellulitis or septicemia but because the legs were useless. That employment of penicillin in cases of compound fracture of the femur does not fully control the incidence of infection or replace accepted fundamental surgical principles was further evident from the reports by Furlong and Clark[27] and by McEwan and Bickerton.[28] Furlong and Clark pointed out that in cases in which penicillin was given there was a definite reduction in mortality and in the number of amputations necessary. This much can be safely said: Penicillin appears to be more effective in the treatment and prevention of severe cellulitis and septicemia in cases of badly infected gunshot fracture than any other therapeutic agent yet available.

ACUTE PYOGENIC ARTHRITIS AND BURSITIS

In the chapter on diffusion of penicillin (p. 77) I have mentioned that when fairly adequate amounts of penicillin are given systemically, according to the studies reported by my colleagues and me, the agent reaches the joint fluid of both normal and infected joints. Likewise, it was evident from the studies of Rammelkamp and Keefer[29] that penicillin could be instilled into joint cavities and the material would remain there for a considerable time. With these facts in mind, and in view of the sensitivity of most of the strains of streptococci and staphylococci, it seemed reasonable to hope that the systemic use of penicillin, as well as the local use of the material, might prove of value in treatment of certain patients with arthritis and bursitis due to susceptible organisms.

Using 20,000 Oxford units of penicillin intramuscularly every four hours for seven days, along with local treatment for ten days, Dawson and Hobby[6] were successful in treatment of suppurative bursitis. Keefer and others,[3] as well as Lyons,[5] Denny and others,[30] Dawson and Hobby,[6] Wollgast[11] and my colleagues and I,[16] have reported on the successful use of penicillin in treatment of acute suppurative lesions of various joints. In some instances, penicillin was instilled into the joint at the time that aspiration was performed. In many instances, local instillation of penicillin has been combined with either intramuscular or intravenous administration. Both staphylococcal and hemolytic streptococcal infections of joints have responded satisfactorily. Bodenham[31] obtained poor results in treatment of two patients with acute staphylococcal arthritis affecting the knee. He administered 10,000 Oxford units of penicillin per day, by needle puncture, for eight days. He was inclined to the opinion that patients with pyogenic arthritis should receive, in addition to local treatment including surgical drainage, large doses of penicillin parenterally. It should be emphasized that long-standing suppurative lesions of joints, with resulting destruction of tissue and irreversible pathologic changes, are not likely to respond satisfactorily to the use of penicillin. The reasons for this are obvious. For treatment of gonorrheal arthritis with penicillin see the chapter on gonorrhea (p. 208).

Plan of Treatment.—In treatment of an acute suppurative lesion of a joint, it is desirable to aspirate fluid from the joint and to instill 10,000 Oxford units of penicillin in 5 or 10 c.c. of physiologic saline solution. This procedure is not necessary oftener than every forty-eight hours because penicillin is slowly absorbed from these joints and will remain in the joint fluid for this length of time. In many instances it is not necessary to resort to intra-articular instillation of penicillin and satisfactory results can be obtained following systemic treatment alone. The quantity of penicillin administered systemically each day should be 80,000 to 100,000 Oxford units, given either by the intramuscular route or by the intravenous drip method. It is my opinion that penicillin should be administered systemically in all cases of the type considered here and that whether intra-articular instillation also should be carried out depends on the nature, the type and the severity of the lesion.

PROPHYLACTIC USE OF PENICILLIN IN ASSOCIATION WITH SURGICAL OPERATION ON THE SKELETAL SYSTEM

Evidence is accumulating that the use of penicillin is of considerable value before, and immediately after, operation on the skeletal system. Ghormley[32] and his colleagues have reported that administration of penicillin has been found of considerable value in preparation of patients for various orthopedic operations, whether or not the patients harbor evident infection. Striking examples are the satisfactory results obtained in cases in which arthroplasty or other surgical procedures on bones and joints have been performed. The risk of infection in association with surgical reduction of compound fractures has been reported to be considerably reduced by employment of penicillin therapy for four or five days before, and for a similar period after, operation.

Earlier in this chapter I have mentioned the experience of Dill,[13] which indicated that penicillin exerted a favorable effect on the postoperative course of certain infections, particularly osteomyelitis, when the material was administered preoperatively and postoperatively.

INFECTIONS OF THE SKELETAL SYSTEM IN WHICH PENICILLIN IS OF DOUBTFUL OR OF NO VALUE

Acute and Chronic Rheumatoid Arthritis.—As has been said of rheumatic fever, many students of rheumatoid infectious arthritis have claimed evidence that the disease is caused by, or is associated with, infections owing to various strains of streptococci. Since most of these organisms are sensitive to the action of penicillin, it seems reasonable that attempts should be made to use penicillin in the treatment of acute, as well as of chronic, rheumatoid arthritis. Preliminary studies by my colleagues and me indicated that penicillin, even when administered in large doses, had little or no effect on the course of rheumatoid infectious arthritis.

TABLE 18

LEUKOCYTES PER CUBIC MILLIMETER OF SYNOVIAL FLUID

Case	Before treatment	After treatment
5	38,000	26,700
6	5,800	5,100
7	5,500	8,200
10	44,500	38,200

From article by Boland, Headley and Hench, Journal of the American Medical Association, November 25, 1944.

This subject has been extensively and carefully investigated by Boland, Headley and Hench.[33] Ten patients suffering with typical rheumatoid arthritis were selected for their clinical investigation. These patients received quantities of penicillin which could be considered adequate for treatment of even the most severe infections. They received penicillin for fourteen to twenty days. The course of the disease was carefully followed with particular reference to changes which might indicate improvement, such as alteration in sedimentation rate and in white cell counts of the synovial fluid before and after treatment (table 18). There was no evidence to suggest that penicillin was of value in treatment of this disease. Since the quantity of penicillin administered was adequate to control infections owing to various strains of Streptococcus pyogenes, the investigators rightfully concluded that it seemed reasonable to assume that rheumatoid arthritis is not caused by any of the bacteria which are already known to be inhibited by the action of penicillin.

Rheumatic Fever.—In chapter X, I have discussed the ineffectiveness of penicillin in treatment of acute rheumatic fever. Penicillin has been found to have little if any effect on the joint manifestations of this disease.

Miscellaneous.—Penicillin is of little or no value in treatment of intermittent hydrops of joints. It is of no value in treatment of tuberculosis involving the skeletal system. Likewise, acute or destructive arthritis of the spinal column, associated with undulant fever or typhoid fever, will not respond to penicillin.

REFERENCES

1. Abraham, E. P., Chain, E., Fletcher, C. M., Gardner, A. D., Heatley, N. G., Jennings, M. A. and Florey, H. W.: Further observations on penicillin. Lancet. *2*:177–188; 189 (Aug. 16) 1941.

2. Florey, M. E. and Florey, H. W.: General and local administration of penicillin. Lancet. *1*:387–397 (Mar. 27) 1943.

3. Keefer, C. S., Blake, F. G., Marshall, E. K., Jr., Lockwood, J. S. and Wood, W. B., Jr.: Penicillin in the treatment of infections; a report of 500 cases. J. A. M. A. *122*:1217–1224 (Aug. 28) 1943.

4. Herrell, W. E. and Nichols, D. R.: The calcium salt of penicillin. Proc. Staff Meet., Mayo Clin. *18*:313–319 (Sept. 8) 1943.

5. Lyons, Champ: Penicillin therapy of surgical infections in the U. S. Army; a report. J. A. M. A. *123*:1007–1018 (Dec. 18) 1943.

6. Dawson, M. H. and Hobby, Gladys L.: The clinical use of penicillin; observations in one hundred cases. J. A. M. A. *124*:611–622 (Mar. 4) 1944.

7. Hageman, P. O., Martin, S. P. and Wood, W. B., Jr.: Penicillin: clinical study of its therapeutic effectiveness. J. A. M. A. *124*:798 (Mar. 18) 1944.

8. Robertson, I. M.: Penicillin in bone infections. Brit. M. J. *1*:519–521 (Apr. 15) 1944.

9. Riddell, Ted: Penicillin in acute osteomyelitis; report of a case. Nebraska M. J. *29*:284 (Sept.) 1944.

10. Altemeier, W. A.: Penicillin in surgery. South. M. J. *37*:494–506 (Sept.) 1944.

11. Wollgast, C. F.: The clinical use of penicillin; a report of 115 cases treated in an army hospital. Texas State J. Med. *40*:225–230 (Aug.) 1944.

12. Christie, R. V.: Discussion on penicillin. Brit. M. J. *2*:655–656 (Nov. 20) 1943.

13. Dill, W. W.: County society reports; Montgomery. Pennsylvania M. J. *47*:63–64 (Oct.) 1943.

14. Williams, H. L. and Nichols, D. R.: Spreading osteomyelitis of the frontal bone treated with penicillin. Proc. Staff Meet., Mayo Clin. *18*:467–469 (Dec. 1) 1943.

15. Iglauer, Samuel: Two cases of osteomyelitis treated with penicillin: Case 1, frontal; case 2, maxillary. Laryngoscope. *54*:150–156 (Mar.) 1944.

16. Herrell, W. E., Nichols, D. R. and Heilman, Dorothy H.: Penicillin; its usefulness, limitations, diffusion and detection, with analysis of 150 cases in which it was employed. J. A. M. A. *125*:1003–1010 (Aug. 12) 1944.

17. Kirby, W. M. M. and Hepp, V. E.: Treatment of osteomyelitis of the facial bones with penicillin. J. A. M. A. *125*:1019–1022 (Aug. 12) 1944.

18. Putney, F. J.: Uses of penicillin in diseases of the nose and throat. J. A. M. A. *126*:620–621 (Nov. 4) 1944.

19. Colbert, R. M.: Osteomyelitis of the frontal bone treated with penicillin. Ann. Otol., Rhin. & Laryng. *53*:522–530 (Sept.) 1944.

20. Mowlem, Rainsford: Surgery and penicillin in mandibular infection. Brit. M. J. *1*:517-519 (Apr. 15) 1944.

21. Johnson, L. F., Weinstein, Louis and Spence, P. S.: Penicillin and primary suture in acute surgical mastoiditis. Tr. Am. Acad. Ophth. (In press.)

22. Swanson, C. A. and Baker, D. C., Jr.: The use of penicillin in diseases of the ear. J. A. M. A. *126*:616–620 (Nov. 4) 1944.

23. Crowe, S. J., Fisher, A. M., Ward, A. T., Jr. and Foley, M. K.: Penicillin and tyrothricin in otolaryngology based on bacteriological and clinical study of 118 patients. Ann. Otol., Rhin. & Laryng. *52*:541–572 (Sept.) 1943.

24. Anderson, D. G., Howard, L. G. and Rammelkamp, C. H.: Penicillin in the treatment of chronic osteomyelitis; a report of forty cases. Arch. Surg. *49*:245–257 (Oct.) 1944.

25. Florey, H. W.: Discussion on penicillin. Brit. M. J. *2*:654 (Nov. 20) 1943.

26. Jeffrey, J. S. and Thomson, Scott: Penicillin in battle casualties. Brit. M. J. *2*:1–4 (July 1) 1944.

27. Furlong, Ronald and Clark, J. M. P.: On the use of penicillin to control infection in open fractures of the femur; interim report. Brit. J. Surg. *32*:147–154 (July Suppl.) 1944.

28. McEwan, R. J. B. and Bickerton, J. G.: Battle casualty fractures of the femur: treatment with penicillin Brit. J. Surg. *32*:154–158 (July Suppl.) 1944.

29. Rammelkamp, C. H. and Keefer, C. S.: The absorption, excretion, and distribution of penicillin. J. Clin. Investigation. *22*:425–437 (May) 1943.

30. Denny, E. R., Shallenberger, P. L. and Pyle, H. D.: Clinical observations in the use of penicillin. J. Oklahoma M. A. *37*:193–205 (May) 1944.

31. Bodenham, D. C.: Discussion on penicillin. Proc. Roy. Soc. Med. *37*:105 (Jan.) 1944.

32. Ghormley, R. K.: Report of orthopedic surgery for year 1943. Proc. Staff. Meet., Mayo Clin. *19*:456–458 (Sept. 6) 1944.

33. Boland, E. W., Headley, N. E. and Hench, P. S.: The effect of penicillin on rheumatoid arthritis. J. A. M. A. *126*:820–823 (Nov. 25) 1944. (Abstr.) Proc. Staff Meet., Mayo Clin. *19*:505–506 (Oct. 18) 1944.

CHAPTER XIV

INFECTIONS OF THE SKIN AND SOFT TISSUES

Local application of penicillin or a combination of local and systemic administration in many instances has resulted in favorable response in cases of certain pyogenic infections of the skin.

ECZEMA

Roxburgh, Christie and Roxburgh[1] have reported on the effectiveness of penicillin in a small group of cases of eczema with secondary infection. For treatment, they used either the sodium or the calcium salt of penicillin in a lanette wax and petroleum jelly base. The preparation contained approximately 400 Oxford units of penicillin per gram. In most of the cases, the organisms recovered from these lesions were Streptococcus pyogenes and Staphylococcus aureus. The duration of the eczema in these cases varied from several weeks even to years. Treatment consisted of one or two local applications per day of the penicillin ointment for as long as two to three weeks. The investigators concluded that there was evidence of improvement and that penicillin should be worthy of trial in cases of eczema, particularly if there was evidence of secondary infection. Likewise, Barron and Mansfield[2] have reported cases of eczema with infection in which treatment with local applications of a cream containing penicillin was successful. In some instances irritation followed use of the cream but it was thought that the irritation resulted from the soft paraffin used as the vehicle. Also, Schoch[3] has reported improvement following local application of penicillin for chronic eczema of the hands. In a case reported by him, the disease was said to have been present for five years and, following local application of penicillin for five days, there was striking clinical improvement and the patient was practically well. It was pointed out by Schoch that in some cases there were mild recurrences but that subsequent local treatment with penicillin resulted in satisfactory response.

Because of the limited supplies of penicillin available in the early period of the investigations on penicillin, sufficient data have not yet been accumulated to justify final statements as to the value of this type of treatment in eczema.

FURUNCULOSIS AND CARBUNCLE

It seemed natural to assume that penicillin would be of value in treatment of furunculosis and carbuncle since the organism of infection is usually rather highly sensitive to penicillin. Striking results have been obtained by most investigators in cases of both furunculosis and carbuncle following local and systemic administration of penicillin. During

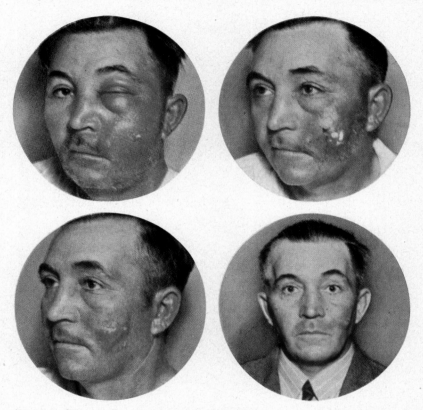

Fig. 27.—Carbuncle of face. *Upper left*, before treatment with penicillin. *Upper right*, forty-eight hours after administration of penicillin started. *Lower left*, after five days of treatment with penicillin; administration of penicillin discontinued. *Lower right*, on dismissal, nine days after penicillin therapy started.

early studies on penicillin, its use for furunculosis and carbuncle was limited for the most part to the more severe cases. The first successful treatment of carbuncle by systemic administration of penicillin was in a case which was included in the first report[4] from Oxford on the clinical studies carried out there (their case 3). The carbuncle was in the region of the scapula of a patient forty-eight years of age. Within four days after the beginning of treatment with penicillin, the lesion had markedly improved and complete resolution occurred in one week. Florey and Florey[5] found that staphylococci were effectively eliminated when penicillin was applied topically to carbuncles. In the majority of cases, both chronic and acute, according to Florey and Florey, healing occurred without any treatment other than use of penicillin.

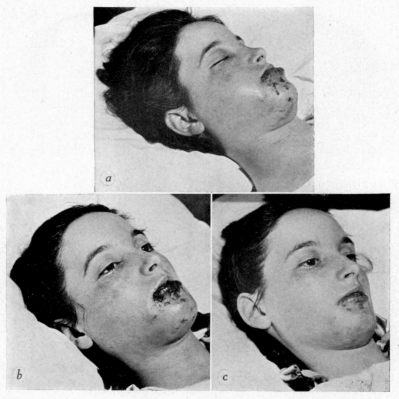

Fig. 28.—*a*, Appearance of patient at onset of penicillin therapy. Extensive cellulitis of mouth and face with extension into the cervical tissues. Staphylococcic septicemia. Patient gravely ill. *b*, Appearance of patient seventy-two hours after treatment with penicillin was started. *c*, Appearance of patient six days after penicillin therapy was started. Edema and cellulitis have practically disappeared. Complete recovery. (From article by Herrell, Nichols and Heilman, Journal of the American Medical Association, August 12, 1944.)

Likewise, Keefer and others[6] reported success with penicillin in treatment of infections of the skin, including multiple abscesses and carbuncles. Robinson and Wallace[7] also reported on the successful local treatment of carbuncles with penicillin.

Since my colleagues and I have reserved penicillin therapy for the more severe infections of this type, practically all of our patients have received the penicillin systemically. It seems unlikely that for very severe carbuncles local application of penicillin is adequate, since the material is not likely to penetrate into the deeper layers of the tissue following its topical use. Results obtained in treatment of an extensive carbuncle involving the face, in which penicillin was administered by the systemic route, are represented in figure 27. Local treatment was not employed in this case. In figure 28 is represented a patient who had a more extensive carbuncle, which was complicated by staphylococcal bacteriemia and in which penicillin also was successfully used; local therapy was not employed.

Many other investigators, including Lockwood, White and Murphy[8] and Coleman and Sako,[9] have reported on the satisfactory use of penicillin in treatment of boils and carbuncles. It has been suggested further by Roxburgh, Christie and Roxburgh[1] that penicillin possibly might be useful in prevention of recurrent boils.

Plan of Treatment.—Penicillin has been administered in some instances by injecting the solutions containing penicillin into the deeper layers of the tissue around furuncles and carbuncles. It is my impression, however, that this method is seldom necessary since most of them will respond satisfactorily to systemic therapy alone. For injection into the tissues, a physiologic saline solution containing 250 to 500 units of penicillin is the one most commonly recommended.

For topical application an ointment made with lanette wax and petroleum base, containing 400 to 500 units of penicillin per gram, is satisfactory.

For systemic treatment, 60,000 to 80,000 Oxford units each twenty-four hours can be given by the intramuscular route or by the intravenous drip method.

IMPETIGO AND SYCOSIS BARBAE

Roxburgh, Christie and Roxburgh[1] have carried out studies to test the value of the local use of penicillin in treatment of a limited number of cases of impetigo. The crusts were removed from the lesions and the penicillin ointment with lanette wax and petroleum jelly base was applied locally once or twice a day. Of twelve patients so treated, eleven were cured. The average time necessary to bring about these results was eight to nine days. The patients selected for treatment were suffering with fairly advanced impetigo. There seemed little doubt that the response to treatment with penicillin was more rapid than that usually experienced following standard forms of treatment, including use of sulfonamides. The organisms most commonly encountered in the cases reported by Roxburgh and his colleagues were Staphylococcus aureus and Streptococcus pyogenes.

At the Mayo Clinic, penicillin has been used successfully in treatment of impetigo affecting a limited number of infants just after birth and later. In these cases, 2,000 to 5,000 units of penicillin was administered intramuscularly every three hours, in 1 or 2 c.c. of physiologic saline solution. The injections usually were made into the buttocks. At times the response to this form of treatment was striking.

Johnson[10] also has used penicillin successfully in treatment of impetigo contagiosa. The penicillin was administered locally and it was concluded that results were considerably better with penicillin than with sulfathiazole ointment or ammoniated mercury ointment. Wollgast,[11] in addition, has experienced satisfactory results with the local use of penicillin in treatment of impetigo.

Roxburgh and others also have reported on the successful use of penicillin ointment applied locally in treatment of sycosis barbae; the organism present usually was Staphylococcus aureus or Streptococcus pyogenes. As in the treatment of impetigo, any crusts that were present were removed and the penicillin was applied locally. Shaving was discontinued in the early stages of treatment. The condition was of long duration and had failed to respond to other standard methods of treatment. In the first six cases in which the treatment was used, the initial response was rather striking; however, in many instances there was a tendency to relapse. The investigators concluded, from the results obtained in the series of fifteen cases in which penicillin was used, that the preparation could not be expected to produce a lasting or permanent cure in all instances. However, in certain cases the results obtained were better than those obtained with other standard measures.

SEVERE CELLULITIS, INCLUDING LUDWIG'S ANGINA AND SINUS THROMBOSIS

Cellulitis.—There seems to be general agreement that penicillin is an effective agent in treatment of severe cellulitis due to organisms sensitive to the action of penicillin. Striking results have been reported following its use in cases of staphylococcal and streptococcal cellulitis. Penicillin also has been found to be effective in treatment of cellulitis associated with anaerobic streptococci as well as that associated with organisms responsible for gas gangrene. Severe and rapidly spreading cellulitis without bacteriemia has been treated satisfactorily by a number of investigators, including Abraham and others,[4] Herrell,[12-14] Herrell and Nichols,[15] Keefer and others,[6] Dawson and Hobby,[16] Lyons,[17] Denny and others[18] and Wollgast.[11] In one group of cases of severe, spreading cellulitis without bacteriemia, in which treatment with penicillin was carried out at the Mayo Clinic, twenty-five recoveries and only three failures occurred in the total of twenty-eight cases.[19] Penicillin was reported by Lyons[17] to be effective in treatment of erysipelas. This also is in agreement with my experience and that of Denny, Shallenberger and Pyle.[18] Certain other infections involving the soft tissues, such as mammary cellulitis and abscess of the breast, were satisfactorily treated by Fraser.[20] For treatment in these cases, the skin was infiltrated with 2 per cent prccaine, pus was evacuated by aspiration and penicillin was injected through the same needle. Quantities varying from 2,000 to 20,000 Oxford units were used, depending on the size of the lesion. This aspiration and injection of penicillin were repeated at intervals of two days. While surgical intervention was necessary in some of these cases, it was pointed out that probably intensive systemic therapy would yield even better results. I favor the latter method of treatment for this type of lesion.

Ludwig's Angina.—Extensive and rapidly spreading cellulitis of the floor of the mouth (Ludwig's angina) always has presented a rather difficult therapeutic problem. Various methods of treatment have been employed in the past, including administration of sulfonamides, with and without radical surgical intervention. According to Taffel and Harvey,[21] the mortality rate in many series of cases is somewhere between 25 and 54 per cent. In cases in which recovery takes place, convalescence usually is slow and often is stormy. It is generally agreed that dental infection is the initiating factor in a high percentage of cases. In fact, it has been reported that the incidence of dental infection as the initial lesion preceding development of this form of cellulitis is as high as 90 per cent. In addition to dental infection, abrasions of the cheek or mouth may precede the onset of Ludwig's angina and this condition may follow extraction of infected teeth. The organisms isolated in these cases include streptococci, staphylococci, Vincent's spirilla, micro-aerophilic streptococci and gas-producing organisms. All of these are known to be sensitive to the action of penicillin. It seems likely that these infections are usually poly-microbial rather than monomicrobial in origin. There is no uniformity of opinion as to the most satisfactory method of treating cellulitis of the floor of the mouth. The local application of heat, roentgen therapy and sulfonamide therapy, together with minimal or radical surgical intervention, have been employed. Some authors have recommended non-surgical treatment; others have advocated immediate radical surgical intervention. It appears that in many instances the systemic administration of penicillin markedly shortens the period of convalescence and in most cases the use of penicillin is effective without resort to radical surgical procedures. If, however, large abscesses form, surgical drainage is indicated in conjunction with the systemic administration of penicillin.

Figure 29 represents a patient whose case previously has been reported by Nichols and me.[15] She was suffering with Ludwig's angina, of which dental infection probably was the initiating factor.

Sinus Thrombosis.—Sinus thrombosis secondary to orbital, nasal and facial cellulitis generally is recognized as one of the gravest infections encountered by those interested in chemotherapy of bacterial infections. The original report by the Oxford investigators[4] included a case of cavernous sinus thrombosis in which penicillin had been used. The patient died of a ruptured aneurysm. On the other hand, in spite of definite clinical and laboratory evidence of the presence of cavernous sinus thrombosis, necropsy revealed that the "infection in the cavernous sinuses had been almost entirely overcome and that the healing processes

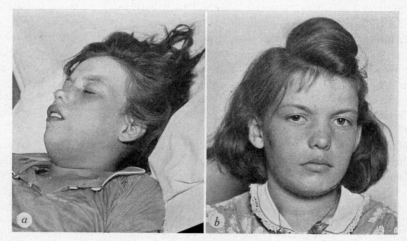

Fig. 29.—Ludwig's angina. *a*, Before administration of penicillin was started; *b*, at time of dismissal from the hospital. (From article by Herrell and Nichols, American Journal of Orthodontics and Oral Surgery, January, 1944.)

were well advanced." Before the vascular accident occurred, this patient had been restored from a moribund condition to what appeared to be convalescence following the use of penicillin.

My colleagues and I[22] subsequently reported a case which appeared to be an example of cavernous sinus thrombosis following severe facial and orbital cellulitis. It seems likely that the use of penicillin was responsible for recovery of this patient (see figure 20, p. 143).

Likewise, Keefer and others[6] reported two cases in which cavernous sinus thrombosis was treated by means of penicillin, with one recovery. Goodhill[23] satisfactorily treated a child five years of age who had bilateral cavernous sinus thrombosis. Before penicillin was used in this case, large amounts of heparin combined with sulfathiazole had been administered for one week but these measures were without effect on the course of the disease. Within twelve hours after administration of penicillin had been started by the intravenous drip method, the temperature began to subside and there was evidence of clinical improvement. As in the case reported from the Mayo Clinic, there was evidence three months later of considerable residual damage to the eyes. According to Goodhill, ophthalmoplegia and optic neuritis were still present although the patient was entirely well otherwise.

Nicholson and Anderson[24] likewise have reported on the successful treatment of cavernous sinus thrombophlebitis affecting a patient suffering with staphylococcal septicemia, Here, again, the use of penicillin appeared to change a hopeless situation into recovery. As in the case reported by my colleagues and me, however, vision in one eye was lost due to optic atrophy. Nicholson and Anderson observed obliteration of the branches of the retinal artery in association with engorgement of the retinal veins and these manifestations were rapidly followed by atrophy of the optic nerve.

In all six cases of sinus thrombosis just mentioned, the organism of infection was Staphylococcus aureus.

Another case of cavernous sinus thrombosis associated with bacteriemia owing to Streptococcus pyogenes has been reported by Wolf.[25] The cavernous sinus thrombosis apparently followed a furuncle on the bridge of the nose. Penicillin was used and its administration was combined with sulfadiazine. The patient recovered.

Hageman, Martin and Wood[26] reported a case of lateral sinus thrombosis which complicated meningitis, petrositis, mastoiditis and bacteriemia due to Diplococcus pneumoniae, type III. Penicillin was administered by the intravenous route and mastoidectomy, with ligation of the jugular vein, was performed. Penicillin also was administered by the intrathecal route and locally into the mastoid wound. The patient was critically ill but recovered.

To my knowledge, it would be difficult to find in the literature, prior to the advent of penicillin, reports of eight consecutive cases of sinus thrombosis, over a period of two years, in which seven recoveries had occurred and in which any one chemotherapeutic agent could be considered responsible solely or in part for the results. Recovery is considered to have taken place in seven cases because death of the patient treated by the Oxford investigators was attributable to aneurysm; the patient apparently had recovered from the sinus thrombosis.

Plan of Treatment.—In cases of severe, spreading cellulitis, including Ludwig's angina and sinus thrombosis (cavernous or lateral), adequate treatment with penicillin should be instituted immediately. If penicillin is available, its use should not be delayed until sulfonamides and other procedures have failed. Whenever possible, penicillin should be administered in these cases by means of the intravenous drip method, at least for the first few days. Each twenty-four hours, 100,000 Oxford units of penicillin should be administered in physiologic saline or glucose solution, and the rate of the intravenous drip should be regulated at 30 drops per minute. If suitable veins for intravenous therapy are not available, 15,000 to 20,000 Oxford units of penicillin should be administered in 3 or 4 c.c. of physiologic saline solution intramuscularly every three hours.

Aside from the use of hot compresses locally, it is probably unnecessary to carry out other procedures, except perhaps occasional ligation of the jugular vein, which may be indicated in cases of lateral sinus thrombosis. It is recommended that the physician refrain from any other local procedures, such as incision and drainage of these lesions when they are about the face and mouth.

POSTOPERATIVE PAROTITIS

Keefer and others[6] and Lyons[17] have reported on the successful use of penicillin in treatment of parotitis. Likewise, my colleagues and I have noted at times the striking clinical response of patients, suffering with severe postoperative parotitis, after penicillin has been administered systemically. It may be necessary to drain the lesion after localization of the process. However, penicillin is easily administered and it does not cause discomfort to the patient, as use of radium and other forms of treatment usually do. Consequently, preliminary results clearly indicate further trials of the use of penicillin in treatment of postoperative parotitis. Epidemic parotitis, as will be mentioned later, is not likely to respond to the use of penicillin.

SCARLET FEVER

Little information is available at present as to the possible value of penicillin in treatment of scarlet fever. Lyons[17] mentioned one case in which the result was not satisfactory. However, in view of the susceptibility of the organism usually associated with scarlet fever, it seems reasonable to assume that use of penicillin would prove effective in treatment of this disease.

INFECTED WOUNDS AND ULCERS

The possible value of penicillin in treatment of infected wounds has been rather intensively studied by a number of investigators, particularly in connection with treatment of infected war wounds. Local application of penicillin in treatment of such wounds was described by Pulvertaft.[27] Although it is generally conceded that the calcium salt of penicillin is more suitable than the sodium salt for local application, the investigator apparently used both preparations in the form of powder, spray or wet dressing. If penicillin is applied locally in the form of the dry powder, the sodium salt may produce irritation of tissue at the site of application. On the other hand, the calcium salt is less likely to do so. From the report by Pulvertaft, it appeared that, within twenty-four hours after penicillin had been applied, a rather uniform reduction occurred in the number of gram-positive pathogens, including clostridia, staphylococci, streptococci and corynebacteria. Gram-negative organisms remained in these wounds and, in some instances, there appeared to be a secondary increase in the number of gram-negative organisms following treatment with penicillin. On the other hand, it was pointed out that the presence of these organisms did not appear to interfere seriously with healing of the wounds.

From the experience of Lyons[17] in the treatment of septic gunshot wounds, it would appear that a combination of systemic and local treatment is the most effective method of treating these wounds. It appears also that removal of devitalized tissue and sequestra is an important part of the successful use of penicillin in these cases.

Other studies on the effectiveness of penicillin in the treatment of infected surface wounds were reported by Bodenham.[28] It is evident from his studies that the tolerance of tissue for penicillin was high and that in no case was there any evidence of local or constitutional untoward reactions following its use. Bodenham combined penicillin with sulfonamides in some instances. He used powdered penicillin and sulfonamides combined. This powder was found satisfactory, particularly if the quantity of exudate from the wound was not great. The penicillin content was approximately 1,000 Oxford units per gram. Bodenham also found that the use of penicillin in amounts up to 20 Oxford units per square centimeter greatly facilitated skin grafting on raw surfaces. I have previously mentioned (Chapter XIII) that Florey found that local and parenteral use of penicillin often permitted primary closure of infected wounds. Local application of penicillin in such cases is carried out by instillation of solution of penicillin through small tubes leading into the depths of the wound.

More extensive studies on the general subject of the use of penicillin, combined with surgical measures, in treatment of superficial and deep flesh wounds have been reported by Bentley[29] and by Brown.[30] In a consecutive series of 200 cases in which flesh wounds were treated by early secondary suture plus local application of penicillin, Bentley reported primary healing in 190, or 95 per cent. Likewise, in the series of cases reported by Brown, 110 wounds were sutured after one insufflation of penicillin-sulfathiazole powder. There were no failures. In this same

7

report, Brown included sixty-eight wounds that were sutured without application of penicillin. Failures occurred in 23 per cent of the cases. Brown further pointed out that recovery was not only rapid in the cases in which penicillin was used but that the nursing care and the number of dressings required were greatly lessened. He also pointed out that penicillin in no way replaced thorough primary surgical treatment.

Penicillin has proved exceedingly effective in treatment of postoperative infection of wounds which have occurred in civilian as well as in military practice. Figure 30 represents a case previously reported by

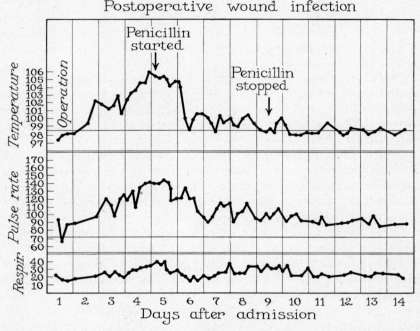

Fig. 30.—Temperature, pulse and respiration in a case of postoperative infection of a wound, in which penicillin was employed.

me.[12] Following left mastectomy, extensive, spreading, postoperative infection of the wound developed; the causative micro-organism was Staphylococcus aureus. Within a few days after administration of penicillin had been started, the infection in the wound receded completely.

According to Dill[31] and to Wollgast,[11] certain types of chronic, indolent ulcers have responded satisfactorily following local use of penicillin. The penicillin was administered in solutions containing approximately 250 Oxford units per cubic centimeter. Biggam[32] has reported that certain tropical ulcers of the legs have become much improved following local application of penicillin.

Hamm and Ouary[33] have reported on the use of penicillin in treatment of phagedenic ulcer (tropical sloughing phagedena). They pointed out that the cause of this ulceration is not entirely clear, although spirochetes and fusiform bacilli are almost invariably present during the active stage of the lesion and frequently these organisms are present in almost pure culture. Many measures have been used in treatment of these ulcerations but, on the whole, treatment has not been satisfactory according to these investigators. They used penicillin in the form of wet dressings in eighteen cases of phagedenic ulcer. For local application of the drug, gauze was soaked in physiologic saline solution containing 2,500 units of penicillin per cubic centimeter. The authors wrote that it was remarkable how quickly the ulcers became clean and the fusiform bacilli and spirochetes disappeared. The investigators further concluded that even better results might have been obtained if the supplies of penicillin had been sufficient to permit intramuscular use of the drug. There seems little doubt, however, but that penicillin was of value in treatment of the ulcers. The result is not surprising in view of the sensitivity of the fusiform bacilli as well as of certain spiral organisms to the action of penicillin.

INFECTIONS OF THE HAND

Mary Florey[34] described excellent results in treatment of infections of the hand by local applications of penicillin combined with surgical measures. In a series of cases of acute infection of the hand, 100 patients were treated surgically and penicillin was administered and in treatment of another 100 (controls) penicillin was not used. Among the patients who received penicillin, organisms and other evidences of infection disappeared more rapidly than among those who did not receive penicillin. Furthermore, healing and restoration of function were reported to be greatly assisted in the group which received penicillin as compared with the control group. In cases of infection of tendon sheaths, the advantages of penicillin were especially striking. A more detailed report on the general subject of the use of penicillin in treatment of infections of the hand was also made by Florey and Williams.[35]

Delaney[36] has reported the successful use of penicillin in treatment of rather severe infections of the hand which followed bites inflicted by man. In the cases reported by Delaney, both patients were dismissed as cured after ten days of treatment with penicillin.

BURNS

Penicillin received some of its greatest publicity in the report on its use in treatment of a number of patients who were victims of the Cocoanut Grove (Boston) fire.[37, 38] Patients who were febrile received penicillin, 5,000 Oxford units administered intramuscularly in 5 c.c. of physiologic saline solution every four hours. Because of the nature of the cases reported, however, as well as the method of treatment, it is difficult to appraise the effectiveness of penicillin.

One of the early reports of an attempt to use penicillin locally in treatment of burns was that of Clark and his colleagues[39] from the Burns Unit, Royal Infirmary, Glasgow. The penicillin was applied locally in the form of a cream which contained 120 Oxford units per gram. Preparation of the cream consisted in adding either sodium or calcium penicillin to a mixture of lanette wax and castor oil. The cream was applied fairly thickly over the wounds and for an inch or so beyond the edge of the wound. The wounds were then covered with gauze. Applications were made twice a day. The investigators subsequently found that the calcium salt was preferable for this form of treatment because it was easier to handle and was not excessively hygroscopic. Of fifty-four cases in which this form of treatment was used in an attempt to eliminate hemolytic streptococci, it was found that the organisms disappeared in 76 per cent within five days and did not reappear. In seven instances the strains of Streptococcus pyogenes which disappeared promptly following use of penicillin were found to be insensitive to the action of sulfonamides. It was the impression of Clark and his coauthors that in no case was application of penicillin without effect. Staphylococci also disappeared quickly from many of the wounds and healing was usually rapid and unattended by any toxic effects. Comparing the use of penicillin in treatment of these wounds with propamidine used in similar burns, the investigators found that healing was fairly good following use of the latter substance but was not as rapid as with penicillin. Neither of these agents was found of value in eliminating Bacillus pyocyaneus or organisms of the genus Proteus.

Keefer and others[6] reported on the successful use of penicillin in treatment of secondary infection in two cases of burns. In three additional cases the treatment was unsuccessful, primarily due to lack of adequate treatment and the presence of severe complications. Likewise, Bodenham,[28] as well as Florey and Cairns,[40] reported that application of penicillin had been effective in eliminating streptococci and staphylococci from infected burned surfaces. It should be emphasized, however, that penicillin is only a part of the successful treatment of these lesions. The importance of toilet of the wound and the use of all the measures at the disposal of the physician are not to be forsaken for penicillin, whether given systemically or locally. This much may be said, however: Penicillin is exceedingly more effective than sulfonamides in eliminating both Streptococcus pyogenes and Staphylococcus aureus from these lesions. The elimination of these organisms is of extreme importance, not only in treatment of the infected burn but in preparation of the patient for skin grafting. As I have already indicated, penicillin is ineffective against Bacillus pyocyaneus or organisms of the genus Proteus although there is some evidence (Florey and Cairns) that free grafts will take satisfactorily in spite of the presence of pus which contains gram-negative organisms. Further reports on the use of penicillin in treatment of infected burns have been made by Galloway and Hobson.[41] For treatment they used dressings of absorbent gauze inoculated with Penicillium notatum. This is essentially the method of Robinson and Wallace for local application of penicillin. As was pointed out in the chapter on methods of administration of penicillin, this method of delivering penicillin to infected areas is not without certain difficulties, including the danger of sensitizing the patient to the mold or to products of the mold which may be present.

Hirshfeld and his colleagues[42] have presented convincing evidence of the value of penicillin in treatment of patients suffering with burns. They experienced gratifying results in the use of penicillin in connection with application of split thickness grafts to these patients. Using penicillin, the procedure of grafting was made possible as soon as slough had separated (three to four weeks after the burn had occurred). Penicillin therapy was begun twelve hours before operation and was continued until the time of the first dressing. The dose administered varied between 5,000 Oxford units every hour and 10,000 Oxford units every two hours, and was given intramuscularly. With one exception in the series of cases reported by Hirshfeld and others, 90 to 100 per cent of the transplanted skin took in every instance. The advantages of penicillin are obviously in the fact that it permits earlier grafting and the split thickness grafts can be applied more successfully as soon as slough has separated; this procedure eliminates the time consuming preparation of granulating areas. It was further evident from these studies that the use of penicillin prevents the loss of skin from infection that ordinarily occurs in about a third of cases in which the split thickness grafts are placed on contaminated recipient areas. Certainly, their experience amply justifies extensive study of the general subject.

CUTANEOUS SYPHILIS

Penicillin has been used successfully in treatment of cutaneous syphilis, both early and late. Its effectiveness in this infection is considered in detail in the chapter on penicillin in treatment of spirochetal infections (p. 218).

INFECTIONS OF THE SKIN IN WHICH PENICILLIN HAS PROVED OF LITTLE OR NO VALUE

In view of the resistance of the virus of vaccinia to the action of penicillin, it is unlikely that the preparation will prove of value in the treatment of smallpox. It also has been of questionable value in treatment of chickenpox (varicella) or herpes. In this connection, however, it should be emphasized that penicillin may play a definite role in treatment of secondary infections complicating these virus diseases. An example is the use of penicillin in treatment of infections due to certain pyogenic organisms which are sensitive to the action of penicillin. That penicillin may have value under the conditions just mentioned is suggested by the report of Jeans, Jeffrey and Gunders[43] on the successful use of penicillin in treatment of what appeared to be almost fatal smallpox but in which the secondary infection of the vesicles was due to Staphylococcus aureus. It seems likely that late toxemia in smallpox, due to secondary infection, may be responsible for many fatalities. Therefore, further attempts to use penicillin under circumstances mentioned are amply justified. It must be remembered, however, that penicillin is unlikely to affect the early course of the disease, due to its feeble virustatic action.

Although the effectiveness of penicillin has not been thoroughly explored in a host of infections of the skin and soft tissues, there is evidence to suggest that penicillin is of no value in certain types of these infections. Penicillin has not been of value in treatment of acne, pemphigus or lupus erythematosus. It has proved to be of little or no value in treatment of blastomycosis. It was also evident, from the report of Michael and others,[44] that penicillin had been of little or no value in treatment of coccidioidomycosis. It has not given evidence of being valuable in treatment of infections with various yeasts and in sporotrichosis. Penicillin likewise has been ineffective in treatment of histoplasmosis. It is unlikely that penicillin will prove of value in treatment of epidemic parotitis (mumps). It is evident from the report of Nelson[45] that penicillin had little or no effect on granuloma inguinale. Thus far, it has proved of no value in the treatment of myositis, dermatomyositis or tularemia Josey[46] has reported a farily typical case of tularemia in which penicillin had little if any effect on the course of the illness.

REFERENCES

1. Roxburgh, I. A., Christie, R. V. and Roxburgh, A. C.: Penicillin in the treatment of certain diseases of the skin. Brit. M. J. 1:524–528 (Apr. 15) 1944.

2. Barron, J. N. and Mansfield, O. T.: The local application of penicillin in soft-tissue lesions. Brit. M. J. 1:521–523 (Apr. 15) 1944.

3. Schoch, A. G.: Local penicillin therapy. Arch. Dermat. & Syph. 50:202 (Sept.) 1944.

4. Abraham, E. P., Chain, E., Fletcher, C. M., Gardner, A. D., Heatley, N. G., Jennings, M. A. and Florey, H. W.: Further observations on penicillin. Lancet. 2:177–188; 189 (Aug. 16) 1941.

5. Florey, M. E. and Florey, H. W.: General and local administration of penicillin. Lancet. 1:387–397 (Mar. 27) 1943.

6. Keefer, C. S., Blake, F. G., Marshall, E. K., Jr., Lockwood, J. S. and Wood, W.

B., Jr.: Penicillin in the treatment of infections; a report of 500 cases. J. A. M. A. *122:* 1217–1224 (Aug. 28) 1943.

7. Robinson, G. H. and Wallace, J. E.: An inoculated penicillin dressing. Science. n.s. *98:*329–330 (Oct. 8) 1943.

8. Lockwood, J. S., White, W. L. and Murphy, F. D.: The use of penicillin in surgical infections. Ann. Surg. *120:*311–344 (Sept.) 1944.

9. Coleman, Rose and Sako, Wallace: Treatment of multiple furunculosis with penicillin. J. A. M. A. *126:*427–429 (Oct. 14) 1944.

10. Johnson, H. M.: Penicillin therapy of impetigo contagiosa and allied diseases: use of penicillium-inoculated dressing. Arch. Dermat. & Syph. *50:*1–5 (July) 1944.

11. Wollgast, C. F.: The clinical use of penicillin; a report of 115 cases treated in an army hospital. Texas State J. Med. *40:*225–230 (Aug.) 1944.

12. Herrell, W. E.: Further observations on the clinical use of penicillin. Proc. Staff Meet., Mayo Clin. *18:*65–76 (Mar. 10) 1943.

13. Herrell, W. E.: The clinical use of penicillin; an antibacterial agent of biologic origin. J. A. M. A. *124:*622–627 (Mar. 4) 1944.

14. Herrell, W. E.: The role of penicillin in the treatment of bacterial infections. South. M. J. *37:*150–156 (Mar.) 1944.

15. Herrell, W. E. and Nichols, D. R.: Penicillin in the treatment of cellulitis of the mouth. Am. J. Orthodont. & Oral Surg. *30:*1–7 (Jan.) 1944.

16. Dawson, M. H. and Hobby, Gladys L.: The clinical use of penicillin; observations in one hundred cases. J. A. M. A. *124:*611–622 (Mar. 4) 1944.

17. Lyons, Champ: Penicillin therapy of surgical infections in the U. S. Army; a report. J. A. M. A. *123:*1007–1018 (Dec. 18) 1943.

18. Denny, E. R., Shallenberger, P. L. and Pyle, H. D.: Clinical observations in the use of penicillin. J. Oklahoma M. A. *37:*193–205 (May) 1944.

19. Herrell, W. E., Nichols, D. R. and Heilman, Dorothy H.: Penicillin; its usefulness, limitations, diffusion and detection, with analysis of 150 cases in which it was employed. J. A. M. A. *125:*1003–1010 (Aug. 12) 1944.

20. Fraser, D. B.: Local treatment of breast abscess with penicillin. Brit. M. J. *1:*523–524 (Apr. 15) 1944.

21. Taffel, Max and Harvey, S. C.: Ludwig's angina; analysis of forty-five cases. Surgery. *11:*841–850 (June) 1942.

22. Herrell, W. E., Heilman, Dorothy H. and Williams, H. L.: The clinical use of penicillin. Proc. Staff Meet., Mayo Clin. *17:*609–616 (Dec. 30) 1942.

23. Goodhill, Victor: Penicillin treatment of cavernous sinus thrombosis. J. A. M. A. *125:*28–30 (May 6) 1944.

24. Nicholson, W. M. and Anderson, W. B.: Penicillin in the treatment of cavernous sinus thrombophlebitis; recovery with unilateral ascending optic atrophy. J. A. M. A. *126:*12–15 (Sept. 2) 1944.

25. Wolf, J. W.: Thrombosis of the cavernous sinus with hemolytic streptococcic bacteremia; treatment by intravenous injection of sulfadiazine and penicillin, with recovery. Arch. Otolaryng. *40:*33–37 (July) 1944.

26. Hageman, P. O., Martin, S. P. and Wood, W. B., Jr.: Penicillin; clinical study of its therapeutic effectiveness. J. A. M. A. *124:*798 (Mar. 18) 1944.

27. Pulvertaft, R. J. V.: Local therapy of war wounds: I. With penicillin. Lancet. *2:* 341–346 (Sept. 18) 1943.

28. Bodenham, D. C.: Infected burns and surface wounds; the value of penicillin. Lancet. *2:*725–728 (Dec. 11) 1943.

29. Bentley, F. H.: The treatment of flesh wounds by early secondary suture and penicillin. Brit. J. Surg. *32:*132–139 (July Suppl.) 1944.

30. Brown, J. J. M.: Early closure of soft tissue wounds with chemotherapeutic agents, a comparative study of sulphanilamide and penicillin. Brit. J. Surg. *32*:140–143 (July Suppl.) 1944.

31. Dill, W. W.: County society reports; Montgomery. Pennsylvania M. J. *47*:63–64 (Oct.) 1943.

32. Biggam, A. G.: Quoted by Hawking, F.: Modern drugs and tropical diseases. Nature. *152*:206 (Aug. 21) 1943.

33. Hamm, W. G. and Ouary, G.: Penicillin therapy in phagedenic ulcer (tropical sloughing phagedena); report of eighteen cases. U. S. Nav. M. Bull. *43*:981–987 (Nov.) 1944.

34. Florey, Mary: Penicillin. Lancet. *2*:639 (Nov. 20) 1943.

35. Florey, M. E. and Williams, R. E. O.: Hand infections treated with penicillin. Lancet. *1*:73–81 (Jan. 15) 1944.

36. Delaney, C. J.: Penicillin in treatment of human bite infections, report of two cases. U. S. Nav. M. Bull. *43*:1020–1022 (Nov.) 1944.

37. Lyons, Champ: Problems of infection and chemotherapy. Ann. Surg. *117*:894–902 (June) 1943.

38. Faxon, N. W. and Churchill, E. D.: The Cocoanut Grove disaster in Boston; a preliminary account. J. A. M. A. *120*:1385–1388 (Dec. 26) 1942.

39. Clark, A. M., Colebrook, Leonard, Gibson, Thomas and Thompson, M. L.: Penicillin and propamidine in burns: elimination of haemolytic streptococci and staphylococci. Lancet. *1*:605–609 (May 15) 1943.

40. Florey, H. W. and Cairns, Hugh: Penicillin in war wounds; a report from the Mediterranean. Lancet. *2*:742–745 (Dec. 11) 1943.

41. Galloway, L. D. and Hobson, A. J.: Penicillin dressings. Nature. *153*:170 (Feb. 5) 1944.

42. Hirshfeld, J. W., Pilling, M. A., Buggs, C. W. and Abbott, W. E.: Penicillin and skin grafting. J. A. M. A. *125*:1017–1019 (Aug. 12) 1944.

43. Jeans, W. D., Jeffrey, J. S. and Gunders, K.: Penicillin and smallpox; report of four cases. Lancet. *2*:44–45 (July 8) 1944.

44. Michael, Paul, McLaughlin, R. F. and Cenac, P. L.: Coccidioidomycosis; report of unsuccessful treatment with penicillin. U. S. Nav. M. Bull. *43*:122–124 (July) 1944.

45. Nelson, R. A.: Penicillin in the treatment of granuloma inguinale. Am. J. Syph. Gonor. & Ven. Dis. *28*:611–619 (Sept.) 1944.

46. Josey, A. I.: Penicillin treatment of a case of tularemia without effect. J. A. M. A. *126*:496–497 (Oct. 21) 1944.

CHAPTER XV

INFECTIONS OF THE GENITO-URINARY SYSTEM EXCLUSIVE OF GONORRHEA

It was evident in consideration of the absorption, diffusion and excretion of penicillin that this substance is rather rapidly excreted in the urine and in fairly large amounts. Analysis of renal tissue also reveals the presence of a considerable quantity of penicillin following its systemic administration. It is not surprising, therefore, that penicillin has proved of value in treatment of infections involving the genito-urinary apparatus due to organisms susceptible to its action.

PERINEPHRITIC ABSCESS AND CARBUNCLE OF THE KIDNEY

Perinephritic abscess and carbuncle of the kidney are not infrequently complications of localized or generalized systemic infections owing to Staphylococcus aureus. Therefore, since penicillin is highly effective against this organism and since adequate therapeutic amounts of penicillin reach the kidney, penicillin has a place in treatment of this type of infection. In some instances it may be possible to treat successfully perinephritic abscess without surgical intervention. On the other hand, once the infection is thoroughly established, penicillin is probably of greatest value in combination with surgical drainage. In one of the reports from the Mayo Clinic,[1] a case was reported in which there was definite evidence of beginning perinephritic abscess following surgical removal of a stone from the kidney. In addition, urine from this kidney was practically purulent. The patient was critically ill and the rectal temperature ranged between 105° and 106° F. Because of the extensive perirenal infection, as well as infection in the wound, it was thought that nephrectomy could not be avoided. Following five days of treatment with penicillin, however, marked improvement occurred and the patient recovered without nephrectomy. It seems likely that the kidney could not have been saved without penicillin therapy.

Lyons,[2] as well as Dawson and Hobby,[3] subsequently reported on the satisfactory use of penicillin in treatment of perinephritic abscess. The reports of these investigators contained one case each of this type. The use of penicillin is indicated in the treatment not only of staphylococcal infections of the kidney but also of infections due to other susceptible organisms, such as Streptococcus pyogenes and certain strains of green-producing streptococci which are sensitive to its action.

Plan of Treatment.—What is to be said here applies in general to all of the infections of the urinary tract which will be dealt with in this chapter. For treatment of these infections, it is rarely necessary to use more than 80,000 to 100,000 Oxford units of penicillin per day. In fact, many of these infections will respond to as little as 40,000 to 80,000 units per day. The penicillin can be administered either by the intravenous drip method or by the intermittent intramuscular method. When the latter method is employed, the twenty-four hour total quantity of penicillin should be divided into eight doses and administered every three hours in 2 or 3 c.c. of physiologic saline solution. If the intravenous drip method is to be employed and there is evidence of renal damage and retention of urea, penicillin should be administered in 5 per cent solution of glucose made up in triple distilled water rather than in the aforementioned saline solution. The intravenous method delivers a more constant flow of penicillin into the kidneys and urine than does the intramuscular method. On the other hand, it may not be desirable to use this method if edema is present and large amounts of fluid are not desired.

PYELONEPHRITIS, PYELITIS AND CYSTITIS

Monovalent and polyvalent pyogenic infections of the renal pelvis and urinary bladder have responded satisfactorily to treatment with penicillin. Included in the first report by the Oxford investigators[4] will be found data which suggested that this type of infection of the urinary tract might be satisfactorily treated with penicillin. In one case reported by them, the patient was seriously ill with an infection of the urinary tract owing to Staphylococcus aureus and Escherichia coli. The patient had been treated with sulfapyridine and apparently the Escherichia coli had disappeared from the urine before administration of penicillin had been started. At that time, however, the urine contained Staphylococcus aureus. The patient received penicillin by mouth along with rather large doses of soda. It was then found that the urine contained strongly bacteriostatic concentrations of penicillin. Within forty-eight hours, steady improvement began. The concentration of urea in the blood, which was elevated when treatment was begun, returned to normal and, at the end of seven days, use of penicillin was discontinued. According to this report, after treatment the urine was sterile and remained sterile.

My colleagues and I[5] likewise have treated successfully coccal infections of the urinary tract with penicillin. If severe renal damage is not present, adequate amounts of penicillin will reach the urine in these cases and frequently effective results can be obtained. In mixed infections of the urinary tract due to sensitive gram-positive cocci and relatively insensitive gram-negative organisms, at times it may be possible to rid the urinary tract of the gram-positive cocci by the use of penicillin and, at the same time, to deal with the gram-negative organisms by combining sulfonamide therapy with the penicillin therapy. In spite of the effectiveness of penicillin in treatment of these conditions, recurrences are almost certain if the physician does not at the same time deal with the associated lesions and mechanical factors such as calculi in the renal pelves, ureters or bladder. Likewise, the presence of obstruction at the vesical neck, with the resulting pooling of urine which favors infection, will lead to recurrence unless these factors are dealt with in addition to administration of penicillin. At least this is my experience in collaborating with urologists in treatment of patients.[6]

The report of Thompson[7] on the use of penicillin in treatment of pyelonephritis and interstitial cystitis is of some interest. He pointed out that the patient may recover spontaneously from acute pyelonephritis and, therefore, that it is difficult to evaluate the effect of penicillin in this type of case. He also was aware that penicillin is of value in eliminating gram-positive cocci from the urine in cases of chronic renal infection but that other chemotherapeutic agents should be combined with penicillin when the infection is of the mixed type (gram-positive cocci and gram-negative bacilli). It was evident from the report of Thompson also that penicillin had proved to be of little or no value in treatment of interstitial cystitis.

NONGONORRHEAL PROSTATITIS, URETHRITIS, PERIURETHRAL ABSCESS, EPIDIDYMITIS AND BALANITIS

Prostatitis, periurethral abscess and epididymitis due to susceptible organisms have responded satisfactorily to the use of penicillin. Sulfonamides together with local, nonspecific therapy, however, still will suffice for treatment of most of these infections. In many cases, however, it will be found that the organism responsible for the infection may resist treatment with sulfonamides as well as local treatment, including hyperthermia. It is in this group of cases that penicillin can be used most effectively. The tendency for such infections as prostatitis to recur, however, and the mechanical factors frequently present, which include localized abscesses and obstruction of the prostatic duct, at times may preclude satisfactory use of penicillin. For that reason, it seems likely that penicillin is of most value when used in combination with local measures directed toward elimination of these factors.

Keefer and others,[8] as well as my colleagues and I, have obtained satisfactory results in treatment of a few patients with prostatitis in which Staphylococcus aureus has been the infecting organism. Likewise, Thompson[7] experienced satisfactory results in treatment of acute nonspecific prostatitis owing to what appeared to be a sensitive strain of nonhemolytic streptococcus. He has pointed out, however, that acute nonspecific prostatitis, including that of staphylococcal origin, does not respond as rapidly as does acute gonorrheal prostatitis. Of further interest is the fact that Thompson reported excellent results in treatment of twenty-four of thirty patients with chronic prostatitis. The organisms isolated in these cases included Staphylococcus albus, Streptococcus pyogenes, Bacillus subtilis, organisms of the genus Micrococcus, diphtheroid organisms and Alcaligenes faecalis.

Thompson further reported that satisfactory results had been obtained in treatment of some patients with nonspecific urethritis. He emphasized, however, the importance of thorough examination in these cases to detect the presence of stricture and other mechanical factors which must be dealt with if penicillin is to be used successfully. My colleagues and I have employed penicillin successfully in treatment of periurethral abscess following such procedures as transurethral prostatic resection.

Acute nonspecific epididymitis, according to Thompson, also has responded well to 20,000 Oxford units of penicillin administered intramuscularly every three hours for ten injections. Prompt relief of pain and rapid reduction of tenderness and swelling were said to occur following use of penicillin. In the small group of cases reported by Thompson, epididymotomy or other surgical procedures were not necessary. Likewise, Thompson successfully used penicillin locally in the treatment of balanitis. Improvement was so striking that dorsal slits were avoided in all cases.

The use of penicillin in treatment of infections owing to Neisseria gonorrhoeae is discussed in chapter XVI.

PELVIC CELLULITIS AND PUERPERAL INFECTION

While sulfonamides have proved of considerable value in treatment of acute and subacute pelvic cellulitis, as well as of puerperal infection, these drugs are not universally nor uniformly effective. Furthermore, sulfonamides have not proved of great value in treatment of certain anaerobic streptococcal infections which follow abortion, delivery or surgical procedures in the pelvis.

It was evident from the report of Keefer and his associates[8] and from the reports of Mitchell and Kaminester,[9] Hellman and Guilfoil,[10] and White[11] that penicillin could be used with remarkable effectiveness in the presence of overwhelming puerperal infection due to Staphylococcus aureus or Streptococcus pyogenes. In some of the cases wherein penicillin was effective, no result had been obtained previously from even heroic doses of one of the sulfonamides.

Likewise, infections with anaerobic streptococci associated with abortion have been treated satisfactorily with penicillin. While my experience is limited to only a few cases of pelvic cellulitis and puerperal infection, I am inclined to believe that penicillin is one of the most effective agents yet available in treatment of these infections. Penicillin will be found highly effective in the presence of cellulitis of pregnant women. Since penicillin is transmitted through the placenta to the fetus, as shown in studies by my colleagues and me (p. 77), I am inclined to believe that the fetal circulation can be protected against blood stream infections. I have seen normal children born while their mothers were under intensive treatment with penicillin for severe, overwhelming infection, including septicemia.

Plan of Treatment.—In treatment of these severe gynecologic infections at least 100,000 Oxford units of penicillin should be administered daily by the intravenous drip method. If the intermittent intramuscular method is used, even larger amounts of penicillin (150,000 to 200,000 Oxford units) should be administered.

INFECTIONS OF THE GENITO-URINARY SYSTEM IN WHICH PENICILLIN IS OF DOUBTFUL OR APPARENTLY OF NO VALUE

It seems clear that penicillin is of little or no value in treatment of infections of the urinary tract due to gram-negative organisms of the colon-typhoid group. In fact, I have seen infections of the urinary tract of this type develop at the very time when patients were receiving adequate amounts of penicillin for infections owing to susceptible organisms. Infections owing to Pseudomonas aeruginosa and to organisms of the genus Proteus likewise have remained unaffected by penicillin therapy.

Infections with certain gram-positive cocci, such as Streptococcus faecalis, have not responded, as a rule, to penicillin. Helmholz and Sung,[12] on the basis of certain studies in vitro, offered the hope that penicillin might prove effective in treatment of infections due to this organism. I have had occasion to treat with penicillin a few cases of infection of the urinary tract owing to Streptococcus faecalis. On the basis of preliminary results, it does not appear that penicillin in the amounts used altered the course of the infection. Whether or not subsequent studies, using large amounts of penicillin, will yield more satisfactory results will depend on further clinical trials.

In my experience, to the time of writing this paragraph, results have not been particularly encouraging after use of penicillin in treatment of that type of cellulitis and peritonitis which may follow radium therapy. The lack of success may be due to the fact that the cellulitis is more on the basis of irritation than of infection. If there is any evidence of bacterial infection, however, penicillin should be used.

It appeared, from the studies of Pereyra and Landy,[13] that penicillin would prove of little or no value in treatment of chancroidal infections.

REFERENCES

1. Herrell, W. E.: Further observations on the clinical use of penicillin. Proc. Staff Meet., Mayo Clin. *18*:65–76 (Mar. 10) 1943.

2. Lyons, Champ: Penicillin therapy of surgical infections in the U. S. Army; a report. J. A. M. A. *123*:1007–1018 (Dec. 18) 1943.

3. Dawson, M. H. and Hobby, Gladys L.: The clinical use of penicillin; observations in one hundred cases. J. A. M. A. *124*:611–622 (Mar. 4) 1944.

4. Abraham, E. P., Chain, E., Fletcher, C. M., Gardner, A. D., Heatley, N. G., Jennings, M. A. and Florey, H. W.: Further observations on penicillin. Lancet. *2*:177–188; 189 (Aug. 16) 1941.

5. Herrell, W. E., Nichols, D. R. and Heilman, Dorothy H.: Penicillin; its usefulness, limitations, diffusion and detection, with analysis of 150 cases in which it was employed. J. A. M. A. *125*:1003–1010 (Aug. 12) 1944.

6. Herrell, W. E. and Nichols, D. R.: The calcium salt of penicillin. Proc. Staff Meet., Mayo Clin. *18*:313–319 (Sept. 8) 1943.

7. Thompson, G. J.: The clinical use of penicillin in genitourinary infections. J. A. M. A. *126*:403–407 (Oct. 14) 1944.

8. Keefer, C. S., Blake, F. G., Marshall, E. K., Jr., Lockwood, J. S. and Wood, W. B., Jr.: Penicillin in the treatment of infections; a report of 500 cases. J. A. M. A. *122*:1217–1224 (Aug. 28) 1943.

9. Mitchell, R. McN. and Kaminester, Sanford: Penicillin; case report of a patient who recovered from puerperal sepsis hemolytic streptococcus septicemia. Am. J. Surg. n.s. *63*:136–140 (Jan.) 1944.

10. Hellman, A. M. and Guilfoil, E. F.: Treatment with penicillin after the failure of sulfa drugs in a case of vaginal plastic followed by blood stream infection. Am. J. Obst. & Gynec. *47*:125–126 (Jan.) 1944.

11. White, R. A.: Puerperal sepsis treated with penicillin; case report. South. M. J. *37*:524–525 (Sept.) 1944.

12. Helmholz, H. F. and Sung, Chieh: The bactericidal effect of penicillin in urine on Streptococcus faecalis and gram-negative bacilli. Proc. Staff Meet., Mayo Clin. *19*:370–374 (July 12) 1944.

13. Pereyra, A. J. and Landy, Simeon: Experimental prophylaxis and treatment of chancroidal infection; inefficacy of penicillin administered intramuscularly. U. S. Nav. M. Bull. *43*:189–191 (July) 1944.

PART III

CLINICAL USE OF PENICILLIN (*Continued*):
EFFECTIVENESS AGAINST VARIOUS DISEASES AND CONSIDERATIONS OF TOXICITY

CHAPTER XVI

GONORRHEA

GENERAL CONSIDERATION

Following the introduction of sulfonamides for treatment of gonorrhea, it was thought that the disease might quickly be brought under control. As experience accrued, it became evident that some strains of Neisseria gonorrhoeae are, or become, resistant to the action of sulfonamides. As a result, many infections owing to Neisseria gonorrhoeae could not be controlled by any of the sulfonamides when used alone or when combined, in some cases, with hyperpyrexia. Although penicillin for the most part is effective against gram-positive pathogens, it was evident from studies made in vitro and reported by Fleming[1] and by the Oxford investigators,[2] that Neisseria gonorrhoeae was susceptible to the action of penicillin. At least most strains examined were susceptible. From studies made in vitro, the Oxford investigators found that six strains were completely inhibited in the presence of dilutions of penicillin as high as 1:2,000,000. The seventh strain examined was inhibited only up to 1:32,000. Further reports on the general subject did not appear until the report from the Mayo Clinic on the use of penicillin in treatment of sulfonamide resistant gonorrhea.

In these studies, reported by my colleagues and me,[3] dilutions of penicillin of 1:100,000 and 1:200,000 were used to test the sensitivity of several strains of Neisseria gonorrhoeae obtained from patients in whom the disease had resisted intensive sulfonamide therapy. Hourly subcultures were made of the preparations containing penicillin and of the controls. Between the first and second hours, there was a sharp decrease in the number of viable organisms of two of the strains that were placed in contact with penicillin. Decrease in the number of viable organisms of another strain occurred between the second and the third hours.

After three or four hours, there were no viable organisms in the tubes which contained penicillin whereas there was moderate growth (table 19) in all the control tubes. Also, five patients who had sulfonamide resistant infections were treated with penicillin. In all cases the patients were cured and prostatic and urinary cultures became negative, in some instances as early as seventeen hours after treatment had been begun. It is possible that prostatic and urinary organisms had been killed sooner than this but, unfortunately, cultures were not taken earlier.

It quickly became evident that if these preliminary studies could be uniformly confirmed in a large series of cases, personnel of the armed forces who were suffering with neisserian infections might be rehabilitated within one day. Many patients had been in hospital for months

TABLE 19

THE ANTIBACTERIAL EFFECT OF PENICILLIN ON NEISSERIA GONORRHOEAE

Strain	Dilution	1 hour	2 hours	3 hours	4 hours
1	1:100,000	+ + +	0	0	0
	1:200,000	+ + +	+	0	0
	Control	+ + +	+ + +	+ + +	+ +
2	1:100,000	+ + +	+ + +	+	0
	1:200,000	+ + +	+ + +	+	0
	Control	+ + +	+ + +	+ + +	+ +
3	1:100,000	+ + +	+ +	+	0
	1:200,000	+ + +	+ +	+	0
	Control	+ + +	+ + +	+ + +	+ +

+ + +, heavy growth; + +, moderate growth; +, slight growth; 0, no growth.

From article by Herrell, Cook and Thompson, Journal of the American Medical Association, May 29, 1943.

without response to sulfonamide therapy. When fever therapy for such patients became necessary, it was impossible to rehabilitate them in less than a week or ten days. Given a thousand such cases, perhaps 240,000 manpower hours could be saved by the use of penicillin. The experience of others following the original report by my colleagues and me on the effectiveness of penicillin in treatment of sulfonamide resistant gonorrhea seems to have more than justified our hopes.

It was later suggested by Miller, Scott and Moeller[4] that the rapidity of the curative action of penicillin had not been emphasized in the early reports. In bacteriologic and cytologic observations of men with gonorrheal urethritis, these investigators noted that the urethral exudate underwent striking changes for the better within two or three hours after initiation of treatment with penicillin. Viable gonococci in the urethra diminished rapidly in number and disappeared altogether in a few hours. The average time from the beginning of treatment until the first negative smear was obtained was three to four hours. This is interesting in view of the fact that viable organisms disappeared between the third and fourth hours of contact with penicillin according to the in vitro studies reported by my colleagues and me.

Possibly the term "sulfonamide resistant gonorrhea," which has been commonly used, is not a good one. I have treated successfully with penicillin patients whose infection had resisted not only sulfonamides but also fever therapy. One could, therefore, speak of "fever resistant gonorrhea." It might be more accurate to consider that, in some instances, the strains of Neisseria that are present are highly virulent. In view of the fact, however, that the term "sulfonamide resistant gonorrhea" has come into general use and is commonly employed by most investigators, no attempt is made to eliminate the term from the following discussion of the effectiveness of penicillin in treatment of gonorrhea.

GONORRHEA IN THE MALE

In the first report on the effectiveness of penicillin in treatment of gonorrhea, all patients represented were males.[3] Also, the next report on the general subject, made by Mahoney and his colleagues,[5] represented only male patients. These workers treated seventy-five patients, none of whom had been cured by sulfonamides or by sulfonamides and fever therapy combined. The total amount of penicillin administered to each of these patients was 160,000 Oxford units. Ten thousand units of penicillin were administered in 2 c.c. of solvent, intramuscularly, every three hours day and night for forty-five hours. Seventy-four of the seventy-five patients were cured and only one represented a therapeutic failure. The duration of the disease at the time when treatment with penicillin was begun, in this group of cases reported from the Marine Hospital at Staten Island, ranged from ten days to 330 days, with an average of forty-five days.

In order to obtain some idea of the effectiveness of penicillin in a large series of cases in which treatment was given under various programs by a large number of different investigators, I have analyzed several reports in the order in which they appeared. These reports represented 7,753 cases. Recoveries which followed the use of penicillin numbered 7,549, giving a recovery rate of 97.4 per cent. The investigators and the number of cases reported by them are as follows: Mayo Clinic[3, 6-8] (sixteen cases); Mahoney and others[5] (seventy-five cases); Dill[9] (six cases); Robinson[10] (ninety-eight cases); Linner[11] (one case); Florey and Cairns[12] (ten cases); Hollenberg[13] (100 cases); Van Slyke, Arnold and Buchholtz[14] (178 cases); Surgical Staff of United States Naval Hospital, San Diego[15] (twenty-one cases); Dawson and Hobby[16] (eight cases);

Barr[17] (1,750 cases); Ferguson and Buchholtz[18] (753 cases); Denny, Shallenberger and Pyle[19] (243 cases); Schwartz and Edge[20] (4,439 cases); Miller, Scott and Moeller[4] (twenty-one cases); Atcheson[21] (four cases) and Page and Heimoff[22] (thirty cases).

It is evident from this collection of cases that penicillin has proved exceedingly valuable in treatment of gonorrhea in the male which had resisted other forms of therapy. More striking is the fact that, with few exceptions, the patients were cured following the first short course of penicillin (usually no more than twenty-four to forty-eight hours). Furthermore, many of the patients were treated very early in the course of studies on the use of penicillin for gonorrhea; many of the 2.6 per cent of failures accordingly were not due to the ineffectiveness of penicillin but to the extremely low doses employed.

When two or three courses of penicillin have been given, in many instances even better results have been obtained. For example, in the report by Sternberg and Turner[23] on the use of penicillin in 1,686 cases, cure resulted in 99 per cent and, in no instance in the series, could resistance to penicillin be proved. Other reports on the general subject have been made by Frisch and others,[24] Riba, Schmidlapp and Bosworth,[25] Menville and Ross,[26] Murphy,[27] Van Slyke and Steinberg,[28] Thompson,[29] Scarcello,[30] and Robinson.[31] When adequate amounts of penicillin are used and the patients receive at least two courses, which are necessary in some instances, it is safe to state that nearly all will respond. I have not encountered a case in which resistance to penicillin could be proved although they undoubtedly will occur.

Striking clinical features attending treatment of gonorrhea in the male by means of penicillin are the rapidity with which viable organisms disappear and the prompt cessation of symptoms. The dysuria and discharge begin to subside often within a few hours following beginning of treatment. Epididymitis and other complications of gonorrheal urethritis in the male abate promptly as a rule following use of penicillin. Pain and local tenderness often disappear within twenty-four hours in cases of epididymitis and prostatitis. Complete disappearance of swelling may take several days. Prostatitis, including prostatic abscess, has been known to subside promptly following initiation of penicillin therapy. One of the cases reported by my colleagues and me[3] was an example of extensive prostatitis and beginning prostatic abscess. Previously urinary retention had developed and severe bilateral lower abdominal pain extended into both flanks. Pain during urination was severe. Bilateral lower abdominal tenderness and muscular spasm were found on physical examination. Five and a half hours after institution of treatment, the abdominal pain and tenderness had subsided. Within forty-eight hours, perineal distress associated with prostatic infection had completely disappeared. At this time, tenderness of the prostate gland was considerably reduced and the gland was approximately half as large as it had been at the beginning of treatment. Fever also subsided within twenty-four hours after penicillin therapy was begun.

Plan of Treatment.—For treatment of gonorrhea in the male, various amounts of penicillin have been recommended. However, on the basis of present knowledge, the most satisfactory total dose appears to be somewhere between 100,000 and 150,000 Oxford units. Ten thousand to 15,000 Oxford units of penicillin should be administered intramuscularly in 2 or 3 c.c. of physiologic saline solution or distilled water every three hours until the total dose has been given. Patients suffering with prostatitis and epididymitis should be hospitalized. In hospital, the penicillin can be administered either intramuscularly or intravenously over a period of twenty-four to forty-eight hours.

Although in some instances gonorrhea can be cured by a single injection of a large dose of penicillin, or by three or four intramuscular injections, each of 20,000 Oxford units of penicillin, I do not favor this procedure. Neither do I favor total doses of less than 100,000 Oxford units because this amount may be subeffective. Therefore resistance to penicillin might develop and the term "penicillin resistant gonorrhea" might take its place along with the term "sulfonamide resistant gonorrhea."

If an attempt is to be made to use the "one shot" treatment for gonorrhea, the material should be incorporated in some substance which will prolong the action of penicillin. For this purpose the beeswax-peanut oil mixture recommended by Romansky and Rittman[32] will prove satisfactory. Two hundred thousand units of penicillin can be administered intramuscularly in 1 c.c. of the beeswax-oil mixture. (See methods of administration, chapter IX.)

GONORRHEA IN THE FEMALE

Results in treatment of women suffering with gonorrhea have been equally as brilliant as those reported in treatment of men. Extensive pelvic inflammatory disease, even of several months' standing, has responded satisfactorily to the preparation. In general, slightly larger amounts of penicillin than are used in treatment of acute gonorrhea in the male should be employed against these infections in women. Although early acute gonorrheal urethritis and cervicitis in the female can be managed satisfactorily while the patient remains ambulatory, penicillin being given meanwhile by the intramuscular route, in a manner similar to that used in treatment of males, this procedure is not recommended for certain types of gonorrheal infections in the female. In the presence of acute or subacute extensive pelvic inflammatory disease, with salpingitis or pelvic cellulitis, it is important to hospitalize the patients. The course of the infection should be followed by means of the sedimentation rate and routine urethral and cervical cultures. As long as the patients should be hospitalized anyway, it is probably preferable to administer penicillin intravenously, although intermittent intramuscular administration will suffice.

Early in the course of our studies, my colleagues and I[6] were impressed by the rapid response to treatment made by a small number of females who were suffering from gonorrhea although in some instances the disease had been present for many months. Patients selected for these therapeutic trials with penicillin had infections which had resisted intensive sulfonamide therapy and, in some instances, fever therapy.

Additional evidence of the effectiveness of penicillin in treatment of gonorrhea in the female was apparent in the article by Cohn, Studdiford and Grunstein.[33] These investigators reported on the use of penicillin in treatment of forty-four women suffering with gonorrhea. The infections of forty-two of these patients had resisted adequate sulfonamide therapy. Forty-three of the forty-four patients became bacteriologically negative after treatment with penicillin and remained negative during the follow-up period. The one patient who failed to respond during the first course of treatment was cured following administration of a second course of 100,000 Oxford units of penicillin. This emphasizes the necessity of treating gonorrhea of females a little more intensively than that of males, and over a longer period of time, in order to insure against failure. Furthermore, as has been said, subeffective doses may result in development of resistance to penicillin. Although Cohn, Studdiford and Grunstein felt that a total dose of 75,000 Oxford units of penicillin was satisfactory for treatment in these cases, and that the total amount could be administered over a period of six hours, my experience would indicate that approximately twice this amount could well be given over a longer period of time in order to obtain the most uniformly satisfactory results.

Further studies on the use of penicillin in treatment of chemoresistant gonorrhea in the female have been made by Greenblatt and Street.[34]

As a rule, the sedimentation rate in cases of pelvic inflammatory disease of women will begin to decline after several days' treatment with penicillin. It is advisable to continue treatment of women for at least four or five days and until at least two negative cultures have been obtained. The sedimentation rate may not have reached normal at the time administration of penicillin is discontinued but, in my experience, it has continued to fall gradually even after administration of penicillin has been discontinued.

Gonorrheal Proctitis.—One case in which gonorrheal proctitis was treated with penicillin has been reported from the Mayo Clinic.[6] The patient had been suffering with severe pelvic inflammatory disease, complicated by gonorrheal proctitis, for eight and a half months. The proctitis was so severe that intense pain and bleeding regularly were associated with defecation. Vesical irritability and pruritus vulvae were severe. A cyst was present in the right Bartholin gland. Cultures of the cervical discharge revealed the presence of Neisseria gonorrhoeae. Furthermore, cultures made from material obtained from the rectal crypts at the time of proctoscopic examination also were positive for Neisseria gonorrhoeae. The patient was cured following administration of penicillin by the intravenous drip method for six days.

Gonorrhea Complicating Pregnancy.—In the previous chapter I have pointed out that penicillin could be used satisfactorily in treatment of various infections of the parturient mother. In the case reported by Strauss,[35] the patient had been entirely refractory to the use of sulfathiazole, sulfadiazine and sulfapyridine. For obvious reasons, intensive fever therapy is not desirable in pregnancy. Penicillin was administered. Delivery was uneventful and the child gave no evidence of infection. Likewise, Cohn, Studdiford and Grunstein[33] reported that the course of pregnancy in four cases of sulfonamide resistant gonorrhea was in no way affected by treatment with penicillin and clinical responses were satisfactory. Wollgast[36] also has reported on the use of penicillin in treatment of a patient who was eight months pregnant. Cure was brought about in three days. Penicillin, therefore, is an exceedingly effective and safe agent for treatment of the pregnant woman suffering with gonorrheal urethritis, cervicitis or other complications including pelvic inflammatory disease.

Gonorrheal Vulvovaginitis.—In view of what has been said concerning the great sensitivity of Neisseria gonorrhoeae to penicillin, and the encouraging results which have been obtained in treatment of a limited number of women who have had gonorrheal infection, including vulvovaginitis, it is not surprising that equally satisfactory results have been reported following use of penicillin in treatment of vulvovaginitis of children.

Sandes[37] mentioned, in a brief communication, that encouraging results were being obtained from local application of filtrates containing penicillin in treatment of this condition. Cohn, Studdiford and Grunstein[33] were also particularly impressed by the effectiveness of penicillin in one case of sulfonamide resistant gonococcal vaginitis in which the patient was five years of age. The patient received four injections of penicillin, each of 10,000 Oxford units, into the gluteal muscles every three hours (total dose 40,000 Oxford units). Cultures apparently became negative promptly and remained negative throughout the follow-up period of twenty-five days.

Estimate of Effectiveness.—From the limited number of reports available, it is evident that penicillin can be used successfully in treatment of gonorrheal infections of women and female children, including such complications as proctitis, vulvovaginitis and diffuse pelvic cellulitis. While some failures undoubtedly will occur, available reports leave little doubt as to the effectiveness of penicillin in these conditions.

GONORRHEAL OPHTHALMIA

Included in the report by Florey and Florey[38] on local administration of penicillin was an account of a case of ophthalmia neonatorum which had not responded to sulfapyridine administered locally for three and a half weeks. A solution of penicillin containing 1,200 Oxford units per cubic centimeter was dropped into the eye every hour. Within twelve hours the discharge had diminished and in forty-eight hours it had disappeared; the eyes were open and the conjunctivae clear. Subsequently, Sorsby[39] reported equally striking results in treatment of this infection. His report, made before the Section on Ophthalmology of the Royal Society of Medicine, November 12, 1943, demonstrated that results with penicillin were more striking than those obtained previously with sulfanilamide. The conjunctivae became completely clear within thirty-six hours following institution of penicillin therapy. Sorsby was inclined to speak with considerable reserve, however, concerning the effectiveness of penicillin in this infection because experience with penicillin until that time had been somewhat limited. Further studies on the effectiveness of penicillin in treatment of ophthalmia were reported by Sievers, Knott and Soloway.[40] In their experience, in four out of five cases the response to systemic administration of penicillin was outstanding. Specific organisms disappeared from smears and cultures in from nine to twenty-four hours following institution of treatment. Gonorrheal complications did not develop in any case. The total dose of penicillin used in these cases varied from 60,000 to 330,000 Oxford units. The penicillin was administered intramuscularly in amounts of 10,000 Oxford units every three hours. Keyes[41] also made brief mention of the effect of penicillin in treatment of gonorrheal ophthalmia although reports of cases were not included in his communication.

Gonorrheal infections of the eyes of adults, including conjunctivitis and iridocyclitis, also have been successfully treated. A striking result was reported by Griffey[42] in treatment of severe gonorrheal conjunctivitis. The patient had been suffering with gonorrheal urethritis, and severe gonorrheal conjunctivitis with copious purulent discharge developed. Although the gonorrheal urethritis subsided considerably under treatment with sulfathiazole, there was apparently no effect on the course of the ocular infection. Penicillin was administered intramuscularly, 25,000 Oxford units every three hours for ten doses, a total dose, therefore, of 250,000 Oxford units. The clinical response was prompt and, within ten hours after beginning of treatment with penicillin, the exudate from the eye had diminished greatly. Likewise, Christie and Garrod[43] reported on successful treatment of these infections following local use of penicillin.

Another instance of successful use of penicillin in treatment of gonorrheal infection of the eye complicating gonorrheal urethritis was reported by Denny, Shallenberger and Pyle.[19] In addition to administration of penicillin into the eye every two hours, relatively large doses were administered intramuscularly (50,000 Oxford units every three hours). The preparation used for local instillation contained 250 Oxford units of penicillin per cubic centimeter.

In the chapter wherein diffusion of penicillin was discussed, it was pointed out that, following systemic administration, very little penicillin reaches the tissues of the eye. However, when fairly large amounts are administered systemically, there is good evidence that some penetration into these tissues occurs. In my experience, therefore, it has proved desirable to use rather large amounts of penicillin for systemic treatment of infections of the eye. It is further suggested that systemic therapy, as a rule, be combined with local instillation.

Plan of Treatment.—*Gonorrheal Ophthalmia of Infants.*—For treatment of gonorrheal ophthalmia of infants and children, it is recommended that at least 40,000 Oxford units of penicillin be administered per day. Five thousand Oxford units in 1 or 2 c.c. of physiologic saline solution should be administered into the gluteal muscles every three hours. This treatment should be continued until at least two negative cultures and two negative smears have been obtained. For local instillation, physiologic saline solutions containing anywhere from 250 to 1,000 Oxford units of penicillin per cubic centimeter should be dropped into the eyes every two hours. Patients should be hospitalized and the same general care should be employed as usually is indicated in these cases.

Gonorrheal Ophthalmia of Adults.—In treatment of gonorrheal ophthalmia of adults it is also recommended that the patients be hospitalized and that fairly large amounts of penicillin be administered. The total daily dose should approximate 120,000 to 160,000 Oxford units per day. To adults, the penicillin can be administered by the continuous intravenous drip method or it can be given intramuscularly in amounts of 15,000 to 20,000 Oxford units every three hours in 3 or 4 c.c. of physiologic saline solution. Likewise, it frequently is desirable to combine local instillation with systemic therapy. For local use, solutions containing as much as 1,000 Oxford units per cubic centimeter should be administered every two hours.

GONORRHEAL ARTHRITIS

Since penicillin is effective against Neisseria gonorrhoeae and since, as was shown by my colleagues and me,[8] when given systemically it is found in the joint fluid in a concentration approximately half that which it attains in the blood, it seemed reasonable to hope that penicillin would be effective in treatment of gonorrheal arthritis. It should be made perfectly clear that there is great difference between treatment of acute gonorrheal arthritis of a few days' to two or three weeks' duration and treatment of gonorrheal arthritis which has been present several weeks or more. In the first instance, prompt treatment may cure the condition before significant or irreparable pathologic changes have damaged the joint. However, in a case of longer duration, irreparable destructive changes may have occurred in the joint and these cannot be expected to be eradicated by penicillin, even though the substance may stop further progress of the infection. I have heard some investigators state that penicillin was totally ineffective in treatment of gonorrheal arthritis. This has not been my experience, nor (as will be shown hereafter) has it been the experience of some other investigators who have had occasion to treat with penicillin patients suffering from acute gonorrheal arthritis. The difference of opinion on this subject may result from the difficulty which always has existed in differential diagnosis of true gonorrheal arthritis and rheumatoid arthritis affecting a patient who has, or has had, an intercurrent gonorrheal infection. Hench[44] has supplied a useful description of gonorrheal arthritis and its differentiation from rheumatoid arthritis precipitated by gonorrhea. According to him:

"The characteristics of *typical* gonorrheal arthritis are as follows: The articular involvement appears acutely or subacutely, generally within one to four weeks (occasionally much later) after the onset of genital gonorrhea. In about 15 per cent of the cases, only one joint is affected; in 85 per cent of cases, two to several joints are affected. There may be: (1) a transient polyarthralgia without actual objective signs of arthritis; (2) a transient polyarthralgia, often migratory, which may soon become a stubborn monarthritis; (3) a polyarthritis; (4) a polyarthritis resolving into a monarthritis or (5) a monarthritis alone. Although several or many joints may be affected subjectively, generally fewer than four or five joints are affected objectively and the articular involvement is commonly asymmetrical. Any joint or joints may be affected; most commonly involved are knees, ankles and wrists. An associated tenosynovitis is common. Articular swelling and redness may be moderate to marked in severity. Tenderness and pain may be moderate but are often very severe.

"Common associated symptoms are fever (99 to 103° F.) and less often, chill or chilliness. Curiously, an acute respiratory infection often precedes the arthritis and in from 10 to 20 per cent of cases there is a sterile nonsuppurative catarrhal conjunctivitis. Gonococcal complement fixation tests on serum or synovial fluid are generally negative for the first two weeks of the gonorrhea but are thereafter positive in about 80 per cent of cases. Synovial fluid cultures are positive for gonococci in only about 30 per cent of cases." These remarks concerning the value of the complement fixation tests and cultures in cases of gonorrheal arthritis are in general agreement with the observations reported by Keefer and Spink.[45]

Hench has stated further: "The articular response to treatment of gonorrheal arthritis by sulfonamides, fever therapy (or penicillin) is generally marked, often dramatic, within a few days; response to salicylates is insignificant. The course of typical gonorrheal arthritis under adequate treatment is generally one of quick healing without residues and occasionally one of slow healing with minor residues. Regardless of treatment, typical gonorrheal arthritis generally 'burns out' in about three or four months. It *generally* does not last indefinitely in the joints initially affected and there is no *general* tendency for the disease later to involve progressively new joints.

"Rheumatoid arthritis precipitated by gonorrhea may (like true gonorrheal arthritis) appear within one to four weeks after the onset of acute genital gonorrhea. Its onset may be acute, subacute or insidious. However, the location of the rheumatoid arthritis precipitated by gonorrhea tends to be more symmetrical than that of gonorrheal arthritis and, in rheumatoid arthritis, the smaller joints are more commonly affected. Fever may or may not be present for a few days. Synovial fluid cultures are negative for gonococci. There is no *unequivocal* response of the joints to antigonococcal therapy. There is usually a gradual progression of the disease; new articular sites may become affected even during antigonococcal treatment and even after the genital gonorrhea is cured; in other words, a picture characteristic of slowly progressive rheumatoid arthritis may develop."

To make a diagnosis of proved gonorrheal arthritis (in contrast to a diagnosis of presumptive or probable gonorrheal arthritis) it is desirable to recover the organism from the joint fluid or, at biopsy, from the joint tissues. According to Hench,[44] gonococci are found in the synovial fluid in only about 30 per cent of cases of gonorrheal arthritis. While other procedures such as gonococcal complement fixation tests are helpful, a more reliable diagnostic procedure is the therapeutic test. In a case of suspected gonorrheal arthritis, if the response is promptly satisfactory following use of either the sulfonamides[46] or penicillin, this is suggestive evidence that the disease was gonorrheal in origin and that it was not rheumatoid arthritis, since the latter disease is unaffected either by sulfonamides or by penicillin. In chapter XIII, I have mentioned the studies reported by Boland, Headley and Hench,[47] which clearly indicated that penicillin had little or no effect on the course of typical rheumatoid arthritis.

It has been pointed out further by Hench[44] that, not infrequently, gonorrheal infection is just one more acute infection which may act as a trigger mechanism on rheumatoid arthritis. In other words, many a patient who is supposed to have gonorrheal arthritis actually does not have the disease but has typical rheumatoid arthritis precipitated by gonorrhea. I am inclined to accept Hench's opinion that many of these cases are examples either of rheumatoid arthritis precipitated by gonorrhea or of old rheumatoid arthritis which has been thrown into exacerbation or recurrence by the acute intercurrent infection (gonorrheal prostatitis). This observation by Hench and his associates is extremely important, especially in determining the "in line of duty" character of the soldier's disability which, of course, materially affects his compensation rights.

Furthermore, Hench[44] has pointed out that a curious viewpoint has been adopted by many as to why penicillin may not be effective in treatment of gonorrheal arthritis. One of the views is based on the fact that penicillin does not diffuse well into synovial fluid. As a matter of fact, penicillin does diffuse fairly well into this fluid (p. 77). Regardless of this fact, however, gonorrheal arthritis is not a disease of the *cavity* of the joint filled with synovial fluid but is a disease of the synovial and periarticular tissues. These tissues are highly vascular and there is no reason why penicillin circulating in these blood vessels should not reach the infected parts. Hench has stated his belief that "when a case of supposed gonorrheal arthritis does not respond promptly and notably to penicillin, one of the following conditions exists: 1. The case is one of gonorrheal arthritis in which the gonococcus is resistant to penicillin; in such a case, penicillin affects neither the arthritis nor the urethritis." I am inclined to believe that this is a rare occurrence. Hench continued: "2. The case is one of gonorrheal arthritis treated so late or so inadequately that irreparable articular damage has already occurred; although in such cases penicillin will probably arrest the articular infection and stop its further progress, there will remain residual symptoms resulting from the articular damage. 3. The case is not, and never was, gonorrheal arthritis but is one either of: (a) rheumatoid arthritis precipitated by gonorrhea or (b) rheumatoid arthritis, old or new, coincident in a patient with old or new gonorrhea, or (c) some other form of nongonorrheal arthritis (e.g., gouty arthritis, rheumatic fever, and so forth) in a patient who also happens to have gonorrhea."

One of the first reports on the effectiveness of penicillin in treatment of gonorrheal arthritis was that of Linner.[11] The arthritis had resisted intensive treatment with sulfonamides and with induced fever. In addition to the arthritis involving the knee, there was the usual complication of suppurative gonococcal myositis, which was drained surgically. Considerable improvement in the knee joint followed intravenous administration of penicillin. Pain and temperature subsided and motion returned, although some slight swelling persisted. Improvement lasted for a week and then an exacerbation occurred. Aspiration of the knee joint still revealed the presence of viable gonococci. Following aspiration, the patient received three intra-articular injections, each of 8,700 Oxford units of penicillin in 15 c.c. of sterile physiologic saline solution. The patient was cured.

Simultaneously, Robinson[10] reported successful treatment in a case of gonorrheal arthritis following intramuscular administration of 200,000 Oxford units of penicillin. The substance was given in amounts of 15,000 Oxford units every three hours. Two patients failed to respond but the failures were due to what are now considered obviously inadequate amounts of penicillin. Robinson did not utilize the intra-articular method of administration of penicillin in combination with the systemic method. Dawson and Hobby[16] likewise successfully treated gonorrheal arthritis with penicillin. In one instance, severe gonorrheal arthritis of the wrist was treated by intramuscular administration of 5,000 Oxford units of penicillin every three hours for six days. Recovery was complete and a normally functioning joint resulted. In another case reported by these same investigators, the arthritis involved the knee joint. In this instance, intra-articular instillations of penicillin were used. Ten thousand units were instilled into the joint cavity daily for three days. The result was striking and the patient was dismissed on the fifth day with a normally functioning joint. In reporting the experiences of Spink, Watson[48] stated that the former had obtained striking results in treatment of gonorrheal arthritis with penicillin.

The experience of my colleagues and me[8] in this field is in agreement with the reports just mentioned. That gonorrheal arthritis can be treated successfully solely by systemic administration of penicillin in some instances was evident from one of the cases which we reported. In this instance, severe gonorrheal arthritis involved the interphalangeal joint of the thumb. There was roentgenologic evidence of a destructive lesion involving the bone and a sinus was present from which Neisseria gonorrhoeae could be cultured (figs. 31a and b and 32a and b).

Two additional cases in which penicillin was successfully used in treatment of gonorrheal arthritis were reported by Anderson.[49] The first case was that of a patient who gave a positive urethral culture for Neisseria gonorrhoeae and who was suffering with an acutely inflamed knee. Cultures of the joint fluid, however, were sterile. The patient received 5,000 Oxford units of penicillin intravenously every four hours for seventy-two hours. Recovery from the urethritis as well as from the

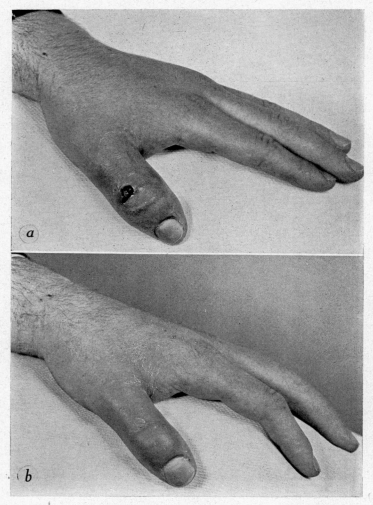

Fig. 31.—*a*, Draining sinus of thumb associated with osteomyelitis of the interphalangeal joint; cultures positive for Neisseria gonorrhoeae; *b*, appearance of thumb after penicillin therapy; sinus completely healed; no limitation of motion of joint. (From Herrell, Nichols and Heilman, Journal of the American Medical Association, August 12, 1944.)

arthritis was complete. In the second case of gonorrheal arthritis reported by Anderson, cultures of the joint fluid revealed the presence of Neisseria gonorrhoeae. Only temporary improvement in the arthritis occurred following intramuscular administration of 160,000 Oxford units of penicillin given over a period of two and a half days. One week later, cultures of joint fluid again were positive and symptoms recurred. The patient then received 10,000 Oxford units of penicillin directly into the joint on three successive days without systemic therapy. The patient made complete recovery.

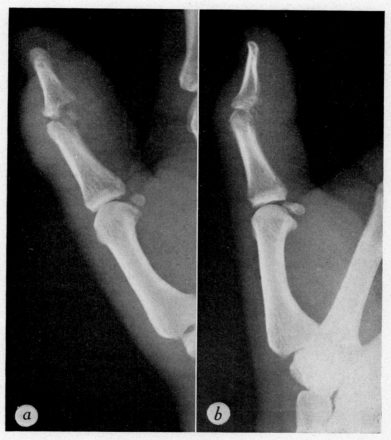

Fig. 32.—Roentgenograms of thumb represented in figure 31. *a*, Before and *b*, after penicillin therapy.

These results following systemic use of penicillin are not surprising in view of the fact that penicillin reaches the joint spaces following its administration. On the other hand, it is evident that in certain cases of gonorrheal arthritis involving large joints, it is probably advisable to combine daily intra-articular instillation of the material with systemic therapy.

Suchet[50] has reported good results of treatment in an unusual case of chronic gonorrheal arthritis following systemic administration of penicillin. The patient was a man, forty-one years of age, who had had gonorrhea in 1923 and again in 1940. Six weeks after the infection in 1940, acute arthritis of the elbow developed and subsequently multiple joints were said to be affected. The patient suffered with arthritis for three and a half years and received intensive sulfonamide therapy. On admission to hospital in May, 1943, gonococci were present in the smears made of the urethral discharge. The gonococcal complement fixation test was strongly positive. Sulfonamide therapy and protein shock treatment resulted in improvement but the arthritis reappeared. At this time, gonococci were not found in the prostatic secretion but staphylococci, which are sensitive to the action of penicillin, were found. One day following commencement of systemic treatment with penicillin, pain in the affected joints was greatly diminished. Improvement continued and the patient was dismissed three weeks after treatment with penicillin had been begun. At the time the report was made, the patient had been observed for nine months after dismissal and had remained perfectly well.

Plan of Treatment.—Although a total dose of 100,000 to 150,000 Oxford units of penicillin, given in about thirty hours, is usually satisfactory in treatment of uncomplicated gonorrhea, it is thought advisable to treat gonorrheal arthritis complicating gonorrheal urethritis a little longer and a little more intensively. Eighty thousand to 100,000 Oxford units of penicillin should be administered each day intramuscularly or intravenously. Administration should be continued in the presence of gonorrheal arthritis until there is evidence of clinical improvement and, if culture of joint fluid has given positive results, until negative cultures are obtained. In treatment of gonorrheal arthritis of small joints, it may not be necessary to combine intra-articular instillation with systemic therapy. If, on the other hand, the initial response in these cases is not satisfactory following use of systemic therapy, aspiration should be performed if possible and this should be followed by intra-articular instillation of 10,000 to 20,000 Oxford units of penicillin dissolved in 10 c.c. of physiologic saline solution. The instillations should be carried out every twenty-four to forty-eight hours for at least three or more doses.

GONOCOCCAL ENDOCARDITIS AND MENINGITIS

Until the time of preparation of this monograph, reports on treatment of gonococcal endocarditis with penicillin had not appeared. If this condition is to be treated successfully with penicillin, I am inclined to recommend that at least 200,000 to 300,000 Oxford units be administered daily by the intravenous drip method and that treatment be continued for at least twenty days. Whether or not patients with this condition can be benefited permanently cannot be stated at the moment. At least, however, attempts should be made to treat them.

The diagnosis of gonococcal meningitis is rarely made. In presence of this disease, however, it is recommended that treatment be fairly intensive and that at least 100,000 Oxford units per day be administered by the intravenous drip method or by the intermittent intramuscular method. In addition, penicillin should be administered by the intrathecal route in amounts of 10,000 to 20,000 Oxford units every twenty-four to forty-eight hours until improvement occurs.

COMMENT

Only time will tell whether or not the intelligent and intensive use of penicillin will result in more nearly complete control of gonorrhea as it affects the armed forces and the civilian population. Certainly, it is one disease in which penicillin has more than justified the enthusiasm attending its introduction.

REFERENCES

1. Fleming, Alexander: On the antibacterial action of cultures of a penicillium, with special reference to their use in the isolation of B. influenzae. Brit. J. Exper. Path. *10:* 226–236 (June) 1929.

2. Abraham, E. P., Chain, E., Fletcher, C. M., Gardner, A. D., Heatley, N. G., Jennings, M. A. and Florey, H. W.: Further observations on penicillin. Lancet, *2:*177–188; 189 (Aug. 16) 1941.

3. Herrell, W. E., Cook, E. N. and Thompson, Luther: Use of penicillin in sulfonamide resistant gonorrheal infections. J. A. M. A. *122:*289–292 (May 29) 1943.

4. Miller, C. P., Scott, W. W. and Moeller, Velma: Studies on the action of penicillin. I. The rapidity of its therapeutic effect on gonococcic urethritis. J. A. M. A. *125:*607–610 (July 1) 1944.

5. Mahoney, J. F., Ferguson, Charles, Buchholtz, M. and Van Slyke, C. J.: The use of penicillin sodium in the treatment of sulfonamide-resistant gonorrhea in men; a preliminary report. Am. J. Syph., Gonor. & Ven. Dis. *27:*525–528 (Sept.) 1943.

6. Cook, E. N., Pool, T. L. and Herrell, W. E.: Further observations on penicillin in sulfonamide resistant gonorrhea. Proc. Staff Meet., Mayo Clin. *18:*433–437 (Nov. 17) 1943.

7. Herrell, W. E. and Nichols, D. R.: The calcium salt of penicillin. Proc. Staff Meet., Mayo Clin. *18:*313–319 (Sept. 8) 1943; Discussion. J. A. M. A. *124:*798 (Mar. 18) 1944.

8. Herrell, W. E., Nichols, D. R. and Heilman, Dorothy H.: Penicillin; its usefulness, limitations, diffusion and detection, with analysis of 150 cases in which it was employed. J. A. M. A. *125:*1003–1010 (Aug. 12) 1944.

9. Dill, W. W.: County society reports; Montgomery. Pennsylvania M .J. *47:*63–64 (Oct.) 1943.

10. Robinson, J. N.: Discussion on penicillin. Brit. M. J. *2:*655 (Nov. 20) 1943.

11. Linner, J. H.: Suppurative myositis and purulent arthritis complicating acute gonorrhea; report of a case. J. A. M. A. *123:*757–759 (Nov. 20) 1943.

12. Florey, H. W. and Cairns, Hugh: Penicillin in war wounds; a report from the Mediterranean. Lancet. *2:*742–745 (Dec. 11) 1943. (Abstr.) The treatment of war wounds with penicillin. Brit. M. J. *2:*755 (Dec. 11) 1943.

13. Hollenberg, H. G.: Letter. J. Arkansas M. Soc. 40:134 (Dec.) 1943.

14. Van Slyke, C. J., Arnold, R. C. and Buchholtz, M.: Penicillin therapy in sulfon-amide-resistant gonorrhea in men. Am. J. Pub. Health. 33:1392–1394 (Dec.) 1943.

15. Staff Surgical Conference, U. S. Naval Hospital, San Diego, California: Summary of experience with penicillin on a surgical service. U. S. Nav. M. Bull. 42:85–86 (Jan.) 1944.

16. Dawson, M. H. and Hobby, Gladys L.: The clinical use of penicillin; observations in one hundred cases. J. A. M. A. 124:611–622 (Mar. 4) 1944.

17. Barr, J. S.: The use of penicillin in the navy. J. Bone & Joint Surg. 26:380–386 (Apr.) 1944.

18. Ferguson, Charles and Buchholtz, Maurice: Penicillin therapy of gonorrhea in men. J. A. M. A. 125:22–23 (May 6) 1944.

19. Denny, E. R., Shallenberger, P. L. and Pyle, H. D.: Clinical observations in the use of penicillin. J. Oklahoma M. A. 37:193–205 (May) 1944.

20. Schwartz, W. H. and Edge, C. O.: Results of penicillin treatment of sulfonamide-resistant gonorrhea; summary of 4,439 cases treated in United States Naval Ho pital July 1943–March 1944. U. S. Nav. M. Bull. 43:193–195 (July) 1944.

21. Atcheson, D. W.: A new source of penicillin in the treatment of chronic gonorrhea. Mil. Surgeon. 95:58–62 (July) 1944.

22. Page, S. G., Jr. and Heimoff, L. L.: One day treatment of sulfonamide-resistant acute gonorrhea with penicillin—a preliminary report. Virginia M. Monthly. 71:423–424 (Aug.) 1944.

23. Sternberg, T. H. and Turner, T. B.: The treatment of sulfonamide resistant gon-orrhea with penicillin sodium: results in 1,686 cases. J. A. M. A. 126:157–160 (Sept. 16) 1944.

24. Frisch, A. W., Behr, Beatrice, Edwards, R. B. and Edwards, M. W.: The suscep-tibility of sulfonamide-resistant gonococci to penicillin. Am. J. Syph., Gonor. & Ven. Dis. 28:627–633 (Sept.) 1944.

25. Riba, L. W., Schmidlapp, C. J. and Bosworth, N. L.: Use of penicillin for gonor-rhea resistant to sulfonamide compounds; report of four hundred and fifty cases. War Med. 6:72–79 (Aug.) 1944.

26. Menville, J. G. and Ross, C. W.: Penicillin in sulfonamide-resistant gonorrhea; pre-liminary report of 154 csases. U. S. Nav. M. Bull. 43:423–428 (Sept.) 1944.

27. Murphy, R. J.: Experimental use of penicillin in treatment of sulfonamide-resistant gonorrhea. Bull. U. S. Army M. Dept. 79:101–105 (Aug.) 1944.

28. Van Slyke, C. J. and Steinberg, S.: Outpatient penicillin treatment of gonococcic infections in males. Ven. Dis. Inform. 25:229–232 (Aug.) 1944.

29. Thompson, G. J.: The clinical use of penicillin in genitourinary infections. J. A. M. A. 126:403–407 (Oct. 14) 1944.

30. Scarcello, N. S.: Penicillin in sulfonamide-resistant gonorrhea; a review of 200 cases. New England J. Med. 231:609–612 (Nov. 2) 1944.

31. Robinson, J. N.: Penicillin therapy in gonorrhoea; a report of 1 000 cases of sul-phonamide-resistant gonorrhoea and 100 cases of acute gonorrhoeae previously untreated. Brit. J. Surg. 32:211–214 (July Suppl.) 1944.

32. Romansky, M. J. and Rittman, G. E.: A method of prolonging the action of pen-icillin. Science. n.s. 100:196–198 (Sept. 1) 1944.

33. Cohn, Alfred, Studdiford, W. E. and Grunstein, Isaak: Penicillin treatment of sulfonamide resistant gonococcic infections in female patients; preliminary report. J. A. M. A. 124:1124–1125 (Apr. 15) 1944.

34. Greenblatt, R. B. and Street, Anita R.: Penicillin for the treatment of chemo-resistant gonorrhea in the female. J. A. M. A. 126:161–163 (Sept. 16) 1944.

35. Strauss, Hyman: Cure by penicillin following repeatedly unsuccessful sulfonamide therapy in a pregnant woman with gonorrhea. Am. J. Obst. & Gynec. *47:*271–272 (Feb.) 1944.

36. Wollgast, C. F.: The clinical use of penicillin, a report of 115 cases treated in an army hospital. Texas State J. Med. *40:*225–230 (Aug.) 1944.

37. Sandes, G. M.: Vulvovaginitis in children. Brit. M. J. *1:*160–161 (Jan. 29) 1944.

38. Florey, M. E. and Florey, H. W.: General and local administration of penicillin. Lancet. *1:*387–397 (Mar. 27) 1943.

39. Sorsby, Arnold: Ophthalmia neonatorum. Brit. M. J. *2:*723 (Dec. 4) 1943.

40. Sievers, J. J., Knott, L. W. and Soloway, H. M.: Penicillin in the treatment of ophthalmia neonatorum. J. A. M. A. *125:*690–692 (July 8) 1944.

41. Keyes, J. E. L.: Recent advances in clinical ophthalmology. Ohio State M. J. *39:* 1110–1112 (Dec.) 1943.

42. Griffey, W. P.: Penicillin in the treatment of gonorrheal conjunctivitis, report of a case. Arch. Ophth. *31:*162 (Feb.) 1944.

43. Christie, R. V. and Garrod, L. P.: A review of the work of a penicillin therapeutic research unit. Brit. M. J. *1:*513–514 (Apr. 15) 1944.

44. Hench, P. S.: Personal communication to the author.

45. Keefer, C. S. and Spink, W. W.: Gonococcic arthritis: pathogenesis, mechanism of recovery and treatment; clinical lecture at Atlantic City session. J. A. M. A. *109:*1448–1453 (Oct. 30) 1937.

46. Coggeshall, H. C. and Bauer, Walter: Treatment of gonorrheal and rheumatoid arthritis with sulfanilamide. New England J. Med. *220:*85–103 (Jan. 19) 1939.

47. Boland, E. W., Headley, N. E. and Hench, P. S.: The effect of penicillin on rheumatoid arthritis. J. A. M. A. *126:*820–823 (Nov. 25) 1944.

48. Watson, C. J.: Discussion. J. A. M. A. *124:*798–799 (Mar. 18) 1944.

49. Anderson, D. G.: Penicillin. Bull. New England M. Center. *6:*145–152 (Aug.) 1944.

50. Suchet, J.: Chronic gonococcal arthritis treated with penicillin. Proc. Roy. Soc. Med. *37:*498 (July) 1944.

8

CHAPTER XVII

SYPHILIS AND OTHER SPIROCHETAL INFECTIONS

GENERAL CONSIDERATION

One of the most fascinating phases of the studies which have been carried out on the possible uses of penicillin was the discovery by Mahoney, Arnold and Harris,[1] of the Venereal Disease Research Laboratory, United States Marine Hospital, Staten Island, that penicillin appeared to possess some spirocheticidal activity. Following preliminary experimental studies, Mahoney and his colleagues examined the effectiveness of penicillin in treatment of four patients with acute, recently acquired syphilis. The course of the disease was followed by means of frequent darkfield examinations and subsequently by extremely carefully conducted serologic tests. Mahoney administered penicillin intramuscularly in amounts of 25,000 Oxford units every four hours day and night for eight days. The total course, therefore, consisted in the use of 1,200,000 units, which were administered in forty-eight intramuscular injections. The spirochetes disappeared from the local lesions within sixteen hours. At the time the report by Mahoney and his colleagues was made, serodiagnostic tests had been carried out for periods varying from eighty-six to 101 days after penicillin therapy had been begun. The results indicated that the reacting substance had disappeared from the blood stream more or less rapidly and completely. This was especially true in cases of early syphilis. The results of the tests carried out by Mahoney and his colleagues are shown in table 20.

EARLY SYPHILIS

Mahoney and his group have continued their studies in a large series of cases and results have continued to be encouraging, especially in treatment of early syphilis. These investigators rightly have conjectured that if prolonged experience confirmed impressions gained from the preliminary study, rebuilding of the structure of therapy for syphilis might well be necessary. Subsequent to their report, the problem of penicillin in the treatment of syphilis was undertaken by the Subcommittee on Venereal Diseases of the National Research Council. Sufficient data have been accumulated to justify certain conclusions.

It appeared from the report of Bloomfield, Rantz and Kirby[2] that penicillin was effective in treatment of early syphilis. Seven cases of early

TABLE 20
RESULTS OF SEROLOGIC REACTIONS
CASE 1—L. W. HOSPITAL NO. 116769. DURATION OF DISEASE—9 DAYS

Days after start of therapy	Qualitative methods							Quantitative methods		
	Kline excl. ppt.	Mazzini floc.	Kline diag. ppt.	Kahn std. ppt.	Hinton floc.	Eagle floc.	Kolmer simp. c. f.	Mazzini floc.	Kahn ppt.	Kolmer comp. fix.
0		4		4	Pos.	Pos.	4	4 4 4 2 1 —	4 4 4 2 ±—	4 4 4 4 1
1		4		4	Pos.	Pos.	4	4 4 4 2 1 —	4 4 4 2 ±—	4 4 4 4 3
9	4	4	4		Pos.	Pos.	4	4 4 4 4 2 —	4 4 4 4 1 —	4 4 4 4 2 —
23	4	4	3	3	Pos.	Pos.	4	4 3 2 — — —	4 4 1 — — —	4 4 4 4 2 —
30	4	4	3	3	Pos.	—	4	4 4 4 2 — —	4 4 3 1 — —	4 4 4 3 ±—
37	4	4	1 Dbt.	3	Dbt.	—	3	4 4 2 1 — —	4 1 — — — —	4 4 4 2 ±—
44	3	4	—	1 Dbt.	—	—	4	4 4 2 1 — —	4 1 — — — —	3 3 2 — —
51	1 Dbt.	4	—	—	—	—	4	4 3 2 — — —	4 ± — — — —	4 4 3 ±—
58	1 Dbt.	4	—	—	—	—	4	4 2 — — — —	1 — — — — —	4 4 4 1 ±—
65	2	2 Dbt.	—	—	—	—	—	4 3 — — — —	1 — — — — —	
72	1 Dbt.	2 Dbt.	—	—	—	—	—	2 1 — — — —	— — — — — —	
80	—	2 Dbt.	—	—	QNS	—	—	2 1 — — — —	— — — — — —	
86	—	2 Dbt.	—	—		—	—	2 ±— — —	±— — — — —	
93	—	1 Dbt.	—	—	—	—	—	2 —	— —	
101	±Dbt.	1 Dbt.	—	—	—	—	—	1 —		

CASE 2—E. D. HOSPITAL NO. 117096. DURATION OF DISEASE—10 DAYS

Days after start of therapy	Kline excl. ppt.	Mazzini floc.	Kline diag. ppt.	Kahn std. ppt.	Hinton floc.	Eagle floc.	Kolmer simp. c. f.	Mazzini floc.	Kahn ppt.	Kolmer comp. fix.
0	3	3	±Dbt.	3	Pos.	Pos.	4	2 1 — — —	4 2 — — —	4 4 3 1 ±—
1	4	4	±Dbt.	3	Pos.	Pos.	4	2 1 — — —	4 1 — — —	4 4 4 3 — —
9		4		3	Pos.	Pos.	4	4 2 — — —	4 2 — — —	4 4 3 ±— —
23	1 Dbt.	2 Dbt.	—	2	—	—	4	2 1 — — —	4 ± — — —	4 3 1 — —
30	1 Dbt.	1 Dbt.	—	±Dbt.	—	—	1	1 — — — —	2 — — — —	1 2 ±— —
37	—	1 Dbt.	—	—	—	—	±Dbt.	1 — — — —	1 — — — —	±± — — —
44	—	—	—	—	QNS	—	4	— — — — —	— — — — —	4 3 2 1 ±—
51	—	1 Dbt.	—	—	—	—	—	1 — — — —	— — — — —	— — — — —
58	—	—	—	—	—	—	—	— — — — —	— — — — —	— — — — —
65	—	—	—	—	—	—	—	— — — — —	— — — — —	— — — — —
72	—	—	—	—	—	—	—	— — — — —	— — — — —	— — — — —
79	—	—	—	—	—	—	—	— — — — —	— — — — —	— — — — —
94	—	—	—	—	—	—	—	— — — — —	— — — — —	— — — — —

CASE 3—H. J. HOSPITAL NO. 117136. DURATION OF DISEASE—8 DAYS

Days after start of therapy	Kline excl. ppt.	Mazzini floc.	Kline diag. ppt.	Kahn std. ppt.	Hinton floc.	Eagle floc.	Kolmer simp. c. f.	Mazzini floc.	Kahn ppt.	Kolmer comp. fix.
0	4	4	2	4	Pos.	Pos.	4	4 3 2 1 — —	4 4 4 4 2 —	4 4 4 4 3 1
1	3	4	2	4	Pos.	Pos.	4	4 4 2 1 1 —	4 4 4 4 2 —	4 4 4 4 4 31
8		4		4	Pos.	Pos.	4	4 4 3 1 1 —	4 4 4 3 2 ±	4 4 4 4 1 ±
15		4		3	Pos.	Pos.	4	3 3 2 1 1 —	4 4 4 2 ±—	4 4 4 4 4 2
22	3	3	1 Dbt.	2	Pos.	—	4	2 1 1 1 — —	4 3 1 1 — —	4 4 4 4 4 ±
29	1 Dbt.	1 Dbt.	—	2	Dbt.	—	4	1 1 1 — — —	2 ±± — — —	4 4 4 4 —
36	—	1 Dbt.	—	—	—	—	4	1 1 1 — — —	2 — — — — —	4 4 4 4 —
43	—	—	—	—	—	—	2	— — — — — —	±— — — — —	2 1 2 ±— —
50	—	—	—	—	—	—	4	— — — — — —	— — — — — —	4 4 4 3 1 —
57	—	1 Dbt.	—	—	—	—	—	1 — — — — —	— — — — — —	— ±1 ±— —
64	—	—	—	—	—	—	—	— — — — — —	±— — — — —	— ±1 — — —
71	±Dbt.	1 Dbt.	—	—	—	—	—	1 — — — —	— — — — —	— — — — —
78	—	—	—	—	—	—	—	— — — — —	— — — — —	— — — — —
85	—	1 Dbt.	—	—	—	—	—	1 — — — —	— — — — —	— — — — —
93	—	—	—	—	—	—	—	1 —	— — — — —	— — — — —

CASE 4—S. I. HOSPITAL NO. 117491. DURATION OF DISEASE—8 DAYS

Days after start of therapy	Kline excl. ppt.	Mazzini floc.	Kline diag. ppt.	Kahn std. ppt.	Hinton floc.	Eagle floc.	Kolmer simp. c. f.	Mazzini floc.	Kahn ppt.	Kolmer comp. fix.
0		1 Dbt.			—			2 1 — — —	3 — — — —	— ±± ±— —
1	4	4	±Dbt.	1 Dbt.	—	Pos.		3 2 — — —	4 4 ±— — —	±± ±— — —
8	4	4		3	—	Pos.	4	3 2 — — —	3 — — — —	— — — — —
15	4	4	1 Dbt.	3	Pos.	Pos.	±Dbt.	4 3 2 1 — —	4 3 1 — — —	4 4 4 2 ±—,
22	4	3	±Dbt.	3	Pos.	Dbt.	±Dbt.	3 1 — — —	4 1 ±— — —	±± ±± — —,
30	1 Dbt.	2 Dbt.	±Dbt.	—	Dbt.	—	±Dbt.	2 1 — — —	1 — — — —	±1 ± — —
36	±Dbt.	2 Dbt.	—	—	—	—	±Dbt.	2 — — — —	1 — — — —	±±1 ± — —
43	—	2 Dbt.	—	—	—	—	—	2 —	— — — —	— — ±± ± —
50	±Dbt.	1 Dbt.	—	—	—	—	—	2 1 — — —	±— — — —	— — — — —
57	—	1 Dbt.	—	—	—	—	—	1 — — — —	— — — — —	— — — — —
64	±Dbt.	1 Dbt.	—	—	—	—	—	1 — — — —	±— — — —	— — ++ — —
71	—	—	—	—	—	—	—	— —	— — — —	— — — — —
86	—	—	—	—	—	—	—	— —	— — — —	— — — — —

From article by Mahoney, Arnold and Harris, Venereal Disease Information, December, 1943.

syphilis were reported by this group of investigators. Some were sero-negative and some were seropositive. A typical case of early seronegative, but darkfield positive, syphilis reported by them is essentially as follows: The patient had noticed a penile lesion fourteen days before he entered the hospital. Two days before his entrance, lymph nodes in the groin had swollen. On examination, he had a typical chancre, 1.2 cm. in diameter, and enlarged inguinal lymph nodes. The Wassermann reaction was negative. On darkfield examination, huge numbers of typical, actively motile spirochetes were seen. The patient received 200,000 Oxford units of penicillin per day by the intravenous drip method for five days—a total dose of 1,000,000 units. Twelve hours after treatment had been begun, only a rare spirochete was seen. At the end of fourteen hours, none were found. This disappearance of spirochetes at the end of fourteen hours was in agreement with the previously reported experience of Mahoney and his colleagues. According to Bloomfield and his colleagues, the chancre underwent rapid involution and the enlargement of the lymph nodes disappeared in ten days.

The next report on the general subject was that by Wise and Pillsbury,[3] who treated with penicillin fifteen patients suffering with early syphilis. Three were examples of seronegative primary syphilis and eight were examples of seropositive primary syphilis; four were examples of so-called secondary syphilis. In thirteen of the fifteen cases, Treponema pallidum could be demonstrated in material from the lesions. In all of these cases the spirochetes disappeared within the first day of treatment. According to the investigators, all types of lesions, including secondarily infected chancres, maculopapular rash and condylomas, healed more quickly than is usual following use of mapharsen. Healing apparently occurred within three to seven days. During the first week of treatment of patients with early syphilis, it appeared that administration of penicillin had the effect in some instances of increasing the serologic titer of the blood as measured by the quantitative Kahn reaction. Later, the serologic test gradually became negative, an observation which was in accord with that of Mahoney and his colleagues.

It was pointed out by Wise and Pillsbury that in two of the fifteen cases a brisk Herxheimer reaction occurred within eight to twelve hours after the initial injection of penicillin. Accompanying this reaction were fever and accentuation of the presenting lesions. In one case in which this accentuation occurred, the patient had a maculopapular eruption and, in the other, a chancre of the lip. These reactions, however, did not interfere with continuation of penicillin therapy.

More comprehensive reports on the use of penicillin in treatment of early syphilis were made subsequently. In a report by Mahoney and his colleagues,[4] follow-up data were presented on the four patients whom they originally had treated. Three of this original group of patients had remained clinically and serologically negative for nearly a year. One patient was considered to be an example of failure of treatment, although the possibility of reinfection was likely. This report also included a series of approximately 100 cases in which treatment was essentially the same as that recommended in the original report by Mahoney and his associates. Patients received no antisyphilitic medication other than penicillin. Treatment consisted of 20,000 Oxford units of penicillin administered intramuscularly every three hours day and night for sixty injections, or a total dose of 1,200,000 Oxford units. It was of some interest that reactions resembling Herxheimer reactions, or therapeutic shock, of varying degrees were observed during the first day of treatment of eighty-six patients. The gratifying feature of this treatment was the lack of any severe toxic reactions, although dermatitis appeared in two instances. Included in this report by Mahoney and others were cases of early darkfield positive but seronegative, and early darkfield positive and seropositive, syphilis, as well as cases of secondary syphilis affecting patients who had been well into the seropositive phase of the disease at the time treatment had been begun. Of the seropositive patients, many gradually progressed, as the investigators put it, to seronegativity following completion of treatment with penicillin. Mahoney and his colleagues have elected to emphasize the fact that syphilis is a disease of chronicity and that any treatment will require a prolonged period of observation before results can be finally evaluated. At all events, it seems well established that penicillin has won a place in the treatment of early syphilis.

Simultaneously with the report by Mahoney and his colleagues, just referred to, there appeared the report of the Penicillin Panel of the Subcommittee on Venereal Diseases of the National Research Council,[5] in which additional information was given on the treatment of early syphilis with penicillin. This report was based on data collected in treatment of 1,418 patients who had early syphilis. Included in this large group of cases were instances of primary syphilis, acute syphilitic meningitis, arsenical resistant early syphilis and infantile congenital syphilis. The results obtained in these cases were, to say the least, encouraging. It is also of interest that of the 1,418 patients treated, 846 (59 per cent) had reactions resembling Herxheimer reactions within the first twenty-four hours of the beginning of treatment. These reactions consisted of fever alone or of exacerbation of the local lesions with or without fever. As in the experience of Wise and Pillsbury,[3] of Bloomfield, Rantz and Kirby[2] and of Mahoney and others,[4] this reaction was never alarming nor did it interfere with continuation of penicillin therapy. Of the patients treated, 4.1 per cent had other mild reactions, such as urticaria, skin rashes or fever. These reactions were considered to be associated with administration of penicillin and not to be a part of the Herxheimer type of reaction.

It would appear from these results that at least 1,200,000 Oxford units of penicillin should be used in treatment of early syphilis. The report by Moore and others[5] contains the statement that relapses appeared to be more frequent after intravenous than after intramuscular administration of penicillin. I am inclined to believe that this was more a coincidence than a fact which could be explained on the basis of the difference in the two methods of administration. If the statement is otherwise significant, it is a most unusual phenomenon in connection with chemotherapy in general. The fact remains, as was pointed out by my colleagues and me,[6] and by White and his associates,[7] that in general nearly twice as much penicillin is required to obtain the same therapeutic effect when the intramuscular method is employed as when the intravenous drip method is used.

O'Leary[8] and his associates at times have used the intravenous drip method for administration of penicillin in treatment of acute syphilis. The course of the infection in darkfield positive cases was followed by repeated darkfield examinations. Spirochetes began to disappear from the local lesions in some instances as early as eight hours, and usually were absent at the end of eighteen hours, following the start of treatment. The question of the method of administration is purely a matter of selecting that method which is most suitable to the individual investigator.

It must be remembered that disappearance of the spirochete from the local lesion does not necessarily mean that the organisms have been completely eradicated from the body. As a matter of fact, it would be surprising if penicillin were found to be spirocheticidal to this degree. Furthermore, all are agreed that long periods of observation are essential to evaluation of the role of penicillin in treatment of early syphilis. Delayed recurrences unquestionably will be encountered, as they have been with other antisyphilitic agents. On the other hand, lack of significant toxic reactions associated with the use of penicillin is a tremendous advantage over the other agents previously available.

Plan of Treatment.—In treatment of early syphilis, penicillin can be administered either by the intermittent intramuscular method or by the continuous intravenous drip method. For the intramuscular method, it would appear that 20,000 Oxford units dissolved in 3 or 4 c.c. of physiologic saline solution should be administered every three hours day and night until 1,200,000 to 1,500,000 units have been administered. Repeated courses may be indicated in some cases.

When the intravenous drip method is employed, the procedure recommended is to administer 100,000 to 150,000 Oxford units per day until the same total dose has been given as that which is employed in the intramuscular method.

LATE SYPHILIS

The use of penicillin for treatment of late syphilis has been investigated in a number of clinics. The data have been reported by Stokes and others.[9] The report (table 21) was based on the use of penicillin for treatment in 182 cases of late and miscellaneous syphilis, including neuro-

TABLE 21

PENICILLIN INVESTIGATION: LATE AND MISCELLANEOUS SYPHILIS;
DISTRIBUTION OF MATERIAL BY SOURCE, DURATION
OF OBSERVATION AND DIAGNOSIS

Diagnosis	Immediate: Less than 20 days	Duration of observation				Total Cases
		20–59 Days	60–99 Days	100–139 Days	140–214 Days	
Paresis and taboparesis...	11	22	15	4	4	56
Tabes, including primary optic atrophy........	6	8	5	2	1	22
Meningovascular neurosyphilis..............	6	3	3	3	1	16
Asymptomatic neurosyphilis..................	2	13	8	1	4	28
Benign late skin and bone.	4	8	3	0	6	21
Interstitial keratitis......	0	5	3	3	2	13
Iritis..................	0	2	1	0	1	4
Miscellaneous	4	6	5	6	1	22
Total.............	....	....	....	....	....	182
Clinic sources						
Bellevue..............	1	3	1	0	0	5
Boston...............	8	8	0	0	0	16
Johns Hopkins........	9	23	10	2	8	52
Mayo...............	7	3	6	1	4	21
Michigan.............	6	2	1	0	0	9
New York Hospital....	1	10	5	0	0	16
Pennsylvania.........	1	18	20	16	8	63
Totals.............	33	67	43	19	20	182

From article by Stokes, Sternberg, Schwartz, Mahoney, Moore, and Wood, Journal of the American Medical Association, September 9, 1944.

syphilis, late syphilis of skin and bone, syphilis involving the eye, and a small group of cases such as visceral syphilis (combined involvement of bone and liver and of liver and spleen for instance).

Neurosyphilis.—Of the 182 cases reported by Stokes and others, 122 were examples of neurosyphilis. The patients had been observed from eight to 214 days after administration of penicillin had been begun. The characteristics of the spinal fluid improved to some degree in 74 per cent of the cases and the improvement was considered definite in at least a third of all the cases. A drop in cell count and in total protein content of the spinal fluid was one of the commonest changes noted and was said to have occurred in 67 per cent of cases. The characteristics of the spinal fluid were said to have improved in 25 per cent of cases of asymptomatic neurosyphilis and in 10 per cent of cases of paresis and taboparesis. Symptomatically, it appeared that 80 per cent of the patients with simple paresis and dementia improved to some degree following the use of penicillin. On the other hand, only one of thirty patients could be considered to have been restored to normal. This, in my opinion, is not a very impressive record. Among patients with paresis and deterioration only two of ten improved as much as 75 per cent; one improved 50 per cent and seven remained unchanged. Of fourteen patients with tabes dorsalis, it appeared that 50 per cent improvement occurred in only a few. Of seven patients suffering with lightning pains, two were completely relieved; one was improved 50 per cent; two were improved 25 per cent; the condition of one was unchanged and one appeared to be made worse. Of patients with meningovascular neurosyphilis, it appeared that the condition of somewhat less than half was improved.

In the chapter on diffusion and distribution of penicillin in the body, it was pointed out that little if any penicillin reaches the structures of the central nervous system following systemic administration of even large amounts of the preparation. This is true not only of the normal subject but also of the patient who is suffering with neurosyphilis. It was obvious from the beginning, therefore, that if anything was to be accomplished in treatment of neurosyphilis, probably intrathecal administration of the material should be combined with systemic therapy. Even then, it is evident that neurosyphilis presents a therapeutic problem quite unlike that presented by acute or early syphilis. In neurosyphilis, destruction of tissue already has occurred and irreparable damage may preclude successful use of an antibacterial agent such as penicillin. It might even be said that in neurosyphilis a situation obtains similar to that which occurs in chronic osteomyelitis. In the latter condition, destruction of tissue has occurred and foci are present which are not easily reached by penicillin. Under such conditions penicillin can be considered only an adjunct to other well established methods of treatment. I am inclined, therefore, to adopt a cautious attitude in evaluation of the results so far obtained in treatment of neurosyphilis. Suffice to say, the results following penicillin therapy have not been particularly exciting. From the experience of O'Leary in treatment of neurosyphilis with rather large amounts of penicillin administered by the intravenous drip or intramuscular method, at times combined with intrathecal administration, it would appear, also, that the results have not been encouraging although, in a few isolated cases of neurosyphilis, progressive reversal of serologic characteristics of the spinal fluid has occurred following intensive use of penicillin. The changes which occurred in the spinal fluid of one such patient are shown in table 22.

TABLE 22

PENICILLIN IN TREATMENT OF ONE PATIENT WITH ASYMPTOMATIC NEUROSYPHILIS*

Tests or observations	Date, 1944			
	February 4	April 5	June 15	September 9
On blood				
Titer	160	160	40	4
Kline	4+	3+	3+	4+
Kahn	3+	4+	2+	4+
Hinton	Positive	Positive	Positive	Positive
Kolmer	44	44	44	44
On spinal fluid				
Kline	3+	Negative	—	Negative
Kahn	44443	41+	—	Negative
Gold	0112110000	0011000000	—	0011000000
Protein content,				
(mg. per 100 c.c.)	70	90	—	75
Cells per cubic millimeter	113	6	—	3
Globulin	Positive	Positive	—	Negative

*120,000 Oxford units per day by intravenous drip for ten days, beginning February 17.

Plan of Treatment.—Rather large amounts of penicillin probably will be required for treatment of neurosyphilis. Penicillin in amounts of 20,000 to 25,000 Oxford units should be administered intramuscularly every three hours, day and night, until a total dose of somewhere between 2,000,000 and 4,000,000 Oxford units has been administered. Penicillin also can be administered by the intravenous drip method in amounts of 100,000 Oxford units per day until the total dose has been administered. To avoid the possible difficulty of therapeutic shock in association with this condition, it is wise to reduce the dose of penicillin during the first twenty-four to forty-eight hours.

For intrathecal therapy, 20,000 Oxford units of penicillin should be administered following spinal drainage. The penicillin should be dissolved in 10 c.c. of physiologic saline solution and the procedure should be carried out at least every forty-eight hours during the period of systemic therapy unless untoward reactions attend the intrathecal therapy. There is no contraindication to simultaneous use of penicillin and other antisyphilitic drugs, nor is there any contraindication to use of penicillin with hyperthermia, including that attending induced malaria or use of the fever cabinet.

Gummatous Syphilis of Skin and Bone.—In view of the fact that cutaneous lesions in general, owing to organisms susceptible to the action of penicillin, have been found to respond satisfactorily to penicillin, it is not surprising that encouraging results have been obtained in treatment of gummatous lesions of the skin. Certainly, if adequate amounts of penicillin are administered, there is very good evidence to support the belief that antibacterial amounts of the substance reach the skin and subcutaneous tissues.

One of the earliest reports on the successful treatment of late cutaneous syphilis with penicillin was that by O'Leary and me.[10] The patient was suffering with a rather extensive nodular syphiloderm of the nose. The lesion had been present for eight months. The patient had had no

TABLE 23

Comparison of Serologic Tests on the Blood and Spinal Fluid Before and After Treatment

Tests or observations	1943		1944	1945
	September 15	November 2	May 1	January 2
On blood				
Kline	4+	4+	4+	4+
Kahn	4+	4+	4+	3+
Hinton	Positive	Positive	Positive	Positive
Kolmer	44	44	44	43
Units of titer	160	200	—	40
On spinal fluid				
Serologic	4442	4442	44 - -	43 - -
Nonne	Negative	Negative	Negative	Negative
Gold	5332000000	1121100000	0111000000	3210000000
Cells per cubic millimeter	31	16	3	2
Protein content (mg. per 100 c.c.)	40	35	30	30

specific treatment other than local measures, which had not brought about improvement. The patient never had been pregnant; she did not know that she had syphilis and she gave no other clinical signs of syphilis than the cutaneous lesion. Penicillin in a total dose of 320,000 Oxford units was administered by the intravenous drip method over a period of eight days. By the end of the eighth day of treatment the lesion had substantially undergone involution and four weeks after treatment had been completed the residual pigmentation was only slightly evident (fig. 33). Results of serologic tests of the blood and spinal fluid before and after treatment are represented in table 23. According to O'Leary, the lesion healed more rapidly and the healing was more nearly complete than it customarily is after use of arsenical drugs for treatment of this type of lesion. No final statements can be made on such results, however, until long periods of observation are possible. On the other hand, the results obtained in this and similar cases amply justify further exploration of the possible effectiveness of penicillin against gummatous syphilis.

Twenty-one cases of gummatous syphilis of skin and bones were included in the report by Stokes and others[9] on the use of penicillin for

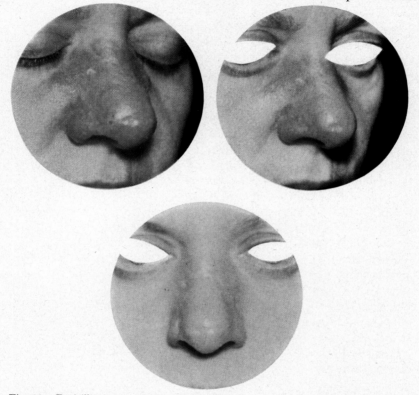

Fig. 33.—Penicillin in the treatment of gummatous syphilis. *Upper left*, before treatment; *upper right*, immediately after treatment; *below*, one month after conclusion of treatment.

treatment of late syphilis. Satisfactory response was said to have occurred almost invariably. Of twenty-one cases, it appeared that in thirteen the results could be rated as 100 per cent; in six, improvement of varying degrees occurred, and failures were experienced in only two. It was pointed out that, in addition to the effect on the primary disease, penicillin was effective in control of the secondary pyogenic infections that frequently are present in these lesions. It seems likely that these secondary infections were responsible for the formerly encountered inability of arsenical drugs to bring about healing of these lesions.

Plan of Treatment.—The total dose of penicillin required to obtain satisfactory results in treatment of gummatous lesions of skin and bone is not as high as that recommended for treatment of neurosyphilis. A total dose of 1,000,000 Oxford units usually is adequate. In fact, satisfactory results have been obtained following the use of as little as 300,000 Oxford units for the entire course of treatment. Ten thousand Oxford units may be administered in 2 c.c. of physiologic saline solution intramuscularly every three hours until the total dose has been given. If the material is to be administered by the intravenous drip method, 80,000 Oxford units per twenty-four hours should be given until the total planned dose has been administered. The clinical response usually determines the duration of treatment.

Late Congenital Syphilis, Including Ocular Lesions.—One of the most important lesions in late congenital syphilis is interstitial keratitis. According to the report of Stokes and others,[9] the complexity of the problem of interstitial keratitis and its behavior is as apparent under penicillin therapy as under other standard forms of treatment. Of fourteen cases, it appeared that varying degrees of improvement occurred in six and that in another six no improvement occurred. In two cases the condition appeared to be made definitely worse. Stokes and his colleagues pointed out that when improvement occurs it is likely to be dramatic.

Other ocular lesions which have been treated with penicillin include optic neuritis, which at times has shown improvement following administration of rather large amounts of penicillin. Included in the report by Stokes also were two cases of iritis in which improvement was striking following the use of penicillin. However, in one of these cases relapse occurred and iridectomy was necessary.

Plan of Treatment.—In treatment of this condition, probably it is wise to administer large amounts of penicillin (100,000 to 200,000 Oxford units per day) by either the intramuscular or the intravenous drip method. Treatment should be continued until at least 2,000,000 to 4,000,000 Oxford units have been given. It may be advisable to combine administration of penicillin with other standard forms of treatment.

Miscellaneous.—Stokes and others have reported on the successful use of penicillin in treatment of gangrenous balanitis. At the time of their report, information on the use of penicillin in various other conditions, including combined involvement of bone and liver and of liver and spleen, was not sufficiently full to justify final conclusions. Doubtful results were obtained following use of penicillin in two cases of eighth nerve deafness and in one instance it appeared that a Charcot joint was unaffected by the use of penicillin.

Therapeutic Shock (Herxheimer Effects).—It should be emphasized that therapeutic shock (Herxheimer effects) may occur in late syphilis as well as in early syphilis. In contrast to the mild and rather insignificant reaction which follows treatment of early syphilis with penicillin, the reaction may be serious in late syphilis. It is therefore to be guarded against. Stokes and others recommended that reduced dosages should be employed during the first twenty-four to forty-eight hours of treatment. According to these investigators, severe symptoms, referable to the cerebrum and spinal cord for example, may develop when patients with neurosyphilis are under treatment with penicillin.

SYPHILIS IN PREGNANCY AND INFANTILE CONGENITAL SYPHILIS

It would appear, from the report of Lentz and others,[11] that penicillin can be safely and satisfactorily used for treatment of syphilis of the pregnant woman and for treatment of infantile congenital syphilis. Most syphilotherapists apparently agree that arsenical therapy for prevention and treatment of congenital syphilis leaves considerable to be desired. Arsenical drugs are relatively toxic and, as usually employed, are not curative of syphilis of the mother. Furthermore, it has been stated that the problem is bound up with the desirability of an antispirochetal agent which readily traverses the placenta. This much can be said: Penicillin is relatively nontoxic and it has been clearly shown by my colleagues and me[6] that it passes through the placenta and reaches the fetal circulation. This is true not only of the normal pregnant mother but also of the mother who is syphilitic. The ratio of the concentration of penicillin in the mother's blood to that in the fetal blood is approximately 2:1. Whether or not penicillin is curative of syphilis of the mother cannot be finally stated as yet; however, the evidence presented by Lentz and others is at least suggestive. These investigators have reported on the use of penicillin in treatment of twelve pregnant women who had symptomatic early syphilis and two who had early latent syphilis. They also have reported on the use of penicillin in treatment of nine infants who had early congenital syphilis. At the time of their report, seven of the fourteen pregnant women had reached term. The serologic response of mother and child would permit the conclusion that penicillin had very favorably affected the course of the disease. Furthermore, the surface lesions of the expectant mothers responded rapidly and spirochetes disappeared from the lesions in less than eight hours after treatment had been begun. Treatment with penicillin in this group of cases had been instituted sometime between the midpoint of pregnancy and one month immediately preceding delivery. Untreated pregnant women with early syphilis almost uniformly give birth to dead or diseased children; however, among the fourteen syphilitic mothers treated with penicillin by Lentz and others, not a single stillbirth or neonatal death occurred and seven of the infants who were delivered were known to have remained physically normal and seronegative for periods of observation as long as 101 days postpartum.

These same investigators expressed the belief that penicillin given to the mother is not recoverable from the blood of the umbilical cord Nevertheless, as I have mentioned (p. 77), penicillin does reach the fetus when given to the mother systemically. The fact that such satisfactory results as have been related were obtained in treatment of this group of pregnant syphilitic women seems explainable primarily on the basis that penicillin does traverse the placenta and is therefore available to the fetus in amounts which are probably therapeutically effective.

According to the report by Lentz and others,[11] infants with congenital syphilis who had been followed long enough to permit a report all became normal to physical examination. The serologic titers of the blood, which initially had been high, dropped sharply to normal or relatively low levels after treatment. Furthermore, two infants who gave roentgenographic evidence of having syphilitic osteochondritis and periostitis resumed almost normal bone development after treatment. In addition, two infants died, which may or may not have been due to penicillin therapy.

On the other hand, it has been observed by some investigators that in a number of cases in which lesions of the skin and mucous membranes of infants underwent favorable involution with treatment, the patients went on to unexplained death a month or so after treatment had been discontinued.

Plan of Treatment.—*The Syphilitic Pregnant Mother.*—A total dose of penicillin ranging between 1,200,000 and 2,400,000 Oxford units is recommended. The penicillin can be administered either by the intravenous drip method or by the intramuscular method. If the intravenous drip method is employed, 100,000 Oxford units per day is sufficient. If the intramuscular method is employed, 15,000 Oxford units of penicillin in 2 or 3 c.c. of solvent should be administered every three hours day and night until the total dose has been given. It has been recommended by Lentz and others that in order to guard against the possibility of therapeutic shock, half the recommended daily dose, or 50,000 to 60,000 Oxford units, should be administered during the first forty-eight hours of treatment.

Infantile Congenital Syphilis.—For treatment of infantile congenital syphilis it is recommended that the patients receive 5,000 Oxford units of penicillin in 1 c.c. of physiologic saline solution, administered intramuscularly into the buttocks, every three hours day and night for ten days. During the first day or two, it is recommended that half this dose be employed, with the idea in mind of protecting the patient against the possibility of therapeutic shock.

PENICILLIN FOR PROPHYLAXIS AGAINST SYPHILIS

The question naturally arises whether penicillin has a possible role in prophylaxis against syphilis and prevention of congenital syphilis has been discussed in connection with the use of penicillin in treatment of the syphilitic pregnant woman. Furthermore, it might be asked: Could a patient be protected by giving him intensive penicillin therapy within the first day or two following exposure to syphilis? Few data are available at present from which answer to this question could be derived.

A report by Carpenter[12] is of some interest in this connection. He described a case in which sulfonamide resistant gonorrhea was treated with 50,000 Oxford units of penicillin twenty-two days after exposure. It was his impression that although the development of syphilis was not prevented, even this amount of penicillin delayed the appearance of a clinically typical, but darkfield negative, chancre. The amount of penicillin used in this instance, however, in light of present knowledge, would be considered totally inadequate either for prevention or treatment of such a lesion. In order to determine the possible effectiveness of such a procedure, 100,000 to 200,000 units of penicillin per day should be administered over a period of eight to ten days following known exposure. Even then interpretation of the results will be fraught with all of the difficulties attending prophylaxis against syphilis.

To be mentioned also in this connection is the masking effect on syphilis which may occur because of treatment with small amounts of penicillin for acute neisserian infections. Given a patient with acute gonorrhea who receives a total of 100,000 to 150,000 Oxford units of penicillin, it is possible that the amount of penicillin given may be enough to delay the appearance of a chancre due to concomitant infection with syphilis. This delay may be of such duration that the patient may have been dismissed by his physician before the chancre appears and systemic syphilis may develop later. This is not a theoretical possibility because it already has occurred in practice. Examples of cases in which early syphilis was masked and its development delayed following the use of penicillin for treatment of gonorrhea have been reported by Shafer and Zakon,[13] by Hailey[14] and by Baier and Pincus.[15] Reports by Ricchiuti[16] and by Boyd, Wagner and Hewson[17] further have emphasized the importance of thorough search for primary and secondary lesions of syphilis prior to administration of penicillin for gonorrhea. They also have directed attention to the fact that subtherapeutic doses of penicillin administered in these cases may modify or obscure the presence of a primary syphilitic lesion.

It should be emphasized that this discussion on the use of penicillin in treatment of syphilis is based on preliminary observations made over a period of only a year and a half. Much work remains to be done. Possibly larger doses and repeated courses of penicillin will be necessary to obtain the most satisfactory result. It is further possible that supplemental therapy, including administration of arsenical preparations, may be necessary in certain cases of syphilis.

YAWS

Because of the possible relationship between syphilis and yaws, attempts have been made to determine the effect of penicillin on the latter disease. As far as I know, the first report on the effect of penicillin in treatment of yaws was that by Whitehill and Austrian.[18] Patients selected for treatment were those with active, primary and secondary yaws, darkfield examinations of whose local lesions revealed spirochetes morphologically identical with Treponema pertenue. The total dose of penicillin was set arbitrarily at 500,000 Oxford units. The penicillin was administered in amounts of 15,000 Oxford units intramuscularly every four hours day and night for five or six days. No other treatment, systemic or local, was employed during the period of penicillin therapy. In every case, whether or not previous treatment had been given, the lesions had been progressing unfavorably before treatment with penicillin was started. In seventeen cases, darkfield examinations revealed that in sixteen the organism had disappeared within sixteen hours after administration of penicillin had been begun. In one case, a single organism was found after this interval of sixteen hours, but none was present after forty hours of treatment. The investigators reported that during the first sixteen hours, the lesions showed definite evidence of healing and thereafter healing progressed with almost spectacular rapidity. Granulomas and ulcers became dry and clean and were soon covered with a firm eschar. Some ulcers were said to heal within one week and all lesions but one were completely healed within three weeks. During the short period of observation, it appeared that use of penicillin had not significantly affected the Kahn reactions of the serum; however, further studies were being undertaken on the general subject by the investigators at the time their preliminary report was submitted.

Subsequent to the report by Whitehill and Austrian,[18] Lofgren[19] also reported on the successful use of penicillin in treatment of yaws. Lofgren's patient apparently was suffering with fairly extensive lesions, including a primary ulcer. Darkfield examinations of serum removed from this ulcer revealed spirochetes which were morphologically typical of Treponema pertenue (Spirochaeta pertenuis). The patient was then given penicillin intramuscularly until a total of 1,500,000 Oxford units had been given over a period of twelve days. A typical local shock reaction occurred four hours after treatment had been started but disappeared eighteen hours after beginning of the treatment. The local lesion, which had been darkfield positive, became darkfield negative eighteen hours after treatment with penicillin had been begun. According to Lofgren's report, all of the lesions except the large primary ulcer on the forearm, were healed within five days. This ulcer on the forearm was completely healed, however, in thirteen days. The Kahn reaction of the blood was positive before treatment and still remained positive when the patient was discharged from the hospital five weeks later; however, by the sixth week the Kahn reaction had become negative. According to Lofgren, when the result obtained in this case was compared with the time required for resolution in cases of yaws treated with mapharsen and bismuth, the more rapid resolution of the lesions under penicillin therapy was impressive. Whether or not subsequent studies on the general subject will lead to more effective treatment in yaws will depend on further clinical trials.

RELAPSING FEVER

Soon after the reports by Mahoney and his colleagues[1] on the antispirochetal effect of penicillin, other reports appeared which suggested that penicillin was effective not only against the spirochete of syphilis but also against the spirochete of relapsing fever. These studies strengthened the idea that penicillin possessed at least some spirocheticidal activity.

The first report to appear on this subject was that by F. R. Heilman and me[20] on the effectiveness of penicillin in treatment of overwhelming experimental infections due to the spirochete of relapsing fever (Borrelia novyi). These studies were described in the chapter on the activity of penicillin in vivo (p. 54). Following this report, other investigators, including Lourie and Collier,[21] Augustine, Weinman and McAllister,[22] and Eagle, Magnuson and Musselman,[23] reported studies which also indicated that penicillin was effective in treatment of this disease.

Relapsing fever has occurred in great epidemics from time to time in Europe, Africa and Asia. In these great epidemics of relapsing fever the disease has been transmitted by the louse. Likewise, louse-borne epidemics of relapsing fever have occurred in the United States. Furthermore, a tick-borne type of relapsing fever has been recorded in many western states of the United States. While the American form of the disease is mild and as a rule not fatal, the louse-borne disease in certain epidemics has been associated with a mortality rate as high as 80 per cent.

Although arsenical preparations have been considered specific in treatment of relapsing fever, relapses have occurred following arsenical therapy and these relapses may at times be associated with severe complications, especially if inadequate doses of neoarsphenamine have been given. If arsenical therapy is instituted in the middle or terminal stages of a febrile paroxysm, or in the afebrile period, relapses are likely to occur with increased frequency. It appears, therefore, that arsenical therapy is most suitably administered only at the onset of a paroxysm. Furthermore, arsphenamine resistant strains of the spirochete have been known to develop following use of this drug. In view of these facts, and in view of the established low toxicity and high tolerance of human subjects for penicillin, it is evident that this drug should prove of value in treatment of this spirochetal infection.

Reports on the clinical use of penicillin in treatment of relapsing fever are not available as yet and for that reason a final statement as to its effectiveness cannot be made at the time of this writing; however, there is every indication that penicillin should prove of value in treatment of this disease.

LEPTOSPIROSIS ICTEROHAEMORRHAGICA (WEIL'S DISEASE)

In view of what has been said concerning the effectiveness of penicillin in treatment of syphilis and relapsing fever, it was natural to suspect that other diseases of spirochetal origin would be favorably influenced by this substance. F. R. Heilman and I,[24] therefore, carried out studies which have been described in the chapter on studies in vivo (p. 56) to test this possibility. There seemed little doubt from these experiments that penicillin would prove effective in treatment of leptospirosis icterohaemorrhagica of man.

Unlike syphilis and relapsing fever, leptospirosis icterohaemorrhagica (Weil's disease) has not been effectively treated with arsenical preparations. Other chemotherapeutic agents, such as sulfonamides, also have appeared useless. In fact, this disease has presented a most difficult problem as far as its successful treatment is concerned. The disease has been reported from nearly every civilized country in the world. The mortality rate at times has been exceedingly high. It is for the most part a rat-borne infection. Rats from all over the world have been examined and the spirochete has been found in at least 10 per cent of them.

Here again, enough data are not available to justify final statements but it is clear from experimental studies that use of penicillin in treatment of the disease should be thoroughly explored.

At the time this is written, the only report on the use of penicillin in the treatment of Weil's disease of man is that by Hart.[25] The patient received penicillin late in the course of the disease and apparently was about to recover at the time penicillin therapy was started. On the other hand, it appeared that administration of penicillin resulted in a rather prompt disappearance of the spirochete from the patient's urine.

REFERENCES

1. Mahoney, J. F., Arnold, R. C. and Harris, Ad: Penicillin treatment of early syphilis; a preliminary report. Ven. Dis. Inform. 24:355–357 (Dec.) 1943; Am. J. Pub. Health. 33:1387–1391 (Dec.) 1943.

2. Bloomfield, A. L., Rantz, L. A. and Kirby, W. M. M.: The clinical use of penicillin. J. A. M. A. 124:627–633 (Mar. 4) 1944.

3. Wise, C. R. and Pillsbury, D. M.: Penicillin in the treatment of syphilis. Proc. Roy. Soc. Med. 37:491–492 (July) 1944.

4. Mahoney, J. F., Arnold, R. C., Sterner, B. L., Harris, Ad and Zwally, M. R.: Penicillin treatment of early syphilis: II. J. A. M. A. 126:63–67 (Sept. 9) 1944.

5. Moore, J. E., Mahoney, J. F., Schwartz, Walter, Sternberg, Thomas and Wood, W. B.: The treatment of early syphilis with penicillin; a preliminary report of 1,418 cases. J. A. M. A. 126:67–73 (Sept. 9) 1944.

6. Herrell, W. E., Nichols, D. R. and Heilman, Dorothy H.: Penicillin; its usefulness, limitations, diffusion and detection, with analysis of 150 cases in which it was employed. J. A. M. A. 125:1003–1010 (Aug. 12) 1944.

7. White, W. L., Flippin, H. F., Lockwood, J. S. and Murphy, F. D.: The indications for penicillin; its dosage and administration. Clinics. 3:309–323 (Aug.) 1944.

8. O'Leary, Paul A.: Personal communication to the author.

9. Stokes, J. H., Sternberg, T. H., Schwartz, W. H., Mahoney, J. F., Moore, J. E. and Wood, W. B., Jr.: The action of penicillin in late syphilis including neurosyphilis, benign late syphilis and late congenital syphilis: preliminary report. J. A. M. A. 126:73–79 (Sept. 9) 1944.

10. O'Leary, P. A. and Herrell, W. E.: Penicillin in the treatment of late cutaneous syphilis: report of case. Proc. Staff Meet., Mayo Clin. 19:20–22 (Jan. 12) 1944.

11. Lentz, J. W., Ingraham, N. R., Jr., Beerman, Herman and Stokes, J. H.: Penicillin in the prevention and treatment of congenital syphilis; report on experience with the treatment of fourteen pregnant women with early syphilis and nine infants with congenital syphilis. J. A. M. A. 126:408–413 (Oct. 14) 1944.

12. Carpenter, C. C.: Failure of penicillin to prevent syphilis. U. S. Nav. M. Bull. 43:389–390 (Aug.) 1944.

13. Shafer, Bertha and Zakon, S. J.: Early syphilis masked and delayed by penicillin in the treatment of gonorrhea. Arch. Dermat. & Syph. 50:200 (Sept.) 1944.

14. Hailey, H. E.: Suppression of syphilis by penicillin therapy of gonorrhea. Arch. Dermat. & Syph. 50:269 (Oct.) 1944.

15. Baier, G. F., III and Pincus, J. A.: The effect of a small dose of penicillin on the diagnosis of early syphilis. Mil. Surgeon. 95:359–360 (Nov.) 1944.

16. Ricchiuti, J. F.: Penicillin therapy in gonorrhea with associated undiagnosed early syphilis. U. S. Nav. M. Bull. 43:1031–1033 (Nov.) 1944.

17. Boyd, G. G., Wagner, J. A. and Hewson, G. F.: Effects of subtherapeutic dose of penicillin on development of primary syphilitic lesion: report of case. U. S. Nav. M. Bull. 43:1034–1035 (Nov.) 1944.

18. Whitehill, Richard and Austrian, Robert: The treatment of primary and secondary yaws with penicillin. A preliminary report. Bull. Johns Hopkins Hosp. 75:232–240 (Oct.) 1944.

19. Lofgren, R. C.: Yaws treated with penicillin; report of case. U. S. Nav. M. Bull. 43:1025–1030 (Nov.) 1944.

20. Heilman, F. R. and Herrell, W. E.: Penicillin in the treatment of experimental relapsing fever. Proc. Staff Meet., Mayo Clin. 18:457–467 (Dec. 1) 1943.

21. Lourie, E. M. and Collier, H. O. J.: The therapeutic action of penicillin in Spirochaeta recurrentis and Spirillum minus in mice. Ann. Trop. Med. 37:200–205 (Dec. 31) 1943.

22. Augustine, D. L., Weinman, David and McAllister, Joan: Rapid and sterilizing effect of penicillin sodium in experimental relapsing fever infections and its ineffectiveness in the treatment of trypanosomiasis (Trypanosomas lewisi) and toxoplasmosis. Science. 99:19–20 (Jan. 7) 1944.

23. Eagle, Harry, Magnuson, H. J. and Musselman, Arlyne D.: The therapeutic efficacy of penicillin in relapsing fever infections in mice and rats. Pub. Health Rep. 59:583–588 (May 5) 1944.

24. Heilman, F. R. and Herrell, W. E.: Penicillin in the treatment of experimental leptospirosis icterohaemorrhagica (Weil's disease). Proc. Staff Meet., Mayo Clin. 19:89–99 (Feb. 23) 1944.

25. Hart, V. L.: A case of Weil's disease treated with penicillin. Brit. M. J. 2:720 (Dec. 2) 1944.

CHAPTER XVIII

MISCELLANEOUS INFECTIONS

GAS GANGRENE

In view of studies made in vitro and in vivo by the Oxford investigators[1, 2] on the sensitivity to penicillin of anaerobic organisms, especially those usually associated with gas gangrene, it seemed reasonable to suspect that penicillin would prove of at least some value in treatment of this infection.

As experience accumulated, however, it was evident that penicillin alone was not the final answer to successful treatment of this disease. Given a well-established infection, necrotic tissue as well as the general circulation may contain toxins already elaborated by the pathogenic organisms and penicillin has little effect on the toxins themselves. The role of penicillin is primarily to rid the diseased tissue of the microorganism and the experience of the British investigators[3, 4] demonstrated that to combine antitoxin with penicillin was essential in treatment of gas gangrene. It is likewise important to use penicillin in fairly large amounts locally whenever possible, as well as to administer it systemically.

The experience of my colleagues and me[5] in treatment of gas gangrene affecting a limited number of civilians is in complete agreement with the recommendations made by Florey and Cairns[4] in connection with their experience in treatment of wounded military personnel in North Africa. They used penicillin systemically in the treatment of severe gas gangrene. The total dose employed was approximately 750,000 Oxford units. Four patients so treated recovered and three died. The infections of all were owing to Clostridium welchii. There seemed little doubt that penicillin was effective in halting the spreading infection. Furthermore, histologic examinations made in these cases revealed extensive macrophage reaction in the zones of necrosis of the muscles. Since spreading gas gangrene is said to produce no cellular reaction, the macrophage reaction can be interpreted as additional evidence of the effectiveness of penicillin against this disease. It was clear from the experience of the investigators, however, that penicillin does not counteract the toxins, as has been said, that dead muscles should be removed surgically and that the neutralizing effect of antitoxin should be combined with penicillin if the best results are to be obtained.

Jeffrey and Thomson[6] have reported on the use of penicillin combined with radical surgical operation and administration of gas gangrene antitoxin in thirty-three cases of the disease as it occurred in Italy in the spring of 1944. The two most striking features in this series of cases, according to the authors, were the arrest of the gangrenous process and the late ill effects that occurred in some cases in which the patients appeared to be recovering from gas gangrene. The arrest of the porgressive myositis was attributed to the effect of penicillin on the microorganisms. The late ill effects were characterized by renal failure. The changes in the kidneys were not unlike those seen in the crush syndrome; that is, tubular degeneration, deposits of pigment and cortical necrosis were present. It was pointed out that these changes probably were toxic effects from retained degenerated and autolyzing muscle. Of this group of thirty-three patients, 63.6 per cent recovered.

Likewise, Cutler and Sandusky,[7] of the United States Army Medical Corps, have reported on the use of penicillin in treatment of clostridial infections of injured flying personnel. While it appears that prophylactic use of penicillin locally and systemically did not prevent development of gas gangrene, satisfactory results were obtained in five of seven cases when administration of penicillin was continued and was combined with surgical extirpation of dead tissue and administration of gas gangrene antitoxin. The investigators also mentioned one patient who had received penicillin in an attempt at cure but had not received it prophylactically, and who died in a state of uremia five days following amputation. This appears to be a type of late ill effect similar to that reported by the British observers.[6] Cutler and Sandusky[7] suggested that their data indicated that surgical débridement is the major factor in both prophylaxis and treatment of gas gangrene. In other words, penicillin is an important part, but not the sole factor, in treatment of this infection.

A few scattered reports by American investigators have appeared on the effectiveness of penicillin in treatment of gas gangrene. McKnight, Loewenberg and Wright[8] reported on the successful use of penicillin in a case of severe gas gangrene which followed compound fracture. All other measures previously used, including surgical amputation, had been unsuccessful. The patient also received antitoxin. Recovery followed the use of penicillin.

Until August, 1944, my colleagues and I[5] had used penicillin in only six cases of gas gangrene. The combination of penicillin with surgical intervention and administration of antitoxin resulted in recovery of four of the six patients. Lyons[9] also reported on the use of penicillin in treatment of two patients suffering with anaerobic cellulitis owing to Clostridium welchii. These infections responded favorably to the use of penicillin. Kepl, Ochsner and Dixon[10] have reported on the successful use of penicillin in two cases of infection with Clostridium welchii. They combined local and systemic administration of penicillin with administration of gas gangrene antitoxin and whatever surgical procedures were indicated. Harvey and Meleney[11] were unsuccessful in the treatment of severe gas gangrene with penicillin. It appears, however, that the patient was extremely ill and was treated late in the course of infection. They were also unsuccessful in treatment of a patient suffering with a mixed infection due to Clostridium sordellii and Clostridium welchii. In this instance the patient received 280,000 Oxford units of penicillin during the last seventeen hours of life. It is possible that the results might have been better had the patient received the benefit of penicillin earlier in the course of the disease.

Penicillin, furthermore, should prove useful in prevention of gas gangrene. If supplies are available, I believe penicillin should be employed if wounds are present from which the infection is likely to develop.

Plan of Treatment.—As soon as the presence of gas gangrene is suspected, or the diagnosis is reasonably certain, adequate amounts of antitoxin should be administered. Whenever surgical procedures are indicated they should be instituted. Penicillin should be applied locally in the form of the powdered substance (the calcium salt is preferred) or it should be applied in a physiologic saline solution containing at least 500 Oxford units per cubic centimeter. If small tubes are inserted into deep wounds, the solution can be instilled into these tubes three to four times a day. In addition, penicillin should be administered systemically by either the intramuscular method or the intravenous drip method. At least 100,000 Oxford units should be given daily and administration should be continued until satisfactory clinical improvement or apparent cure has been obtained.

ACTINOMYCOSIS

Nearly all strains of Actinomyces bovis have been found to be fairly sensitive to the action of penicillin. On the other hand, treatment of actinomycosis with penicillin or any other agent presents some rather difficult problems. Although penicillin may be effective against the causative organism, at times it may be difficult for the agent to reach the organisms which are walled off in certain regions where the blood supply is poor. In treatment of chronic actinomycosis of long standing, therefore, it may be difficult or even impossible at times completely to eradicate the disease from the body. Actinomycosis with involvement of bone, associated with walled-off foci, presents a therapeutic problem not unlike that of chronic osteomyelitis, wherein the successful use of penicillin is dependent on adequate drainage and removal of foci. On the other hand, early actinomycosis frequently can be successfully treated when adequate amounts of penicillin are administered. In certain early cases it may be possible to effect cure without surgical intervention.

The Floreys[12] reported on the use of penicillin in two cases of actinomycosis. The results were not particularly impressive; however, the amounts of penicillin used and the method of administration employed probably would be considered inadequate in the light of present knowledge. Likewise, the Committee on Chemotherapeutic and Other Agents[13] reported three cases of actinomycosis in which treatment was with penicillin. In one case, the patient was said to have recovered or his condition to have improved but in two cases treatment was said to have resulted in failure. The report contained no details as to type of case or method of treatment. Lyons[9] reported four cases in which penicillin was used in treatment of actinomycosis and at least temporary improvement followed its use. Christie and Garrod[14] were unsuccessful in treatment of extensive pulmonary actinomycosis in one case. This is not surprising because, in my experience, recovery from extensive systemic infections due to actinomycosis, including pulmonary actinomycosis, is not the rule although there may be a favorable temporary response.

My colleagues and I[5] have reported on the use of penicillin in treatment of twelve patients with actinomycosis. Since our report was issued, other patients with this disease have been treated with penicillin at the clinic. Patients of both groups had, for the most part, early maxillofacial actinomycosis although, in a few cases, the disease was of the abdominal, pulmonary or generalized type. Satisfactory results have been obtained in many of the cases of maxillofacial actinomycosis, not only in early cases but also in several cases of long standing. Although I already have indicated that at times it is possible to bring about recovery of these patients without surgical drainage, this procedure frequently is carried out. In many instances, however, the incision has been made primarily to obtain material for direct examination and for culture.

An example of maxillofacial actinomycosis of long standing, in which penicillin appeared to bring about recovery, is the following case, which was encountered at the Mayo Clinic. The patient had been suffering for more than two years with maxillofacial actinomycosis involving not only the soft tissues but also bone. Multiple sinuses persisted in spite of many attempts at surgical drainage, use of iodides and intensive roentgenologic treatment. After three courses of penicillin, recovery occurred (fig. 34). Although this patient recovered in the presence of evident involvement of bone, it is almost essential that surgical drainage still form part of the plan of treatment.

Another interesting example of the effectiveness of penicillin in treatment of maxillofacial actinomycosis is the following case: The patient had received his first course of penicillin for rather extensive maxillofacial actinomycosis. Shortly thereafter, evidence developed of intracranial spread of the disease. This may occur in about one of 200 cases of actinomycosis. The patient became critically ill, with severe headache, mental confusion and high fever. Physical examination gave evidence of meningeal irritation. The spinal fluid pressure was 170 mm. of water and microscopic examination of the fluid revealed 500 lymphocytes and 7,000 polymorphonuclear leukocytes per cubic millimeter. Intensive treatment with penicillin was begun, using the intravenous drip method, and daily

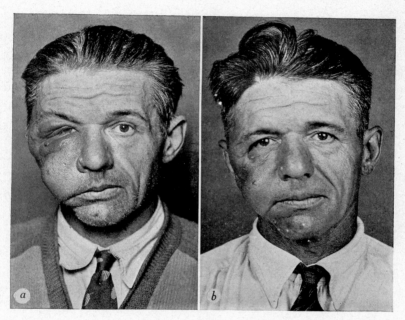

Fig. 34.—Actinomycosis. *a*, Before treatment with penicillin. The multiple draining sinuses which were present are not visible in the photograph. Deformity and edema of the right eye are evident. Cultures were positive for Actinomyces bovis. *b*, After completion of third course of penicillin.

intrathecal instillations of penicillin following spinal taps were continued for ten days. The patient recovered (fig. 35).

Abdominal actinomycosis has been treated successfully in a few cases in which the diagnosis was made early and intensive treatment with penicillin was carried out. Abdominal actinomycosis of long standing, however, associated with multiple sinuses and inaccessible foci, is not likely to respond satisfactorily. Likewise, extensive pulmonary actinomycosis complicated by multiple metastatic lesions or disseminated systemic infections is unlikely to respond satisfactorily. On the other hand, I have observed a practically moribund patient who made satisfactory temporary response and lived for nearly a year following intensive treatment with penicillin.

Plan of Treatment.—Surgical drainage is indicated in most cases of actinomycosis. Because of the difficulty in reaching the foci which usually are present, administration of rather large amounts of penicillin is advisable. My colleagues and I have adopted the following plan: At least three courses of penicillin, each of ten to fourteen days' duration, are administered. Although a few patients have responded to as little as 60,000 Oxford units of penicillin per day, in view of present knowledge, administration of at least 100,000 Oxford units, and in some instances 200,000 Oxford units, per day is indicated; the intravenous drip method

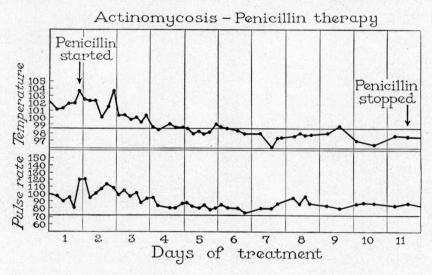

Fig. 35.—Temperature and pulse chart of a patient who had maxillofacial actinomycosis with intracranial involvement and was treated with penicillin.

or the intermittent intramuscular method may be used. Between the first and second and the second and third courses we have allowed a rest period of two to four weeks. Patients should be followed for a long time before they are finally pronounced cured. However, the plan of treatment just outlined has resulted in satisfactory results in many instances.

VIRUS INFECTIONS

There seems to be general agreement among most investigators that penicillin is not particularly effective against most virus infections. This is especially true of infections with the smaller viruses, such as the virus of *influenza* and the virus of *poliomyelitis*. Certain larger viruses, however, more nearly approach the bacterial scale and there is evidence that penicillin should prove of some value against them. In the chapter on studies in vivo, the effectiveness of penicillin in treatment of certain experimental virus infections was mentioned. It was evident from the experiments of Moragues and his colleagues[15] that penicillin exhibited a definite protective effect against experimental *murine typhus*.

From studies reported by F. R. Heilman and me,[16, 17] there seemed reason to believe that adequate doses of penicillin would prove effective in treatment of *ornithosis* and *psittacosis*. Although clinical data are lacking on which to base final statements, it appears that penicillin has been used satisfactorily in treatment of these diseases. Whenever the diagnosis can be established, penicillin should be employed in treatment

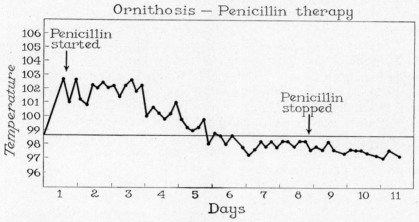

Fig. 36.—The temperature in a case of ornithosis in which penicillin was used. (From article by Turgasen, Journal of the American Medical Association, December 30, 1944.)

of either of these infections as it occurs in human beings. Since no other form of treatment has proved of great value, there is everything to be gained and nothing to be lost by making clinical trials with penicillin.

Turgasen[18] used penicillin for treatment in a proved case of ornithosis of man and the results suggest that penicillin was of value. The patient was a white man, forty-three years of age. He had maintained a loft of homing pigeons for a number of years and had taken care of them himself. Some of the birds had died of illness. Seven days before the patient became ill he had cleaned out the loft and had inhaled a considerable amount of dust. He complained of generalized aching, fever, abdominal discomfort and indigestion. At the time of his admission to hospital, the patient was troubled by photophobia and lack of mental co-ordination. There was evidence of pneumonia on the left and roentgenograms revealed an unusual type of pneumonia. The spleen was palpable. Leukocytes numbered 9,200 per cubic millimeter of blood and the degree of eosinophilia was 4 per cent. The blood, according to Turgasen, was found by Karl Meyer to give a positive complement fixation; this manifestation usually is present in cases of ornithosis and psittacosis. Pigeons from the loft were examined by F. R. Heilman and, from the spleen of one of them, he recovered the virus of ornithosis. The patient received 100,000 Oxford units of penicillin per day for seven and a half days. Improvement was rapid; the temperature reached normal after five days of treatment and remained normal. Penicillin seemed to have a favorable influence on the course of the disease in this case (fig. 36).

Judging from the reports of Keefer and others,[13] of Lyons,[9] and of Dawson and Hobby,[19] penicillin does not appear to be of value in treatment of *so-called primary atypical (virus) pneumonia*. At variance with the reports just mentioned, however, is that of Short,[20] who used penicillin in nine cases of so-called primary atypical pneumonia. Commenting on his results, Short pointed out that in this small series of cases the average number of days from onset of penicillin therapy until the temperature became normal was 3.5, which is decidedly less than is usually required to produce this result when a patient is under supportive treatment. Short was inclined to the opinion that the results were definite and striking. The possible value of penicillin in treatment of this disease probably has not been finally evaluated and its possible or probable value against the viruses of ornithosis and psittacosis makes it necessary to keep in mind that these agents may be causative in some cases of atypical pneumonia.

Data are lacking on which to base any statement as to the possible effect of penicillin in treatment of *lymphogranuloma venereum*.

RAT-BITE FEVER

It is now well established that rat-bite fever is due to infection by either Spirillum minus or Streptobacillus moniliformis. It was evident from the experimental studies of Lourie and Collier,[21] as well as from studies[22] reported from the Mayo Clinic, that infections owing to Spirillum minus could be satisfactorily treated with penicillin. It was further evident, from the report by F. R. Heilman and me,[22] which has been discussed in the chapter on the activity of penicillin in vivo, that the other pathogenic organism associated with rat-bite fever, namely, Streptobacillus moniliformis, was exceedingly susceptible to the action of this chemotherapeutic agent. Although arsenicals have proved of some value in treatment of rat-bite fever owing to Spirillum minus, their use at times has been followed by undesirable reactions. Furthermore, arsenicals have not been of value in treatment of rat-bite fever due to

Streptobacillus moniliformis. Although gold is somewhat effective in treatment of infections owing to Streptobacillus moniliformis, its use is not without certain well-known hazards. Penicillin, however, is exceedingly effective against both organisms that are responsible for rat-bite fever and, at the same time it is of exceedingly low toxicity. Patients with rat-bite fever, therefore, have been treated successfully with penicillin.

In the three cases reported by Altemeier,[23] for example, the organism of infection was Streptobacillus moniliformis. In two of these instances administration of penicillin was followed within twenty-four hours by permanent disappearance of Streptobacillus moniliformis from the blood stream. The cutaneous lesions promptly faded and clinical improvement occurred. In a third case the blood stream was sterilized following administration of an inadequate amount of penicillin but later became positive. It seems reasonable to conjecture that if adequate amounts of penicillin had been administered the result would have been as satisfactory as that obtained in the other cases.

Another case of bacteriemia owing to Streptobacillus moniliformis has been reported by Robins.[24] Two days before admission, the patient had been bitten by a rat on the left wrist. Twenty-four hours later malaise and lassitude had appeared. Following this, chills, nausea, vomiting and fever developed. Sulfonamides were administered intensively without benefit. Penicillin then was administered intravenously and intramuscularly. Blood cultures became negative and the patient recovered after receiving a total of 1,922,000 Oxford units of penicillin.

Kane[25] also has successfully used penicillin in treatment of a child, fifteen years of age, severely ill with rat-bite fever owing to Streptobacillus moniliformis. The patient had been in the hospital for a long time and had had nine relapses. Gold therapy apparently had not resulted in satisfactory response. Within twelve hours following the beginning of administration of penicillin, however, the temperature returned to normal and the patient apparently made a complete recovery.

At the Mayo Clinic[26] we have had occasion to use penicillin in only one case of suspected rat-bite fever. Unfortunately, attempts to isolate Spirillum minus or Streptobacillus moniliformis from the blood of this patient were unsuccessful. All the clinical evidence for a diagnosis of rat-bite fever was present but laboratory confirmation of the diagnosis was lacking. The patient was an infant, two years of age, who had been bitten on the finger by a rat four days before admission. Three days before admission at the clinic, the patient had been bitten again, and this time on the lip. On the fourth day following the initial bite by the rat, which was the day of admission, the temperature was 104° F. On this day, the child had begun to shake and obviously was having chills.

The lesion on the finger and that on the lip were similar to those usually seen in cases of rat-bite fever. Also, a maculopapular rash of the sort usually seen in rat-bite fever developed. The patient received 5,000 Oxford units of penicillin intramuscularly every three hours day and night for nine days. Recovery was prompt and uneventful. At the time of the patient's dismissal, after nine days of treatment with penicillin, both of the local lesions were completely healed and the child was well.

Haverhill Fever.—In view of the high degree of sensitivity of Streptobacillus moniliformis to the action of penicillin, it seems reasonable to assume that penicillin should prove effective in treatment of this disease. The disease is essentially a bacteriemia owing to Streptobacillus moniliformis, with symptomatic manifestations owing to the infection. However, the infection is not associated with the bite of a rat.

Plan of Treatment.—If patients are infants or young children, 5,000 Oxford units of penicillin dissolved in 1 or 2 c.c. of physiologic saline solution should be administered intramuscularly every three hours and administration should be continued for at least seven to ten days. To adults it probably is advisable to give at least 100,000 Oxford units per day, by the intravenous drip method or by the intermittent intramuscular method, and to maintain administration for a period similar to that recommended for infants and children.

INFECTIONS DUE TO BORRELIA VINCENTII (VINCENT'S SPIRILLUM)

In view of the effectiveness of penicillin against Spirillum minus, it is not surprising that evidence already has accumulated to suggest that the substance is also effective against another spirillum; namely, Borrelia vincentii. My colleagues and I have successfully used systemic administration of penicillin in a few cases of infection with this organism. In some instances, necrotic lesions of the mouth, in which the spirillum has been found, have healed within twenty-four to forty-eight hours after the beginning of treatment.

Likewise, Denny, Shallenberger and Pyle[27] have reported on the effectiveness of penicillin in treatment of infections owing to Vincent's organisms. A solution containing 250 Oxford units of penicillin per cubic centimeter was swabbed on the infected areas four times daily. Treatment was continued for three days and, according to the report, smears negative for Vincent's spirillum were obtained at the end of two and a half days of treatment. Edema of the mucous membranes rapidly subsided and disappeared. Furthermore, rapid improvement in appearance of the gums, tonsils and pharynx followed use of penicillin. These investigators also used penicillin systemically in some cases of Vincent's angina. The investigators concluded that penicillin was the most effective agent yet known in treatment of this infection.

Moreover, Strock[28] has reported striking results from treatment of ulceromembranous gingivitis (Vincent's infection). This investigator administered the penicillin intramuscularly and locally.

I am inclined to the opinion that if penicillin is to be used in the treatment of this type of infection, it should be administered systemically as well as locally. It is difficult, following local application, to retain adequate concentrations of the drug in the mouth for a period of time long enough to permit the action of penicillin to be completed.

Plan of Treatment.—For local application, a solution of penicillin containing 1,000 Oxford units per cubic centimeter is recommended. For systemic treatment, a total daily dose of 80,000 Oxford units usually will prove satisfactory. Treatment should be continued until clinical improvement occurs and negative smears have been obtained.

ERYSIPELOID

The occupational disease, erysipeloid, at times may be rather serious and debilitating. It is now well established that the etiologic agent of this disease is the organism Erysipelothrix rhusiopathiae. It is the organism responsible, in swine, for the so-called "diamond-back" disease, or swine erysipelas. Persons who work with the bones of infected swine or who come in contact with the disease for any other reason may acquire erysipeloid. Serious outbreaks among swine, with great loss, have occurred from time to time in Europe and in this country. Other than antiserum, no form of treatment has been effective either for man or swine. Sulfonamides have been ineffective.

In the chapter on the activity of penicillin in vivo I have mentioned the report by F. R. Heilman and me[29] on the effect of penicillin against experimental infections due to the organism of swine erysipelas. Results were encouraging and various investigators are now carrying out studies to determine the possible usefulness of penicillin in treatment of this disease.

ANTHRAX

Although the incidence of anthrax and the fatalities among human beings from anthrax have decreased in recent years, the disease is still an important one. Antiserum, arsenical preparations and sulfonamides have proved of some value in treatment of the disease but none of these agents is ideal. In the chapter on the activity of penicillin in vivo I have described the results obtained by F. R. Heilman and me[30] when penicillin was used in treatment of anthrax of experimental animals. At least half of the animals which received 10,000 lethal doses of the organism survived when penicillin was administered.

The first report on the use of penicillin in treatment of patients suffering with anthrax was that by Murphy, La Boccetta and Lockwood.[31]

The clinical response in three cases of uncomplicated cutaneous anthrax of man, without bacteriemia, was rapid and definite. In each instance, the lesions promptly underwent regression and involution. The clinical response, according to these investigators, was paralleled by the disappearance of Bacillus anthracis from the lesions. A total of 100,000 Oxford units of penicillin appeared to be the minimal effective dose in these cases. A total of at least 400,000 Oxford units of penicillin, administered at the rate of 100,000 Oxford units per twenty-four hours, was recommended for treatment in the average case of this type in which the patient was an adult. It was thought that larger doses of penicillin probably would be indicated for treatment in severe cases in which bacteriemia was present. According to the investigators named, continuous intravenous infusion probably is the most efficient method of administration of penicillin in these cases.

Plan of Treatment.—On the basis of the experience reported by Murphy and his colleagues in the treatment of anthrax, it can be said that patients suffering with this disease should receive at least 100,000 Oxford units of penicillin per day until improvement or cure has occurred. Probably the most effective method of administering penicillin in these cases is by means of the continuous intravenous drip, as has been said; however, satisfactory results may be obtained by using the intramuscular method of administration.

TETANUS

In view of the fact that penicillin is effective against Clostridium tetani, it seems reasonable to hope that this agent will prove of value in treatment of tetanus. As in the case of gas gangrene, penicillin is primarily effective against the micro-organism and is not effective against toxins already present in the tissues. Hence, it is recommended that penicillin be combined with antitoxin in treatment of tetanus. The first relevant report is that of Buxton and Kurman.[32] Both patients whose cases were reported by these investigators recovered following administration of large doses of antitoxin combined with penicillin. Enough data are not available at the time of this writing to make any final statements on the value of penicillin in this condition although use of the agent should be thoroughly studied.

PERITONITIS

In view of the fact that satisfactory results have been obtained from intraperitoneal application of sulfanilamide or sulfathiazole in treatment of already established peritonitis and in prophylaxis of peritonitis; in view of the fact, also, that not infrequently certain intestinal micro-organisms which are insensitive to the action of penicillin are responsible for the disease, very little data are available concerning the possible value of penicillin in this condition. There is reason, however, to make use of penicillin for treatment in these cases, particularly if sulfonamide therapy and other measures have failed. There are certain types of peritonitis, particularly pneumococcal peritonitis, which should respond satisfactorily to systemic administration of penicillin. If the physician is dealing with severe peritonitis, it may be wise to combine penicillin with sulfonamide therapy in the hope that organisms which are insensitive to the action of sulfonamides could be eliminated by the action of penicillin.

REFERENCES

1. Chain, E., Florey, H. W., Gardner, A. D., Heatley, N. G., Jennings, M. A., Orr-Ewing, J. and Sanders, A. G.: Penicillin as a chemotherapeutic agent. Lancet. *2*:226–228 (Aug. 24) 1940.

2. Abraham, E. P., Chain, E., Fletcher, C. M., Gardner, A. D., Heatley, N. G., Jennings, M. A. and Florey, H. W.: Further observations on penicillin. Lancet. *2*:177–188; 189 (Aug. 16) 1941.

3. Royal Society of Medicine: Discussions on penicillin. Lancet. *2*:638–639 (Nov. 20) 1943.

4. Florey, H. W. and Cairns, Hugh: Penicillin in war wounds; a report from the Mediterranean. Lancet. *2*:742–745 (Dec. 11) 1943. (Abstr.) The treatment of war wounds with penicillin. Brit. M. J. *2*:755 (Dec. 11) 1943.

5. Herrell, W. E., Nichols, D. R. and Heilman, Dorothy H.: Penicillin; its usefulness, limitations, diffusion and detection, with analysis of 150 cases in which it was employed. J. A. M. A. *125*:1003–1010 (Aug. 12) 1944.

6. Jeffrey, J. S. and Thomson, Scott: Gas gangrene in Italy; a study of 33 cases treated with penicillin. Brit. J. Surg. *32*:159–167 (July Suppl.) 1944.

7. Cutler, E. C. and Sandusky, W. R.: Treatment of clostridial infections with penicillin. Brit. J. Surg. *32*:168–176 (July Suppl.) 1944.

8. McKnight, W. B., Loewenberg, R. D. and Wright, Virginia L.: Penicillin in gas gangrene; report of a successfully treated case. J. A. M. A. *124*:360 (Feb. 5) 1944.

9. Lyons, Champ: Penicillin therapy of surgical infections in the U. S. Army; a report. J. A. M. A. *123*:1007–1018 (Dec. 18) 1943.

10. Kepl, Maxwell, Ochsner, Alton and Dixon, J. L.: Two cases of Clostridium welchii infection treated with penicillin. J. A. M. A. *126*:96–98 (Sept. 9) 1944.

11. Harvey, H. D. and Meleney, F. L.: A case of infection with Clostridium sordellii and a case of gas gangrene treated by penicillin. Surgery. *15*:622–627 (Apr.) 1944.

12. Florey, M. E. and Florey, H. W.: General and local administration of penicillin. Lancet. *1*:387–397 (Mar. 27) 1943.

13. Keefer, C. S., Blake, F. G., Marshall, E. K., Jr., Lockwood, J. S. and Wood, W. B., Jr.: Penicillin in the treatment of infections; a report of 500 cases. J. A. M. A. *122*:1217–1224 (Aug. 28) 1943.

14. Christie, R. V. and Garrod, L. P.: A review of the work of a penicillin therapeutic research unit. Brit. M. J. *1*:513–514 (Apr. 15) 1944.

15. Moragues, Vicente, Pinkerton, Henry and Greiff, Donald: Therapeutic effectiveness of penicillin in experimental murine typhus infection in dba mice. J. Exper. Med. *79*:431–437 (Apr. 1) 1944.

16. Heilman, F. R. and Herrell, W. E.: Penicillin in the treatment of experimental ornithosis. Proc. Staff Meet., Mayo Clin. *19*:57–65 (Feb. 9) 1944.

17. Heilman, F. R. and Herrell, W. E.: Penicillin in the treatment of experimental psittacosis. Proc. Staff Meet., Mayo Clin. 19:204–207 (Apr. 19) 1944.

18. Turgasen, F. E.: Human ornithosis treated with penicillin. J. A. M. A. 126:1150–1151 (Dec. 30) 1944.

19. Dawson, M. H. and Hobby, Gladys L.: The clinical use of penicillin; observations in one hundred cases. J. A. M. A. 124:611–622 (Mar. 4) 1944.

20. Short, J. J.: Penicillin in the treatment of primary atypical pneumonia; report of nine cases. U. S. Nav. M. Bull. 43:974–980 (Nov.) 1944.

21. Lourie, E. M. and Collier, H. O. J.: The therapeutic action of penicillin on Spirochaeta recurrentis and Spirillum minus in mice. Ann. Trop. Med. 37:200–205 (Dec. 31) 1943.

22. Heilman, F. R. and Herrell, W. E.: Penicillin in the treatment of experimental infections with Spirillum minus and Streptobacillus moniliformis (rat-bite fever). Proc. Staff Meet., Mayo Clinic. 19:257–264 (May 17) 1944.

23. Altemeier, W. A.: Penicillin in surgery. South. M. J. 37:494–506 (Sept.) 1944.

24. Robins, George: Haverhill fever following rat bite treated with penicillin; report of a case. Clinics. 3:425–426 (Aug.) 1944.

25. Kane, F. F.: Rat-bite fever due to Streptobacillus moniliformis. Lancet. 2:548 (Oct. 21) 1944.

26. Herrell, W. E. and Kennedy, R. L. J.: Penicillin: its use in pediatrics. J. Pediat. 25:505–516 (Dec.) 1944.

27. Denny, E. R., Shallenberger, P. L. and Pyle, H. D.: Clinical observations in the use of penicillin. J. Oklahoma M. A. 37:193–205 (May) 1944.

28. Strock, A. E.: Relationship between gingivitis and penicillin administration; preliminary report. J. Am. Dent. A. 31:1235–1236 (Sept. 1) 1944.

29. Heilman, F. R. and Herrell, W. E.: Penicillin in the treatment of experimental infections due to Erysipelothrix rhusiopathiae. Proc. Staff Meet., Mayo Clin. 19:340–345 (June 28) 1944.

30. Heilman, F. R. and Herrell, W. E.: Penicillin in the treatment of experimental infections with Bacillus anthracis. Proc. Staff Meet., Mayo Clin. 19:492–496 (Oct. 4) 1944.

31. Murphy, F. D., La Boccetta, A. C. and Lockwood, J. S.: Treatment of human anthrax with penicillin; report of three cases. J. A. M. A. 126:948–950 (Dec. 9) 1944.

32. Buxton, Russell and Kurman, Rachelle: Tetanus: a report of two cases treated with penicillin. J. A. M. A. 127:26 (Jan. 6) 1945.

CHAPTER XIX

CONSIDERATION OF THE TOXICITY OF PENICILLIN AND OF ITS LACK OF TOXICITY FOR BLOOD CELLS

TOXICITY

It has been emphasized repeatedly by most investigators that use of penicillin is very infrequently followed by serious toxic reactions. This is remarkable when it is considered that most of the penicillin used in the early studies was relatively impure and contained fairly large amounts of products other than penicillin itself. Part of what will be read in the following paragraphs will appear familiar to those who have read the chapter on "Methods of administration and dosage."

Pain at the Site of Intramuscular Injection.—Immediately following injection of penicillin into gluteal or other muscles, pain or a burning sensation may be experienced occasionally. This reaction, however, has not been particularly troublesome. Of 500 cases, in many of which injections were into the gluteal muscles, and which were reported by the Committee on Chemotherapeutic and Other Agents,[1] pain and tenderness in the region occurred in only five. However, these manifestations may occur more frequently in other series. Furthermore, different batches of penicillin have been found to vary somewhat in their tendency to cause pain at the site of local injection. It was evident from the report of Herwick[2] and his colleagues that there was a significant reverse correlation between purity of the preparation and irritation following intramuscular injection; the more nearly pure was the substance, the less was the irritation.

The most helpful suggestion for prevention of irritation on injection is to keep the amount of solvent in which the penicillin is dissolved as small as it can be. If possible, the penicillin for a single intramuscular dose should be given in no more than 3 to 4 c.c. of physiologic saline solution or distilled water. If 10 or 15 c.c. are used, the mere mechanical distention of the muscle fibers may play some part in the reaction. Frequently application of an ice bag for half an hour at the site of injection before penicillin is administered will greatly decrease pain.

Venous Irritation at the Site of Injection.—Local venous irritation at the site of injection of penicillin may occur following repeated venipuncture or following administration of the material by the continuous

251

intravenous drip method. In my experience this reaction also varies considerably with different batches of penicillin. On the other hand, in a fairly large series of cases the reaction does not occur in more than 5 to 10 per cent. This so-called penicillin phlebitis is more an irritative phenomenon than genuine phlebitis if the word "phlebitis" is to be used in its true sense. I have repeatedly administered as much as 200,000 Oxford units of penicillin per day by the intravenous drip method, for as long as eight to ten days, without changing the site of the original injection. To be mentioned in this connection also is the fact that the solvents used may play some part in this reaction. For example, if patients receive penicillin in glucose solution over a long period of time, the solvent may favor venous irritation. Furthermore, if the needle is not carefully seated in the vein and adjusted so as to be kept away from the wall of the vein, venous irritation may occur.

When irritation of the vein occurs at the site of injection, the site of administration should be changed immediately. It is also desirable, when restarting the intravenous drip, to use an entirely new set of tubing and a new needle.

According to Lyons,[3] the so-called phlebitis does not occur at the site of intermittent single injections. In support of this contention he has reported that 500 intravenous injections were given to a single patient without development of thrombosis.

It is generally agreed that veins of the arm should be used for continuous intravenous administration of penicillin, since if thrombosis should occur in a vein of the leg it would be more likely to be followed by embolism. On the other hand, penicillin can be safely administered through veins of the lower extremities. When local irritation or thrombosis develops, the reaction usually will subside promptly after the site of injection has been changed. It is my practice, when irritation or thrombosis appears, immediately to change the site of injection to the other arm or to a vein of the leg and to apply moist, hot packs to the area of irritation. Embolic phenomena have been reported following venous thrombosis in cases in which penicillin has been employed; however, in a fairly large series of cases I have not seen this occur. Whether or not incorporation of small amounts of heparin in the infused material, as recommended by Martin,[4] will prevent development of venous thrombosis will not be known until further trials have been made.

Chills and Fever.—Most of the penicillin now available is pyrogen free and chills and fever following its administration are not commonly encountered. Chills and fever may occur during the course of administration of penicillin, however, for reasons which are not in any way connected with the substance itself. Improperly sterilized apparatus used for administration of penicillin favors conditions which may be followed by chills and fever, just as may occur in association with any intravenous medication if proper care has not been taken in preparation of the tubing and the rest of the intravenous apparatus. Furthermore, any bacterial contamination such as may occur owing to the relatively non-pathogenic "water organisms" may be responsible for chills and fever during administration of penicillin. On several occasions it has been found that chills and fever attributable to penicillin therapy apparently were due to the presence of one of these organisms in the apparatus. These organisms, to be sure, are not highly pathogenic and they disappear rather rapidly from the blood stream of patients; however, their introduction into the blood stream will be followed by chills and fever. The "Herxheimer reaction," with chills and fever, has been mentioned in chapter XVII.

Chills and fever in general have not been encountered in more than 5 to 10 per cent of cases in which penicillin has been used, even including those cases in which treatment was administered in the very early days of use of penicillin, when the substance available was relatively impure. In some series of cases this reaction has not been encountered at all. Here again the reaction may vary somewhat with different preparations. In any event, the reaction does not preclude the continued use of penicillin in a given case. Little or no harm is done the patient by its occurrence. If it occurs during the course of administration of penicillin by the intravenous drip method, the entire apparatus should be discarded for cleaning and sterilization, another set of apparatus secured and the site of injection changed.

Cutaneous Toxic Manifestations.—It is not surprising that a limited number of persons are sensitive to penicillin or to preparations containing mold products other than penicillin. Many individuals are known to be sensitive to certain molds and to substances elaborated by these molds. The cutaneous reactions which have been observed following use of penicillin in a limited number of cases may take the form of either an urticarial type of reaction or true irritative dermatitis.

Urticaria.—There is nothing particularly unique or specific about the type of urticaria which sometimes appears subsequent to administration of penicillin. Furthermore, the reaction may occur following either local or systemic administration of the substance. It may appear within the first few days of the start of penicillin therapy or it may occur late in the course of treatment. It may even occur several days to a week after administration of penicillin has been discontinued. Another interesting aspect of this reaction is that administration of penicillin at times may be continued, or the preparation may be administered again to the same patient after an interval during which it has not been used, without the urticaria developing again. The urticaria usually will disappear, at least temporarily, following administration of epinephrine. At times the urticaria may be accompanied by slight fever and other relatively mild reactions, such as abdominal cramps.

Dermatitis.—Dermatitis or cutaneous eruptions occasionally may develop following local or systemic administration of penicillin, or they may occur in the process of preparing the material, as a result of contact with finished penicillin or with the mold, Penicillium notatum. Penicillin dermatitis, therefore, may be an occupational disease. Although administration of penicillin may be continued in the presence of urticaria, to force its use in the presence of severe dermatitis might result in the development of a more severe, exfoliative lesion.

Graves, Carpenter and Unangst[5] reported two cases in which administration of penicillin was followed by the development of vesicular eruptions on the hands and feet. In one instance, the vesicular eruption appeared within three hours after the patient had received a first injection of 15,000 Oxford units of penicillin. In another case, an itching, vesicular eruption developed on the fingers and palms twenty-four hours after the patient had received the first injection. In the first case, each succeeding injection of 15,000 Oxford units of penicillin was followed by the development of new lesions on the hands, feet and groins. In this case, administration of penicillin was continued in spite of the vesicular eruption and, at the completion of a course of administration of 360,000 Oxford units of penicillin, petechial lesions appeared in profusion on the feet, legs and forearms. The whole process quickly subsided after administration of penicillin had been discontinued. However, all of the involved parts underwent superficial desquamation. It is of some interest that both of the patients had had similar lesions before penicillin had been used and gave histories of positive reactions to trichophytin. A similar type of reaction following the administration of penicillin was observed in a case reported by Binkley and Brockmole.[6]

An interesting example of contact dermatitis from penicillin (dermatitis venenata of the face and genitalia) was reported by Pyle and Rattner.[7] In the case of a medical officer who prepared and administered penicillin to patients, blepharitis, conjunctivitis and some blurring of vision developed. Glasses were prescribed but, according to the investigators, the blepharitis persisted and dermatitis soon appeared on the bridge of the nose and on the forehead. The glasses were then discarded but the dermatitis became worse and the fingers and penis became involved. It was then evident that the patient had a contact dermatitis and an assistant was delegated to handle the penicillin, following which the medical officer's lesions disappeared. Sometime later, when the assistant was not available, the medical officer again was forced to handle solutions of penicillin and, within twenty-four hours, the dermatitis recurred. A patch test with penicillin was performed on this patient and the result was strongly positive. A patch test made with only the medium in which the penicillin was grown gave no reaction. Several weeks later, a patch test was done with crystalline penicillin and a strongly positive reaction occurred. It was therefore concluded that the dermatitis in this case was produced by penicillin itself.

In contrast to the case of dermatitis reported by Pyle and Rattner,[7] is the case reported subsequently by Silvers.[8] Patch tests showed that the skin of Silvers' patient reacted only to the impure penicillin whereas pure white, crystalline penicillin produced no reaction on the skin. Silvers, therefore, concluded that the contact dermatitis in his case was caused by the impurities present in the amorphous sodium penicillin. Binkley and Brockmole[6] have reported another case of proved contact dermatitis due to sodium penicillin. In this instance there occurred a strongly positive skin reaction to a solution of sodium penicillin as measured by intradermal and patch tests.

Even in the presence of these skin reactions, if the infection which is being treated endangers life, and if other forms of treatment are not effective, it is justifiable to continue the use of penicillin. However, the warning which I have already mentioned must be kept in mind; namely, the possibility that an extensive exfoliative lesion may develop.

Interesting studies on the possibility of penicillin allergy have been reported by Feinberg.[9] By means of intracutaneous and scratch tests with various amounts of penicillin, he studied ten patients who were sensitive to various Penicillia and who gave positive reactions to extracts of Penicillium notatum as well as to extracts of Penicillium rubrum and of Penicillium digitatum. All subjects who gave positive scratch reactions to Penicillium notatum failed to react positively either to 500 Oxford units of relatively pure penicillin given intracutaneously or to a scratch test made with a solution containing 5,000 units per cubic centimeter of the same relatively pure preparation. This study would suggest that persons who are sensitive to Penicillium may be safe from allergic reactions to penicillin. Also, it seems to suggest that, not infrequently, certain local reactions probably are not due to penicillin itself but to the mold or other mold products present in some of the penicillin as it is prepared at the present time for clinical use.

Abdominal Pain.—Occasionally, patients who were receiving penicillin have had abdominal colicky pains. The pain is not severe and is of no great importance. The physician should keep it in mind, however. Patients have been encountered whose complaint of this type of pain had caused surgeons seriously to consider the possibility of appendicitis being its cause. As a rule, however, the patient is not sufficiently ill to justify a diagnosis of acute abdominal surgical disease. This lower abdominal pain probably is more frequently encountered among females than among males.

Miscellaneous.—Various other inconsequential reactions have been attributed to administration of penicillin. Included are mild headache, flushing of the face and muscular aches and pains. All of these symptoms are characteristic of any group of patients suffering with bacterial infection and, therefore, it is difficult to state conclusively that any of the symptoms result from penicillin.

Moreover, transient azotemia has been mentioned by the Floreys[10] and by Lyons.[3] According to Lyons, temporary elevations in nonprotein nitrogen of 5 to 10 mg. per 100 c.c. of blood have occurred following administration of penicillin. In view of lack of evidence of renal irritation as measured by other standard procedures, I am inclined to regard such a minimal rise in nonprotein nitrogen as being of little or no significance.

LACK OF TOXICITY FOR BLOOD CELLS

Another remarkable fact in connection with the use of penicillin is the complete lack of evidence of any damage to erythrocytes and leukocytes in the circulating blood of patients who are being treated with the material. In striking contrast to sulfonamides and some other chemotherapeutic agents, penicillin can be administered safely in the presence of marked leukopenia or even of complete agranulocytosis. Repeatedly, among patients with various infections, whose leukocyte counts were extremely low, or from whose blood streams polymorphonuclear leukocytes were absent, I have observed progressive rise in the counts and return of the blood picture to normal following treatment with penicillin. I do not wish to leave the impression that I believe penicillin to be a specific therapeutic agent for agranulocytosis. I do wish to emphasize, however, that penicillin therapy is exceedingly effective in treatment of that type of suppression of bone marrow, with resulting leukopenia, which occasionally is associated with severe overwhelming infection. An example of such improvement in the blood is recorded in the lower part of figure 37. The patient had a severe systemic infection and previously had received sulfonamides. One of the first patients treated with penicillin by the Oxford investigators[11] also demonstrated profound suppression of polymorphonuclear leukocytes and was treated satisfactorily with penicillin. Reports on the successful use of penicillin in treatment of patients with agranulocytosis, which followed sulfonamide therapy for mixed infections, have been made by Sprague and Ferguson[12] and by Meredith, Douglas and Fink.[13]

In this connection also might be mentioned the transient eosinophilia which was reported by Keefer and others,[1] and by Lyons,[3] to occur occasionally in the course of treatment with penicillin. I have not had occasion to see this reaction and I do not know that it is of any great significance.

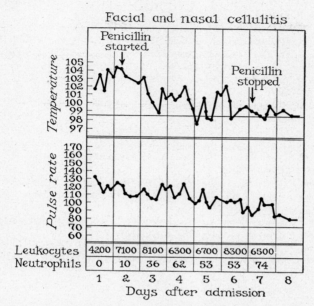

Fig. 37.—The rising leukocyte count and the return of the percentage of neutrophils to normal under penicillin therapy.

COMMENT

The toxic reactions which have been considered in this chapter; namely, pain or irritation at the site of injection, the cutaneous toxic manifestations, chills and fever, as well as other miscellaneous toxic reactions, are all easily recognized and easily controlled. None endangers life and none, for all practical purposes, requires a great deal of the intelligent physician in its management. Some of these reactions are unquestionably due not to penicillin itself but to impurities present in some of the preparations which to date have been available for clinical use. No chemotherapeutic agent yet available presents such a wide margin between therapeutic effectiveness and toxicity.

REFERENCES

1. Keefer, C. S., Blake, F. G., Marshall, E. K., Jr., Lockwood, J. S. and Wood, W. B., Jr.: Penicillin in the treatment of infections; a report of 500 cases. J. A. M. A. *122*:1217–1224 (Aug. 28) 1943.

2. Herwick, R. P., Welch, Henry, Putnam, L. E. and Gamboa, A. M.: Correlation of the purity of penicillin sodium; with intramuscular irritation in man. J. A. M. A. *127*:74–76 (Jan. 13) 1945.

3. Lyons, Champ: Penicillin therapy of surgical infections in the U. S. Army: a report. J. A. M. A. *123*:1007–1018 (Dec. 18) 1943.

4. Martin, Peter: Heparin in intravenous infusions, including penicillin therapy. Brit. M. J. *2*:308 (Sept. 2) 1944.

5. Graves, W. N., Carpenter, C. C. and Unangst, R. W.: Recurrent vesicular eruptions appearing during administrations of penicillin. Arch. Dermat. & Syph. *50*:6–7 (July) 1944.

6. Binkley, G. W. and Brockmole, Arnold: Dermatitis from penicillin; report of two cases. Arch. Dermat. & Syph. *50*:326–327 (Nov.) 1944.

7. Pyle, H. D. and Rattner, Herbert: Contact dermatitis from penicillin. J. A. M. A. *125*:903 (July 29) 1944.

8. Silvers, S. H.: Contact dermatitis from amorphous sodium penicillin. Arch. Dermat. & Syph. *50*:328–329 (Nov.) 1944.

9. Feinberg, S. M.: Penicillin allergy: on the probability of allergic reactions in fungus-sensitive individuals; preliminary experiments. J. Allergy. *15*:271–273 (July) 1944.

10. Florey, M. E. and Florey, H. W.: General and local administration of penicillin. Lancet. *1*:387–397 (Mar.) 1943.

11. Abraham, E. P., Chain, E., Fletcher, C. M., Gardner, A. D., Heatley, N. G., Jennings, M. A. and Florey, H. W.: Further observations on penicillin. Lancet. *2*:177–188; 189 (Aug. 16) 1941.

12. Sprague, H. B. and Ferguson, L. K.: Agranulocytosis treated with penicillin; report of case. U. S. Nav. M. Bull. *43*:1014–1016 (Nov.) 1944.

13. Meredith, W. C., Douglas, A. H. R. and Fink, Harold: Penicillin in malignant granulocytopenia; report of case. U. S. Nav. M. Bull. *43*:1017–1019 (Nov.) 1944.

PART IV

OTHER ANTIBIOTIC AGENTS

CHAPTER XX

INTRODUCTION

Although the theory of bacterial antagonism has been known since 1877, it is only in recent years that the therapeutic possibilities associated with this phenomenon have been extensively explored. According to Chain and Florey,[1] Pasteur and Joubert[2] in 1877 described the antagonistic effect of certain contaminating organisms on the growth of Bacillus anthracis. Even at this early date, Pasteur and Joubert were aware that this phenomenon of bacterial antagonism possessed therapeutic possibilities.

Since the days of Pasteur, many investigators from time to time have been interested in the general subject of bacterial antagonism. To obtain some idea of the enormous amount of data which already have accumulated, the reader will do well to examine the extensive review of this subject published by Waksman[3] in 1941. Waksman and others,[4] in 1942, suggested the terms "antibiotic" and "antibiotic effect" in connection with antibacterial agents of microbial origin. These terms are now generally accepted as descriptive of these agents or of their action. The term "antibiotic" therefore is herein used in connection with the description of these agents and their properties.

CHRONOLOGIC CONSIDERATION

It is evident from a clinical standpoint that the most important antibiotic agent yet available is penicillin, which has been considered in detail in previous parts of this monograph. It should be emphasized, however, that penicillin was not the first antibiotic agent discovered. The first attempt to employ an antibiotic agent for treatment of infections was made by Emmerich and Loew[5] who, in 1899, used for this purpose a culture medium containing what they believed to be an enzyme, "pyocyanase." That the organism Pseudomonas pyocyanea was antagonistic to other bacterial species had been discovered by Bouchard[6] in 1889; on the other hand, he did not name the antibacterial substance. Emmerich and Loew further reported that experimental anthrax could be cured by pyocyanase and, according to Chain and Florey,[1] these investigators suggested its use for local treatment of diphtheria as well as of certain other infections. In light of subsequent experience, however, it seems evident that this enzyme did not find great usefulness in treatment of bacterial infections. Of some interest, nevertheless, is the fact that Wrede and Strack[7] later found that the organism Pseudomonas aeruginosa elaborated at least one other substance in addition to pyocyanase. This other substance was called "pyocyanin."

In 1913, another antibiotic substance was described by Alsberg and Black.[8] To this was given the name "penicillic acid" and the substance was reported to be produced by Penicillium puberulum. According to the investigators, this agent was found to be effective against both gram-positive and gram-negative pathogens. This same substance, penicillic acid, was studied more intensively in 1942 by Oxford, Raistrick and Smith.[9]

The next antibiotic agent to be seriously considered was described by Gratia and Dath[10] in 1924. This substance was produced by strains of Actinomyces and to it was given the name "actinomycetin." It was found also to be effective against certain gram-positive, as well as gram-negative, organisms.

It is well known that five years later, in 1929, penicillin was discovered by Fleming.[11] It is also well known that this important antibiotic agent was derived from a strain of mold, Penicillium, later identified as Penicillium notatum. In this section no further description will appear concerning the isolation, purification or clinical use of penicillin.

In 1931, citrinin, another antibiotic substance, was reported by Hetherington, Raistrick and their colleagues.[12,13] The source of citrinin was a species of Penicillium identified as Penicillium citrinum, Thom. The agent was later found to be effective primarily against gram-positive bacteria. The investigators reported rather extensive studies of the molecular structure of this substance.

The next antibiotic agent described was gliotoxin, which was reported by Weindling and Emerson[14] in 1936. The source of gliotoxin was Trichoderma lignorum and the substance was said to be effective against both gram-positive and gram-negative organisms. Two years later (1938) Anslow and Raistrick[15] described another antibiotic substance, fumigatin, a heretofore undescribed metabolic product elaborated by Aspergillus fumigatus. This substance was subsequently found to possess antibacterial activity against certain gram-positive pathogens.

Widespread new interest and revival of interest in antibacterial agents of microbial origin followed the report on gramicidin by Dubos[16] in 1939. The source of this antibiotic substance was Bacillus brevis and the agent was found to be predominantly effective against gram-positive pathogenic organisms. To this substance was given the name "gramicidin" but it was later to be called "tyrothricin" since Hotchkiss and Dubos[17] found that what had been called "gramicidin" in the beginning was a mixture of two different substances now known as (1) pure gramicidin and (2) tyrocidine.

The following year (1940) Waksman and Woodruff[18] reported on the isolation of actinomycin A and B from the organism Actinomyces antibioticus. These substances were said to be bacteriostatic for many gram-positive bacteria and only weakly active against gram-negative organisms. Several other antibiotic agents were described in 1942. During this year, the isolation of streptothricin was reported by Waksman and his associates.[19, 20] The source of this antibiotic substance was Actinomyces lavendulae. The agent appeared to be somewhat polyvalent in its activity since both gram-positive and gram-negative organisms were sensitive to its action. In this same year, penicillic acid, derived from Penicillium cyclopium and Penicillium puberulum was reinvestigated by Oxford, Raistrick and Smith.[9] Also, in 1942, claviformin,[21] described later as "patulin,"[22] another agent effective against both gram-positive and gram-negative organisms, was described. Claviformin was derived from Penicillium claviforme and was described by Chain, Florey and Jennings.[21]

Two other antibiotic agents were described by Waksman and his colleagues[23] in 1942. One of these substances, fumigacin, was derived from Aspergillus fumigatus, the same organism from which Anslow and Raistrick[15] had obtained fumigatin in 1938. The other agent reported by Waksman and his associates was derived from Aspergillus clavatus and was named "clavacin." This agent was said to be effective also against both gram-positive and gram-negative organisms.

In 1943, another antibiotic substance, named "aspergillic acid" was described. This substance was obtained from Aspergillus flavus. According to White and Hill,[24] who described the substance, it was effective against both gram-positive and gram-negative pathogenic organisms. It should be pointed out, however, that the bactericidal property of filtrates of the media in which Aspergillus flavus had been grown had been mentioned previously by White,[25] in 1940. Also in 1943, Bush and Goth[26] described flavicin, which also was obtained from Aspergillus flavus. This substance, according to the investigators, behaved in some ways like penicillin and, in fact, appeared to be somewhat more active than penicillin against certain gram-positive organisms. Another antibiotic agent reported in 1943 was helvolic acid. This agent was obtained from Aspergillus fumigatus and was reported by Chain, Florey, Jennings and Williams[27] to be effective against gram-positive organisms. Also in 1943, Philpot[28] reported on gigantic acid, an antibiotic agent similar to penicillin. The substance was obtained from Aspergillus giganteus. It appeared to Philpot, therefore, that production of antibiotic agents chemically similar to penicillin was not limited to the genus Penicillium since it was shown by her work, as well as by that of others, that at least two different species of Aspergillus were capable of producing such substances.

It is evident, therefore, that approximately a dozen antibiotic agents were described in the five years (1939–1943) which immediately followed the report on gramicidin by Dubos.

In January, 1944, a new antibiotic substance which may prove of considerable importance was described by Schatz, Bugie and Waksman.[29] To this substance was given the name "streptomycin" by the group of investigators at Rutgers University because the substance was produced by one of the aerial-mycelium producing and sporulating group of actinomycetes. To this group of actinomycetes Waksman and Henrici,[30] in 1943, had given the generic name "Streptomyces." Streptomycin was obtained from two strains of Actinomyces griseus. These strains of Actinomyces were similar in cultural characteristics as well as morphology to a strain of Actinomyces griseus which had been described some twenty-five years before by Waksman. While streptomycin resembles in some respects the previously described antibiotic agent, streptothricin (from Actinomyces lavendulae), it was evident that streptomycin differed from streptothricin in that streptomycin possessed greater activity against various gram-negative organisms. Furthermore, streptomycin appears to possess little, if any, toxicity for animals.

Another antibiotic agent was described in 1944 to which was given the name "flavacidin." This substance was isolated by McKee, Rake and Houck[31] from Aspergillus flavus. Their studies gave good evidence that the biologic characteristics of flavacidin and penicillin are similar. The similarity between these substances will be mentioned again later.

It is now agreed by all students of the general subject that the phenomenon of bacterial antagonism and the existence of many antibiotic agents are rather widespread in nature. The entire field is being extensively explored and hundreds of such agents probably will be described. I have attempted, therefore, to enumerate the more important antibiotic substances which were isolated between the time of the initial studies on the general subject in 1877 and the time of preparation of this monograph in 1944.

CONSIDERATION FROM THE STANDPOINT OF ORIGIN

From a general standpoint, I have found it practical to follow the suggestion of Waksman and Woodruff[32] of classifying antibiotic agents produced by microbes according to their origin. Antibiotic agents obtained from sources other than microbes (lysozyme, chlorellin and so forth) are not included in this classification but will be discussed in the chapter on antibiotic substances originating from sources other than microbes (Chapter XXV). In the present classification, antibiotic agents of microbial origin may be said to be derived from three general sources: (1) nonspore-forming or spore-forming bacteria; (2) molds and fungi and (3) actinomycetes.

In the foregoing classification, group 1 includes, as I already have mentioned, antibacterial agents obtained from bacteria, either non-spore-forming or spore-forming. Examples of these agents of bacterial origin are listed in table 24.

Group 2 includes the antibacterial agents obtained from molds and fungi. Examples are listed in table 25, from examination of which it is evident that the two most important sources of antibiotic substances in this group are species of Penicillium and species of Aspergillus. While

TABLE 24

ANTIBIOTIC AGENTS OF BACTERIAL ORIGIN

Antibiotic agent	Organism from which derived	Author who described agent and date of report	Organisms sensitive to agent
Pyocyanase	Pseudomonas aeruginosa	Emmerich and Loew, 1899	Gram-positive and gram-negative
Pyocyanine	Pseudomonas aeruginosa	Wrede and Strack, 1924	Mainly gram-positive
Tyrothricin Gramicidin Tyrocidine	Bacillus brevis Bacillus brevis Bacillus brevis	Dubos, 1939 Hotchkiss and Dubos, 1940 Hotchkiss and Dubos, 1940	Gram-positive Gram-positive Gram-positive; some gram-negative

some of the antibiotic substances shown in the table have not been isolated in pure form, they have been fairly well recognized by their chemical and biologic properties. Further, it is now evident that several of the agents obtained from fungi are at least similar and they may be identical. It seems probable, for example, that claviformin, clavacin and patulin are identical substances, isolated and named differently by different groups of investigators. Likewise, it appears that fumigacin and helvolic acid, both of which are obtained from Aspergillus fumigatus, are similar if not identical.

Group 3 includes those antibacterial agents which originate from actinomycetes (table 26).

Of the antibiotic agents of bacterial origin, tyrothricin (crude grami-cidin) has proved to date to be the most important as far as possible clinical application is concerned. It seems clear, also, that at the moment

TABLE 25
ANTIBIOTIC AGENTS DERIVED FROM MOLDS AND FUNGI

Antibiotic agent	Organism from which derived	Author who described agent and date of report	Organisms sensitive to agent
Penicillic acid	Penicillium puberulum	Alsberg and Black, 1913	Gram-positive and gram-negative
Penicillin	Penicillium notatum	Fleming, 1929	Gram-positive and some gram-negative
Citrinin	Penicillium citrinum	Hetherington, Raistrick and others, 1931	Gram-positive
Gliotoxin	Trichoderma lignorum	Weindling and Emerson, 1936	Gram-positive and gram-negative
Fumigatin	Aspergillus fumigatus	Anslow and Raistrick, 1938	Gram-positive
Claviformin*	Penicillium claviforme	Chain, Florey and Jennings, 1942	Gram-positive and gram-negative
Fumigacin†	Aspergillus fumigatus	Waksman, Horning and Spencer, 1942	Gram-positive
Clavacin*	Aspergillus clavatus	Waksman, Horning and Spencer, 1942	Gram-positive and gram-negative
Aspergillic acid	Aspergillus flavus	White and Hill, 1943	Gram-positive and gram-negative
Flavicin	Aspergillus flavus	Bush and Goth, 1943	Gram-positive
Helvolic acid†	Aspergillus fumigatus	Chain, Florey, Jennings and Williams, 1943	Gram-positive
Patulin*	Penicillium patulum	Raistrick and others, 1943	Gram-positive and gram-negative
Gigantic acid	Aspergillus giganteus	Philpot, 1943	Gram-positive
Flavacidin	Aspergillus flavus	McKee, Rake and Houck, 1944	Gram-positive

* Claviformin, clavacin and patulin are similar if not identical.
† Fumigacin and helvolic acid are similar if not identical.

the most important antibiotic agent derived from molds and fungi is penicillin, which has been considered in the previous sections of this book. It appears likely, moreover, that penicillin is not only the most important antibiotic substance from this source but also the most important of any of the antibiotic substances available to date. Of the antibiotic agents originating from actinomycetes, it seems reasonable to state that the most important are streptothricin and streptomycin.

TABLE 26

ANTIBIOTIC AGENTS DERIVED FROM ACTINOMYCETES

Antibiotic agent	Organism from which derived	Author who described agent and date of report	Organisms sensitive to agent
Actinomycetin	Actinomyces	Gratia and Dath, 1924	Gram-positive and gram-negative
Actinomycin A	Actinomyces antibioticus	Waksman and Woodruff, 1940	Gram-positive
Actinomycin B	Actinomyces antibioticus	Waksman and Woodruff, 1940	Gram-positive
Streptothricin	Actinomyces lavendulae	Waksman and Woodruff, 1942	Gram-negative and gram-positive
Streptomycin	Actinomyces griseus	Schatz, Bugie and Waksman, 1944	Gram-negative and gram-positive

This monograph is designed primarily to deal with the clinical application of antibiotic agents and for that reason only those antibiotic agents (tyrothricin, streptothricin and streptomycin) which appear to possess possible clinical application will be considered in detail in this part of the book. The properties of those antibiotic substances which, at the time of this writing, do not appear to be of great importance from a clinical standpoint will be discussed in the chapter on miscellaneous antibiotic agents (p. 321).

REFERENCES

1. Chain, E. and Florey, H. W.: Penicillin. Endeavour. vol. 3, no. 9 (Jan.) 1944.
2. Pasteur, L. and Joubert: Quoted by Chain, E. and Florey, H. W.[1]
3. Waksman, S. A.: Antagonistic relations of microörganisms. Bact. Rev. 5:231–291 (Sept.) 1941.
4. Waksman, S. A., Horning, E. S., Welsch, M. and Woodruff, H. B.: Distribution of antagonistic actinomycetes in nature. Soil Sc. 54:281–295, 1942.
5. Emmerich, R. and Loew, C.: Quoted by Chain, E. and Florey, H. W.[1]
6. Bouchard, L.: Quoted by Chain, E. and Florey, H. W.[1]
7. Wrede, F. and Strack, E.: Quoted by Waksman, S. A.[3]
8. Alsberg, C. L. and Black, O. F : Quoted by Chain, E. and Florey, H. W.[1]
9. Oxford, A. E., Raistrick, H. and Smith, G.: Antibacterial substances from moulds. II. Penicillic acid, a metabolic product of Penicillium puberulum Bainier and Penicillium cyclopium Westling. Chem. & Ind. 61:22 (Jan. 10) 1942.
10. Gratia, A. and Dath, S.: Quoted by Chain, E. and Florey, H. W.[1]
11. Fleming, Alexander: On the antibacterial action of cultures of a penicillium, with special reference to their use in the isolation of *B. influenzae*. Brit. J. Exper. Path. 10:226–236 (June) 1929.
12. Hetherington, A. C. and Raistrick, H.: Studies in the biochemistry of micro-organisms. Part XIV. On the production and chemical constitution of a new yellow colouring

matter, citrinin, produced from glucose by Penicillium citrinum, Thom. Tr. Roy. Soc. London. s.B., *220*:269–295, 1931. (Abstr.) Chem. Abstr. *26*:2486 (May 10) 1932.

13. Coyne, F. P., Raistrick, Harold and Robinson, Robert: Studies in the biochemistry of micro-organisms. Part XV. The molecular structure of citrinin. Tr. Roy. Soc. London. s.B., *220*:297–300, 1931. (Abstr.) Chem. Abstr. *26*:2486 (May 10) 1932.

14. Weindling, R. and Emerson, O. H.: Quoted by Chain, E. and Florey, H. W.;[1] Waksman, S. A.[3]

15. Anslow, W. K. and Raistrick, Harold: Studies in the biochemistry of micro-organisms. LVII. Biochem. J. *32*:687–696, 1938.

16. Dubos, R. J.: Studies on a bactericidal agent extracted from a soil bacillus. I. Preparation of the agent, its activity in vitro. J. Exper. Med. *70*:1–10 (July) 1939.

17. Hotchkiss, R. D. and Dubos, R. J.: Bactericidal fractions from an aerobic sporulating bacillus. J. Biol. Chem. *136*:803–804 (Dec.) 1940.

18. Waksman, S. A. and Woodruff, H. B.: Bacteriostatic and bactericidal substances produced by a soil Actinomyces. Proc. Soc. Exper. Biol. & Med. *45*:609–614 (Nov.) 1940.

19. Waksman, S. A., Woodruff, H. B. and Horning, Elizabeth S.: The distribution of antagonistic properties among actinomycetes. J. Bact. *42*:816 (Dec.) 1941.

20. Waksman, S. A. and Woodruff, H. B.: Streptothricin, new selective bacteriostatic and bactericidal agent, particularly active against gram-negative bacteria. Proc. Soc. Exper. Biol. & Med. *49*:207–210 (Feb.) 1942.

21. Chain, E., Florey, H. W. and Jennings, M. A.: An antibacterial substance produced by Penicillium claviforme. Brit. J. Exper. Path. *23*:202–205 (Aug.) 1942.

22. Raistrick, Harold and others: Patulin in the common cold. Collaborative research on a derivative or *Penicillium patulum* Bainier. Lancet. *2*:625–635 (Nov. 20) 1943.

23. Waksman, S. A., Horning, Elizabeth S. and Spencer, E. L.: The production of two antibacterial substances, fumigacin and clavacin. Science. n.s. *96*:202–203 (Aug. 28) 1942.

24. White, E. C. and Hill, Justina H.: Studies on the antibacterial products formed by molds. I. Aspergillic acid, a product of a strain of Aspergillus flavus. J. Bact. *45*:433–442 (May) 1943.

25. White, E. C.: Bactericidal filtrates from a mold culture. Science. n.s. *92*:127 (Aug. 9) 1940.

26. Bush, M. T. and Goth, Andres: Flavicin; an antibacterial substance produced by an Aspergillus flavus. J. Pharmacol. & Exper. Therap. *78*:164–169 (June) 1943.

27. Chain, E., Florey, H. W., Jennings, M. A. and Williams, T. I.: Helvolic acid, antibiotic produced by Aspergillus fumigatus, mut. helvola Yuill. Brit. J. Exper. Path. *24*:108–119 (June) 1943.

28. Philpot, Flora J.: A penicillin-like substance from Aspergillus giganteus Wehm. Nature. *152*:725 (Dec. 18) 1943.

29. Schatz, Albert, Bugie, Elizabeth and Waksman, S. A.: Streptomycin, a substance exhibiting antibiotic activity against gram-positive and gram-negative bacteria. Proc. Soc. Exper. Biol. & Med. *55*:66–69 (Jan.) 1944.

30. Waksman, S. A. and Henrici, A. T.: The nomenclature and classification of the actinomycetes. J. Bact. *46*:337–341 (Oct.) 1943.

31. McKee, C. M., Rake, Geoffrey, and Houck, C. L.: Studies on Aspergillus flavus. II. The production and properties of a penicillin-like substance—flavacidin. J. Bact. *47*:187–197 (Feb.) 1944.

32. Waksman, S. A. and Woodruff, H. B.: Selective antibiotic action of various substances of microbial origin. J. Bact. *44*:373–384 (Sept.) 1942.

CHAPTER XXI

TYROTHRICIN (GRAMICIDIN AND TYROCIDINE)

DUBOS' DISCOVERY

Dubos[1,2] (1939), and Dubos and his colleagues,[3-5] deserve great credit for having isolated from bacteria specific chemical antibacterial agents. The organism which Dubos studied and from which he obtained these substances was the gram-positive, spore-forming bacterium, Bacillus brevis, which was isolated from soil that had been enriched with various pathogens. It was evident to Dubos that this organism elaborated an antibiotic substance into the medium in which the organism grew.

After Bacillus brevis had been grown in 1 per cent tryptone broth for four days at 37° C. the active principle, first named "gramicidin," was found to be present in the medium. Incubation was carried out in shallow layers. Isolation of the substance was effected by adjusting the whole culture to a pH of 4.5 by addition of concentrated hydrochloric acid. A heavy precipitate formed which contained cellular material and the active bactericidal substance. The precipitate was obtained by filtration and the clear filtrate discarded. The precipitate then was taken up in acetone which contained hydrochloric acid and was allowed to stand for twenty-four hours. The acetone soluble fraction was then obtained by filtration and the acetone removed by distillation. The residue in the distillation flask then was thrown into water to which had been added hydrochloric acid. A heavy precipitate formed and the mixture was then filtered through a Büchner funnel. The filtrate was discarded and the precipitate desiccated in vacuo over phosphorus pentoxide. By certain other refinements in the process of extraction, Dubos and Cattaneo[3] were able to obtain a very active, purified, protein-free preparation of the material which had been isolated from the soil bacillus and which appeared to exert marked antibacterial effect on gram-positive micro-organisms.

This substance later was found by Hotchkiss and Dubos[4,5] to consist of two separate fractions and, therefore, what was earlier known as "gramicidin" henceforth was known as "tyrothricin." The two separate substances are tyrocidine and pure gramicidin. The relationship of gramicidin and tyrocidine to the parent substance, tyrothricin, can be better understood from table 27, which was published by Dubos and Hotchkiss.[6]

Henceforth in this chapter the word "tyrothricin" is used to describe the antibiotic substance obtained from Bacillus brevis which, as I have said, is a mixture of both gramicidin and tyrocidine. For certain experimental studies, each of these two substances has been used in its pure state; however, for clinical purposes practically all of the material used is tyrothricin. Tyrothricin, gramicidin and tyrocidine are fairly stable substances which in their final form exist as powders or in crystalline form. Purified gramicidin is obtained by extraction from the crude material. The crystals appear as colorless platelets (fig. 38). The em-

TABLE 27

PREPARATION OF TYROTHRICIN, GRAMICIDIN AND TYROCIDINE

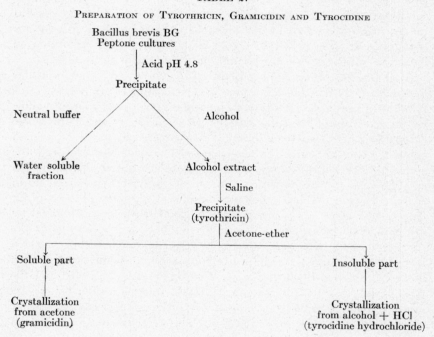

pirical formula suggested by Dubos and Hotchkiss is: $C_{74}H_{105}N_{15}O_{13}$ (molecular weight, 1,413). The substance appears to have no free carboxyl or amino groups, although it is composed of amino acids.

Tyrocidine, the second fraction present in tyrothricin, appears to be a basic polypeptide (fig. 39). In contrast to gramicidin, tyrocidine, according to Dubos and Hotchkiss,[6] contains many amino acids suitable for quantitative estimation. The investigators named have suggested that the approximate formula for tyrocidine is: $C_{126}H_{166}N_{26}O_{26} \cdot 2HCl$ (molecular weight 2,534).

Unlike the antibiotic agent, penicillin, tyrothricin and its fractions are not soluble in many ordinary solvents. Tyrothricin itself is soluble in alcohol but is insoluble in water, chloroform, sulfuric ether, petroleum ether, benzol or toluol. By dissolving tyrothricin in alcohol, however,

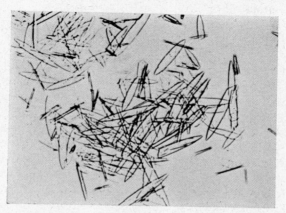

Fig. 38.—Photomicrograph of crystals of gramicidin ($\times$ 225). (From article by Dubos and Hotchkiss, Transactions and Studies of the College of Physicians of Philadelphia, April, 1942.)

suspensions suitable for experimental or clinical use can be made by adding this alcohol stock solution to physiologic saline solution or triple distilled water. Both gramicidin and tyrocidine are stable in alcohol

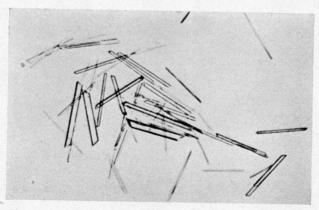

Fig. 39.—Photomicrograph of crystals of tyrocidine hydrochloride ($\times$ 320). (From article by Dubos and Hotchkiss, Transactions and Studies of the College of Physicians of Philadelphia, April, 1942.)

solutions even when maintained at high temperatures. Both gramicidin and tyrocidine are only feebly soluble in water; however, fairly stable colloidal emulsions of either substance can be made in distilled water.

Both gramicidin and tyrocidine behave as surface active substances (this is especially true of tyrocidine) and it has been suggested by Dubos and Hotchkiss[6] that tyrocidine increases appreciably the stability of emulsions of gramicidin.

ANTIBACTERIAL ACTIVITY OF TYROTHRICIN AND ITS COMPONENTS IN VITRO

In the first studies reported by Dubos[1] (February, 1939) tyrothricin, which later was to be found to contain both gramicidin and tyrocidine, was used. It was evident from experiments of Dubos that this crude material (tyrothricin) was highly antibacterial. One milligram of the material added to a medium containing 10^9 pneumococci resulted in lysis of the bacterial cells after incubation at 37° C. for one hour. Further, staphylococci and streptococci would undergo lysis under the same conditions but at a somewhat slower rate. Minute amounts of the extract added to broth also would prevent growth of other gram-positive cocci. According to studies made by Dubos, 0.0001 mg. of the crude substance was sufficient to inhibit growth when 5 c.c. of broth was inoculated with 10^7 pneumococci. These studies were extended by Dubos[2, 7] and by Dubos and his colleagues[3] and reports of them appeared in subsequent communications.

Further studies on the antibacterial activity of tyrothricin and its two fractions in vitro were reported by Dorothy Heilman and me.[8] In our work, the tissue culture method was used to test the antibacterial activity of these agents. This method has two advantages: 1. The effect of the substance on pathogenic bacteria growing in the presence of tissue, serum and tissue extract can be observed. 2. Also, it is possible to observe the effect of the substance on the growth and maintenance of various types of cells, as well as on erythrocytes suspended in the tissue culture clot.

The tissue culture method used in the studies of bactericidal effect was similar to the modified Maximow technic described by King, Henschel and Green.[9] The tissue culture was planted on a 22 mm. round coverslip and consisted of a drop of heparinized plasma from the blood of a rabbit and three drops of tissue extract made by extracting seven-day chick embryos with rabbit serum. To the preparation was added an explant from a mesenteric lymph node of a rabbit; each explant measured approximately 1.5 mm. across. The total volume of each culture was approximately 0.2 c.c. Bacterial cultures used in this study were grown in dextrose-brain broth. One cubic centimeter of rabbit serum was added to a brain broth culture of pneumococci and hemolytic streptococci. Dilutions of young dextrose-brain broth cultures were made in plain broth and added to the tissue extract in the proportion of one part of a suspension of bacteria in plain broth to forty parts of tissue extract. The final concentration of the original bacterial culture in the tissue culture clot was 1:10,000,000. This inoculum resulted in the appearance of twenty or more bacterial colonies in each tissue culture preparation, with the exception of certain strains of hemolytic streptococci which grew only in the vicinity of the fragment of tissue. It was necessary to use a dilution of 1:1,000,000 of these strains.

TABLE 28

AMOUNTS OF BACTERICIDAL SUBSTANCE CAUSING INHIBITION

Organism	Number	Tyrothricin	Gramicidin	Tyrocidine
		µg. per c.c.	µg. per c.c.	µg. per c.c.
Diplococcus pneumoniae				
Type I		2.5	1.0	100
Type III	1	1.0	0.5	20
Type III	2	1.0	1.0	20
Type XIX			2.5	40
Hemolytic streptococcus	1	10	5.0	80
(Group A Lancefield)	2		5.0	100
	3		10.0	80
	4		5.0	100
	5		20.0	120
Streptococcus viridans	1		10	60
group	2		60	120
Streptococcus faecalis	1	20	40	300
	2		60	– – –*
	3		20	260
	4		60	300
Staphylococcus aureus	1		100	140
	2		– – –*	– – –*
	3		300	– – –*
	4		– – –*	– – –*
	5		– – –*	– – –*
	6		300	300

* Not inhibited by 300 µg. of bactericidal substance.
From article by Herrell and Heilman, Journal of Clinical Investigation, September, 1941.

Three fractions of the substance elaborated by the soil bacillus were used: the crude bactericidal substance, tyrothricin, and the two fractions, gramicidin and tyrocidine. Since all three of these products of the soil bacillus are insoluble in saline solutions, each material was dissolved in 95 per cent alcohol, and the resulting solution was suspended in Tyrode's solution. Such suspensions, containing varying amounts of bactericidal substance, were added in the ratio of 1:10 to plasma and to tissue extract which, in turn, were used in preparing the tissue culture clot. The greatest amount of bactericidal substance used was 300 micrograms per cubic centimeter of medium. Similar mixtures of 95 per cent alcohol and Tyrode's solution, but without bactericidal substance, were added to plasma and to tissue for use in tissue culture clots, as controls. Four cultures were prepared for each experimental condition. Cultures were incubated at 37° C. in a specially constructed circulation type incu-

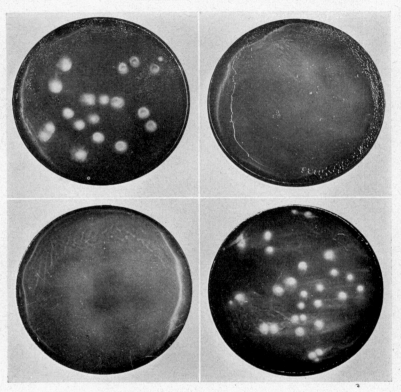

Fig. 40.—Tissue culture clots containing Diplococcus pneumoniae type I after forty-eight hours' incubation at 37° C. *Upper left*, control. *Upper right*, clot treated with 2.5 micrograms tyrothricin per cubic centimeter media. Complete inhibition. *Lower left*, clot treated with 1 microgram gramicidin per cubic centimeter. Complete inhibition. *Lower right*, clot treated with 40 micrograms tyrocidine per cubic centimeter. No inhibition. (From article by Herrell and Heilman, Journal of Clinical Investigation, September, 1941.)

bator,[10] and final readings were made after the culture had been incubated for forty-eight hours. The cultures were examined by using a magnification of seven diameters. The least amount of bactericidal substance which would completely prevent the appearance of bacterial colonies in all four cultures after incubation for forty-eight hours was determined for each bacterial strain tested.

Tissue cultures to which bactericidal substances and bacteria had been added, but which showed no evidence of bacterial growth in forty-eight hours, were put into tubes of dextrose-brain broth to which 1 c.c. of horse serum or rabbit serum had been added. These cultures were incubated at 37° C. for five days in order to determine whether or not any viable bacteria were present.

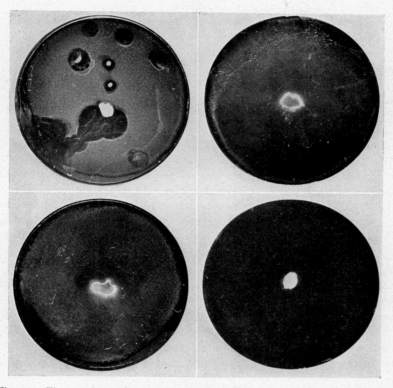

Fig. 41.—Tissue culture clots containing hemolytic streptococcus and lymph node explants after forty-eight hours' incubation at 37° C. *Upper left,* control. Note liquefaction of plasma around colonies. *Upper right,* clot treated with tyrothricin 10 micrograms per cubic centimeter. Complete inhibition. *Lower left,* clot treated with 5 micrograms gramicidin per cubic centimeter. Complete inhibition. *Lower right,* clot treated with 100 micrograms tyrocidine per cubic centimeter. Complete inhibition. (From article by Herrell and Heilman, Journal of Clinical Investigation, September, 1941.)

The results of the bactericidal tests are recorded in table 28. There was a considerable degree of species resemblance in the reaction of the various strains to gramicidin. Dubos also observed this in his in vitro experiments. The amount of gramicidin necessary to inhibit the growth of all representatives of each species was as follows: Diplococcus pneumoniae, 0.5 to 2.5 micrograms per cubic centimeter; hemolytic strepto-coccus, 5 to 20 micrograms per cubic centimeter; Streptococcus faecalis, 20 to 60 micrograms per cubic centimeter; Streptococcus salivarius, 10 to 60 micrograms per cubic centimeter; and Staphylococcus aureus, 100 to 300 micrograms per cubic centimeter. Three strains of Staphylococcus aureus were not inhibited by 300 micrograms of gramicidin per cubic centimeter. For the most part, a slightly greater amount of tyrothricin had to be used to cause inhibition of bacterial growth as compared to gramicidin. In general, it was necessary to use a much greater concen-tration of tyrocidine than of gramicidin to obtain the same degree of inhibition (figs. 40 and 41).

Although no bacterial growth occurred in cultures containing a suffi-cient amount of bactericidal substance, not all of the bacteria were killed. When such cultures were placed in brain broth, serum added, and incubated at 37° C. for several days, an occasional tube would show growth of the organism originally introduced into the tissue culture. This occurred when any of the bactericidal fractions were used and for all species except Staphylococcus aureus. In experiments with this species, however, there were few negative clots available for study.

It was further evident from the report of Rodaniche and Palmer[11] that Streptococcus faecalis and related fecal streptococci were sensitive to the action of tyrothricin. It is clear, therefore, that tyrothricin, like most of the other antibiotic agents, tends to exhibit a rather selective antibacterial activity. Observations on the general subject of activity of tyrothricin in vitro were subsequently reported by Rammelkamp[12] who studied the effectiveness of tyrothricin against various strains of Staphylococcus aureus. From his report it appeared that various strains of Staphylococcus aureus were somewhat resistant to the action of this antibiotic agent. It was further evident that the resistance to tyrothricin could be increased by growing the organisms in the presence of increasing concentrations of the bactericidal substance. Downs[13, 14] also investi-gated the activity in vitro of gramicidin and tyrocidine on a variety of pathogenic organisms. It was evident from these studies that gramicidin and tyrocidine both were fairly active substances when tested against gram-positive coccal forms. There was also some evidence from the studies of Downs that both gramicidin and tyrocidine would inhibit the growth of Neisseria intracellularis and Neisseria gonorrhoeae. However, at least fifty times more was required to inhibit certain gram-negative pathogens than was required to inhibit Diplococcus pneumoniae, type I. It was further evident that either of these substances might, under certain conditions, be bactericidal but, for the most part, they should be considered bacteriostatic agents.

In view of the fact that Neisseria gonorrhoeae was only slightly sensitive to the action of tyrothricin or its two components, Stokinger, Ackerman and Carpenter[15] recommended the routine use of tyrothricin in concentrations of 1:15,000 in chocolate blood-agar cultures used to isolate Neisseria gonorrhoeae. The amount used was for the purpose of inhibiting the growth of contaminating pathogens. While this procedure may be of some value, it is exceedingly important to keep the amount of tyrothricin small in order not to get into the range which might also result in inhibition of Neisseria gonorrhoeae and thus yield false-negative cultures from clinical material studied as a routine in the bacteriologic laboratory.

Further studies on the activity of gramicidin and tyrocidine in vitro, made by Dubos, Hotchkiss and Coburn,[16] suggested that the latter substance inhibited the oxidation-reduction system of Staphylococcus aureus and Streptococcus pyogenes; however, there was some evidence that gramicidin only partially injured the cells and could either depress or stimulate metabolism, depending on the conditions of the experiment.

The studies of Robinson and Graessle[17] on tyrothricin, gramicidin and tyrocidine seemed to indicate that tyrothricin exerted bactericidal action on aerobic and anaerobic gram-positive bacteria. Gramicidin, according to the investigators, appeared to be only bacteriostatic. From their studies it was further suggested that tyrothricin and tyrocidine lose their bactericidal properties in the presence of blood or serum, whereas gramicidin retains its activity under similar conditions.

In connection with the studies on antibacterial action of gramicidin and tyrocidine against rhizobia, it appeared from the report of Trussell and Sarles[18] that gramicidin and tyrothricin may be bacteriostatic or bactericidal depending on the conditions of the experiment and that tyrocidine is usually bactericidal. I am inclined to believe that neither tyrothricin nor its two components can be considered as bactericidal agents except under conditions wherein large amounts of the material are present.

While gramicidin and tyrocidine are fairly active against most gram-positive coccal pathogens, with the possible exception of strains of Staphylococcus aureus which are somewhat resistant, it was evident from the studies of Dubos,[2] as well as from those of subsequent investigators, that gramicidin exerted little if any effect against gram-negative bacteria. Neither the viability nor the growth of most gram-negative organisms appears to be affected by even large amounts of this agent. Tyrocidine, on the other hand, according to Dubos and Hotchkiss,[6] appeared under certain conditions to exert antibacterial activity against both gram-positive and gram-negative species. Neither tyrothricin, gramicidin nor tyrocidine appears to inhibit the growth of Mycobacterium tuberculosis.

ANTIBACTERIAL ACTIVITY OF TYROTHRICIN AND ITS COMPONENTS IN VIVO

The first report on the activity in vivo of the crude bactericidal extract from Bacillus brevis (tyrothricin) was that by Dubos.[1] A single intra-abdominal injection of 2 mg. of the extract was found to protect mice against 10,000 to 100,000 fatal doses of five different strains of pneumococci. With repeated treatments, death from even larger bacterial inoculations could be prevented. Furthermore, administration of this material to mice several hours after the bacterial inoculation was said to exert a curative effect. Dubos also mentioned that preliminary experiments, carried out with Lancefield, indicated that the substance was protective for mice which had been infected with Streptococcus pyogenes.

TABLE 29

PROTECTIVE EFFECT OF REPEATED TREATMENTS WITH THE BACTERICIDAL AGENT

Infective dose of pneumococcus		Treatment on 3 consecutive days			Number of mice	Results†					
	c.c.	mg.	mg.	mg.							
Type I	0.1	2	1	1	6	D 22	S	S	S	S	S
"	0.01	2	1	1	6	D 22	S	S	S	S	S
"	0.000,000,01	0	0	0	1*	D 40					
Type II	0.1	2	1	1	6	D 26	S	S	S	S	S
"	0.01	2	1	1	6	D 22	S	S	S	S	S
"	0.000,000,01	0	0	0	1*	D 72					
Type III	0.1	2	1	1	6	D 72	D 72	D 72	D 72	S	S
"	0.01	2	1	1	6	D 72	D 72	S	S	S	S
"	0.000,000,01	0	0	0	1*	D 60					
Type V	0.1	2	1	1	6	D 72	S	S	S	S	S
"	0.01	2	1	1	6	S	S	S	S	S	S
"	0.000,000,01	0	0	0	1*	D 72					
Type VIII	0.1	2	1	1	6	D 22	D 22	D 40	D 48	S	S
"	0.01	2	1	1	6	D 22	S	S	S	S	S
"	0.000,000,01	0	0	0	1*	D 40					

* The untreated control animals inoculated with 0.000,000,1 and 0.000,001 c.c. of culture died within 44 hours.
† D = died and numerals after D indicate the number of hours after inoculation when death took place. S = survived. W. E. H.
From article by Dubos, Journal of Experimental Medicine, July 1, 1939.

In a subsequent and more detailed report by Dubos,[19] it was evident that in some instances five of six mice survived ordinarily fatal infections owing to Diplococcus pneumoniae after receiving intra-abdominal injections of the bactericidal agent for three consecutive days (table 29).

It was further evident (table 30) that animals could not be protected against infections owing to Klebsiella pneumoniae (Friedländer's bacillus), which in general agreed with the evidence, obtained in vitro, of the lack of effectiveness of this agent against gram-negative organisms. When the crude material, tyrothricin, was subsequently separated into its two components, gramicidin and tyrocidine, it was apparent from the reports of Hotchkiss and Dubos[5] and of Dubos and Hotchkiss[20] that both gramicidin and tyrocidine would protect mice infected intra-peritoneally with pneumococci; however, gramicidin appeared to be considerably more effective than tyrocidine.

Following these reports, all students of chemotherapy became hopeful that a bactericidal agent was about to be made available for the systemic treatment of severe coccal infections. Unfortunately, for reasons which will be mentioned in the section of this chapter which will deal with toxic effects (p. 282), this was not the case.

Subsequent studies on the activity in vivo of tyrothricin, gramicidin and tyrocidine were reported by Weinstein and Rammelkamp.[21] Although they had found that Lactobacillus acidophilus was susceptible to the action of tyrothricin in vitro, tyrothricin had no effect on this organism when the material was administered orally to mice in amounts which

TABLE 30

EFFECT OF THE BACTERICIDAL AGENT UPON EXPERIMENTAL INFECTION OF MICE WITH KLEBSIELLA PNEUMONIAE

Infective dose of Klebsiella pneumoniae type B	Treatment	Number of mice	Results*			
c.c.	mg.					
0,000,1	2	4	D 17	D 17	D 17	D 17
0.000,01	2	4	D 17	D 17	D 17	D 72
0.000,001	2	4	D 17	D 17	D 17	D 48
0.000,000,1	0	2	D 48	D 72		
0.000,000,01	0	2	D 72	D 72		

* D = died and numerals after D indicate the number of hours after inoculation when death took place. W. E. H.

From article by Dubos, Journal of Experimental Medicine, July 1, 1939.

could be considered adequate for investigation. This result, according to the investigators, is explainable on the basis that tyrothricin and its two fractions were probably destroyed in the intestinal tract. Further studies made in vivo were reported by Rammelkamp[22] on the subject of the effectiveness of tyrothricin in treatment of experimental hemolytic streptococcal empyema. This condition was experimentally produced in rabbits. Tyrothricin, in amounts varying from 3 to 40 mg., was administered as a single injection, either at the time of infection or at varying intervals up to eighteen hours after infection. The tyrothricin was administered into the pleural cavity. Although some of the animals died if treatment was delayed (due to extension of the infection), the treated pleural cavity was found to be sterile at the time of necropsy. It was also evident from these studies that staphylococcal infections of the pleural cavity were somewhat more resistant to this form of treatment than were infections owing to hemolytic streptococci. This is not surprising in view of the fact that Dorothy Heilman and I,[8] and subsequently Rammelkamp,[12] found most strains of staphylococci to be somewhat resistant to the action of this antibacterial agent. Rammelkamp,[22] however, was on occasions able to sterilize the pleural cavities of rabbits infected with Staphylococcus aureus by using large doses of tyrothricin. It should be pointed out, however, that amounts of 10 mg. or more of the substance, introduced into the pleural cavity, at times produced thickening of the pleura as well as certain other evidences of local irritation. No significant systemic pathologic changes were said to occur. These results, therefore, suggested that gramicidin might prove of some value in treatment of empyema. According to Rammelkamp,[22] staphylococcal infections of the knee joints of rabbits were found to be resistant to tyrothricin, whereas knee joints infected with Streptococcus pyogenes could be sterilized following treatment with tyrothricin.

Tillett, Cambier and Harris[23] reported certain studies carried out to test the relationship of sulfonamide resistance of certain organisms to activity of tyrothricin against the same organisms. These experiments, carried out on mice, yielded results which suggested that the protection afforded by tyrothricin against sulfonamide resistant pneumococci was rather variable. On the other hand, there was no evidence to indicate any definite relationship between the presence of sulfonamide resistance and the effectiveness, or lack of effectiveness, of tyrothricin. That tyrothricin was unlikely to afford protection unless the material was placed in direct contact with the infecting organism seemed evident from studies made in vivo and reported by Robson and Scott.[24] When pneumococci were injected into the cornea of the rabbit and local administration of tyrothricin was begun one hour after inoculation, only slight beneficial effect was noted and development of ulceration was not prevented. Obviously, the rather insoluble tyrothricin did not penetrate the deeper layers of the tissue where the infection had been established.

Robinson and Graessle[17] also carried out studies which indicated rather clearly that tyrothricin and its components are effective only when placed in direct contact with infecting bacteria. For example, when animals were infected intraperitoneally with organisms susceptible to the action of tyrothricin, oral, subcutaneous or intravenous administration of the substance did not protect the animals. Moreover, if the infection was established by means of intravenous administration of bacteria and the antibacterial substance was administered intraperitoneally, no protection resulted. It is probable that the high degree of insolubility of the substance, and its low diffusibility, made it impossible for the substance to reach the infecting organism; therefore, in order to obtain protection, the antibacterial substance must be placed in direct contact with the pathogenic organism. These studies, therefore, cast some further doubt as to the future role of tyrothricin and its components in the treatment of systemic infections. On the other hand, these as well as other studies indicated that, as a local agent placed in direct contact with the infecting pathogen, tyrothricin or its components might prove of some value.

MODE OF ACTION

It is difficult to make final statements concerning the exact mode of action of tyrothricin or its components, gramicidin and tyrocidine. Among the first reports on the general subject was that by Dorothy

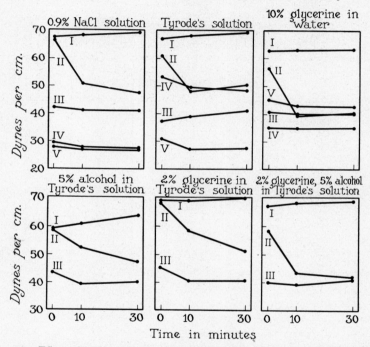

Fig. 42.—Effect of gramicidin, tyrocidine, sodium oleate and aerosol OT on surface tension of various solutions at 25° C. Key to curves (type of solution concerned in each chart is given in its caption) is as follows: I, solution with 0.5% alcohol added; II, solution same as I, gramicidin added 1 to 10,000; III, solution same as I, tyrocidine added 1 to 10,000; IV, solution same as I, sodium oleate added 1 to 10,000; V, solution same as I, aerosol added 1 to 10,000. (From article by Heilman and Herrell, Proceedings of the Society for Experimental Biology and Medicine, June, 1941.)

Heilman and me.[25] From our studies it was evident that these substances possess ability to depress the surface tension of aqueous solutions. Tyrocidine was found to be more active than gramicidin in this regard (fig. 42). However, the ability of gramicidin to depress surface tension was increased by the addition of certain organic solvents, such as glycerin. Since serum is known to inhibit the activity by virtue of which certain detergents depress surface tension, the effect of serum on the ability of these antibiotic substances to depress surface tension was examined by Dorothy Heilman and me (table 31). It was found that the inhibitory effect of increasing amounts of serum appeared to be proportionately about the same for gramicidin and the detergent, aerosol OT. Tyrocidine showed considerable ability to depress surface tension even in the presence of large amounts of serum. Furthermore,

TABLE 31

EFFECT OF RABBIT'S SERUM ON DEPRESSION OF SURFACE TENSION OF SALINE
SOLUTIONS BY 1:5,000 CONCENTRATIONS OF GRAMICIDIN, TYROCIDINE,
TYROTHRICIN, SODIUM OLEATE AND AEROSOL OT

	Gramicidin	Tyrocidine	Tyrothricin	Sodium oleate	Aerosol OT
0.9% NaCl solution	18*	26	26	40	41
1% serum in .9% NaCl sol.	14	20	21	31	31
5% serum in same	10	19	18	18	24
10% " " "	8	17	17	10	17
20% " " "	4	14	16	4	10
40% " " "	3	18	17	1	6
Tyrode's solution	20	28	27	19	40
1% serum in Tyrode's sol.	12	19	21	13	32
5% serum in same	6	17	19	9	24
10% " " "	4	15	16	8	16
20% " " "	4	15	15	4	10

* Values indicate the difference in dynes between the surface tension of the original solution and that of the same solution to which the various substances have been added. Determinations were made at 10 minutes. Temperature 25° C. All solutions were adjusted to pH 7.6.

From article by Heilman and Herrell, Proceedings of the Society for Experimental Biology and Medicine, June, 1941.

tyrothricin appeared to retain somewhat more ability to depress surface tension in the presence of serum than would be expected from its content of gramicidin.

In the report by Dorothy Heilman and me it was pointed out, therefore, that the effectiveness of gramicidin against bacteria appeared to depend on its partial solubility and that the ability of gramicidin and tyrocidine to depress the air-liquid interfacial tension was not proportional to their respective bactericidal action. The fact that tyrocidine was more active than gramicidin in depressing surface tension under all conditions studied suggested that the greater bactericidal action of gramicidin on gram-positive organisms depended on a more specific activity than mere depression of surface tension. This further seemed likely in view of the fact that heating destroyed the bactericidal property of gramicidin but did not alter its ability to depress surface tension.

Gramicidin exhibits definite specificity of bacterial action. As pointed out by Dorothy Heilman and me, the growth of Diplococcus pneumoniae and Streptococcus pyogenes is inhibited by extremely small amounts of the substance. Larger amounts were found necessary to inhibit staphylococci. Gram-negative bacteria in general are not affected. A similar type of bacterial selectivity has been shown for detergents, such as soaps of unsaturated fatty acids. Reports on this general subject have been made by Lamar,[26] Avery,[27] Walker,[28] Eggerth,[29] and Bayliss and Halvorson.[30] Baker, Harrison and Miller[31] also pointed out that anionic synthetic detergents display the same kind of specificity in their inhibitory effect on the metabolism of various bacterial species.

In connection with the studies on mode of action, it was pointed out by Dorothy Heilman and me[8] that as much as 10 mg. per cubic centimeter of para-aminobenzoic acid in tissue culture preparations did not inhibit the action of gramicidin on pneumococci. We[32] showed, further, that certain cationic detergents would inactivate gramicidin, which substance appeared to us to behave somewhat as an anionic detergent behaves. It was evident from the report of Pittman[33] that certain anionic detergents, on the other hand, in suitable concentrations could also inactivate gramicidin. Subsequent work carried out in our laboratories at the Mayo Clinic has confirmed this observation by Pittman.

It was suggested in the report of Dubos and Hotchkiss,[6] on the mode of action of these substances, that in certain respects the effect of tyrocidine could not be differentiated from that of cationic detergents, which must be considered as general protoplasmic poisons, and it seems now generally agreed that both gramicidin and tyrocidine are surface active. Although Dubos and Hotchkiss were willing to accept the idea that tyrocidine acts as cationic detergents act, they were inclined to the opinion that the effect of gramicidin on susceptible cells is of a little more complex nature. They were further of the opinion that gramicidin could hardly be considered a gross protoplasmic poison but that it more likely behaved as a specific inhibitor, blocking one or several metabolic reactions. Studies on the effect exerted by tyrocidine and gramicidin on the oxidation-reduction system of certain pathogenic organisms have been mentioned in the section of this chapter which deals with activity in vitro (p. 275).

The mode of action of gramicidin and of tyrocidine may differ in degree or kind and may involve different combinations of interference with normal cellular metabolism; however, there seems little doubt that both substances behave biologically in a manner similar to that of certain detergents.

CONSIDERATION OF TOXICITY

What is now to be said relates to the statement which was made in connection with the activity of tyrothricin, gramicidin and tyrocidine in vivo (p. 277). Although, under some conditions, animals could be protected against certain coccal infections, it quickly became evident that tyrothricin possessed certain toxic effects when administered to experimental animals. I consider that the most important and significant toxic effect of tyrothricin pertains to its high degree of hemolytic activity, which was first pointed out by Dorothy Heilman and me.[34]

Hemolytic Effect of Tyrothricin, Gramicidin and Tyrocidine.—Early in the course of the tissue culture studies carried out by Dorothy Heilman and me on tyrothricin, it was observed that there was a strong hemolytic effect on rabbit erythrocytes suspended in the tissue culture medium to which had been added extremely small amounts of tyrothricin. It was further evident that 1 per cent suspensions of washed sheep cells containing 0.01 mg. of tyrothricin per cubic centimeter were completely hemolyzed after one hour in a water bath at 37.5° C. Hemolysis of suspensions of red cells was complete in twenty-four hours in tubes containing as little as 0.001 mg. of tyrothricin per cubic centimeter. Addition of serum did not alter this hemolysis, nor did the presence or absence of complement appear to affect the process. In subsequent reports from the Mayo Clinic[8,35] as well as from elsewhere,[6] it was evident that both fractions of tyrothricin, gramicidin and tyrocidine, would cause hemolysis. Although the rate of hemolysis caused by tyrocidine is more rapid than that caused by gramicidin, gramicidin ultimately causes a greater degree of hemolysis than tyrocidine. All attempts by Dorothy Heilman and me[36] to nullify the hemolytic effect of these substances resulted in loss of antibacterial activity. Furthermore, although it has been suggested that the presence of 5 per cent solution of dextrose would prevent hemolysis due to gramicidin, it was obvious that the concentration of glucose necessary to prevent this phenomenon is far in excess of what would normally be present in the blood of animals or human beings. Moreover, this effect of glucose is in no way specific, since glucose in a concentration of 5 per cent will protect erythrocytes from hemolysis by a number of hemolytic agents. There can be little doubt but that this hemolytic effect precludes the successful use of either of these agents where they may come in direct contact with the circulating blood. It is not surprising, therefore, in view of the studies just mentioned, that animals could not tolerate intravenous administration of therapeutic amounts of these substances. MacLeod, Mirick and Curnen,[37] for example, described effects on animals which seem likely to have been due to the hemolytic activity of these agents.

Likewise, Robinson and Molitor[38] reported that daily intravenous ad-

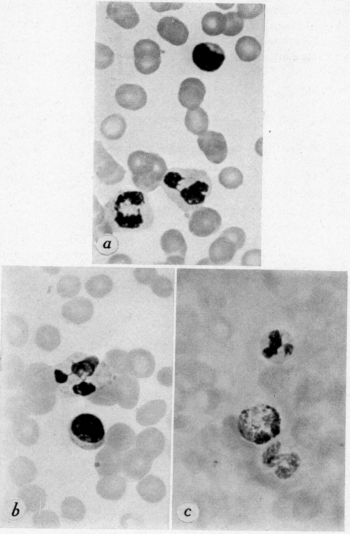

Fig. 43.—Whole human blood treated with tyrocidine and gramicidin 100 micrograms per cubic centimeter. Smears shown made after four hours' water bath incubation at 37° C. (× 1,000). *a*, Control blood smear. *b*, Tyrocidine treated blood. Minimal change in erythrocytes. Granulocytes appear normal. *c*, Gramicidin treated blood. Marked agglutination of erythrocytes but no evidence of toxicity of granulocytes. (From article by Herrell and Heilman, Journal of Clinical Investigation, September, 1941.)

ministration of 2 mg. of gramicidin or tyrothricin per kilogram of body weight caused death of dogs within two to eight days. During this period the animals lost appetite for food, lost weight and the erythrocyte counts fell in some instances from 6,000,000 to 3,500,000 per cubic millimeter of blood. All three agents proved definitely toxic on intraperitoneal and intravenous administration; however, gramicidin and tyrothricin (probably due to its content of gramicidin) were considerably more toxic than tyrocidine. None of the components was toxic when administered orally but this is explainable on the basis that destruction of the substances occurred in the intestinal tract or that they were not absorbed into the blood stream. Single doses were tolerated without any marked toxic effect, which explains the apparent lack of toxicity evident in the early reports by Dubos[1] in which, for therapeutic purposes, single injections were used.

Effect of Tyrothricin, Gramicidin and Tyrocidine on Cellular Elements Other than Erythrocytes.—Most investigators seem to agree that tyrothricin and its components do not produce any serious toxic effects on cellular elements, excluding erythrocytes, in the presence of concentrations of the substance which will result in inhibition of bacterial growth. In a study of the possible toxic effects of gramicidin and tyrocidine for leukocytes of whole human blood, Dorothy Heilman and I[8] found no significant morphologic changes in these cellular elements in the presence of as much as 100 micrograms of either gramicidin or tyrocidine per cubic centimeter of blood (fig. 43). According to Clapp,[39] however, tyrothricin and tyrocidine in high concentrations caused cytoplasmic and nuclear disintegration of polymorphonuclear leukocytes; however, it was evident from her studies that when no apparent microscopic injury occurred to cells, phagocytosis of pneumococci occurred as would be expected. Other studies on the general subject were reported by Rammelkamp and Weinstein.[40] From their report it appeared that there was considerable difference between the effect of tyrocidine and gramicidin on leukocytes. According to them, tyrocidine exhibited considerable leukocytolytic action and gramicidin, in the amounts used, caused little or no change in the total number of leukocytes. Dubos and Hotchkiss[6] also reported that even high concentrations of gramicidin did not affect the oxygen uptake of polymorphonuclear cells, whereas similar concentrations of tyrocidine caused cessation of respiration and disintegration of white cells.

Using the tissue culture method, it appeared from studies carried out by Dorothy Heilman and me[32, 41, 42] that gramicidin, on the other hand, was more toxic than tyrocidine and that the cytotoxicity of tyrothricin was largely due to its content of gramicidin. It was evident that migration of lymphocytes was decreased in the presence of 100 micrograms per cubic centimeter of gramicidin, whereas the same amount of tyrocidine had no appreciable effect on the migration of these cells. Likewise, migration of macrophages was considerably reduced in the presence of 10 micrograms per cubic centimeter of gramicidin or tyrothricin whereas 100 micrograms of tyrocidine were required to produce a similar effect. It should be emphasized, however, that when the cytotoxicity of gramicidin or tyrocidine is compared with that of other germicides commonly used for local application, such as merthiolate, zephiran or phemerol, these antibiotic agents will be found to be considerably less toxic under the same conditions. In figure 44, the cytotoxicity of gramicidin is compared with that of certain other bactericidal agents. In this connection, the report by Henle and Zittle,[43] of a comparison of the activity of tyrothricin, gramicidin and tyrocidine on the motility of spermatozoa is of some interest. According to their report, the oxygen consumption and motility of spermatozoa were markedly reduced or

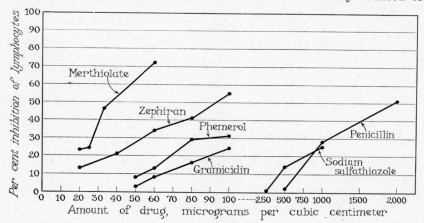

Fig. 44.—Cytotoxicity of various concentrations of bactericidal agents. (From article by Herrell and Heilman, American Journal of the Medical Sciences, August, 1943.)

destroyed in the presence of 10 micrograms per cubic centimeter of tyrothricin or gramicidin. On the other hand, only a small reduction in the oxygen consumption of spermatozoa was observed with the same amount of tyrocidine.

Toxicity for Experimental Animals.—In a preceding paragraph I have mentioned the acute toxicity for animals of tyrothricin and its fractions, which was reported by Robinson and Molitor.[38] Either tyrothricin, gramicidin or tyrocidine, when administered intravenously to rabbits or dogs, usually resulted in death within a period of one to a few days. Likewise, reports of Robinson and Molitor demonstrated that mice would not tolerate any of the substances when administered intravenously. Following single intravenous doses of 5 mg. of tyrothricin, 25 mg. of tyrocidine, or 3.75 mg. of gramicidin per kilogram of body weight, 100 per cent of mice died. Likewise, intraperitoneal injection of fairly large

10

amounts of these substances into mice and rats was found to result in death.

Although these substances may be administered orally without toxic effect, there is little evidence to suggest that any therapeutic effect is attainable from oral administration.

Comment.—It seems apparent, from what has been said, that tyrothricin and its two fractions are fairly active antibacterial agents and that serious toxic effects are not likely to occur following local use of antibacterial amounts of these agents. Because of their hemolytic properties and because of their known toxicity for experimental animals, however, none of these agents can be administered intravenously, intramuscularly or subcutaneously in treatment of bacterial infections. For the following reasons, tyrothricin (often incorrectly referred to as gramicidin) is the most suitable preparation of the three for local use: 1. Tyrothricin is fairly easily prepared and fairly easily attainable. 2. There is some selective difference between the action of gramicidin and tyrocidine, tyrocidine being slightly effective against gram-negative organisms. Tyrothricin contains both gramicidin and tyrocidine. 3. The presence of tyrocidine in the mixture which composes tyrothricin increases the stability of emulsions of gramicidin and, therefore, aids in keeping gramicidin in suspension.

PREPARATIONS FOR CLINICAL USE

In the preceding paragraph I have emphasized that some of the properties of tyrothricin, together with its toxicity for experimental animals, limit use of this substance to topical application or local injection into certain infected portions of the body.

Preparations for Local Use.—*Alcoholic Solutions.*—Rammelkamp[44] found a 95 per cent alcohol solution, containing 50 mg. of tyrothricin per cubic centimeter, satisfactory for local application to certain ulcerated areas. The amount of a single application may range from 1 to 100 mg. The alcoholic solution is allowed to dry, leaving a thin film of tyrothricin covering an area. After this, dry, sterile dressings are applied.

Aqueous Suspensions.—Tyrothricin usually is dispensed as a mixture in alcohol or in alcohol and glycerin. These stock solutions are stable and do not deteriorate. For local application, a suitable preparation may be made as follows: Enough of the stock solution is added to 1 liter of triple distilled water so that the final suspension contains at least 0.5 mg. (500 micrograms) per cubic centimeter. This can be applied frequently, or by a constant spray, to local lesions. In aqueous suspension, the material should be used within a period of seven to ten days. Deterioration and certain other undesirable changes may occur if the preparation is held in the aqueous phase for a longer time.

Dry Preparations.—At the Mayo Clinic, dry preparations are made as follows: 20 c.c. of an alcoholic stock solution, containing 500 mg. of tyrothricin, is added to 100 gm. of dry, powdered boric acid. The mixture is ground in a mortar and the alcohol allowed to evaporate. This dry preparation, containing 500 mg. per 100 gm. of boric acid, is satisfactory for insufflation into certain regions. It is particularly suitable for vaginal insufflation in treatment of localized infections.

CLINICAL RESULTS WITH TYROTHRICIN

Infected Ulcers and Wounds.—It was evident in reports from the Mayo Clinic,[8, 45] as well as in the reports of Rammelkamp and Keefer[46] and of Rammelkamp,[44] that tyrothricin might prove of value in local treatment of certain infected stasis ulcers and wounds. It has been my practice to use the aqueous suspension of tyrothricin, containing 500 micrograms per cubic centimeter, for treatment in these cases. The area of infection is kept bathed with tyrothricin by frequent local application. Rammelkamp used the alcoholic solutions which contained 50 mg. of tyrothricin per cubic centimeter. This alcoholic solution was allowed to dry, leaving a film of tyrothricin coating the ulcer.

The most satisfactory responses I[45] secured were in cases in which ulcers were infected with Streptococcus pyogenes. In treatment of infections attributable to Staphylococcus aureus, results were a little less satisfactory. Results were not at all encouraging in the presence of gram-negative organisms. This was to be expected on the basis of experimental studies. Rammelkamp's observations are in general agreement with these statements. It was further evident from his studies that lesions from which both gram-negative and gram-positive bacteria were isolated failed to respond to the use of tyrothricin. Rammelkamp[44] attributed these failures to the production of inhibitory substances by gram-negative bacteria. He reported that twelve of sixteen ulcers infected with gram-positive organisms were sterilized shortly after institution of treatment with tyrothricin. In some instances, healing of the lesion was rapid. In one of the cases reported by Rammelkamp, ulcerations which had been present for six weeks healed following two applications of tyrothricin. The strain of Staphylococcus aureus isolated from this patient's ulcer was found to be especially susceptible to the action of tyrothricin. I likewise have seen ulcers of this type respond promptly to treatment with tyrothricin (fig. 45).

It was further evident, in my experience and in the experience of Rammelkamp,[44] that ulcers secondary to poor circulation, or ulcers associated with damage to tissue, healed comparatively slowly although, in some instances, it was possible to eliminate the bacteria from the lesion. In one series of cases reported from the Mayo Clinic,[45] tyrothricin was used in treatment of ninety-three patients suffering with infected ulcers and wounds. Failures occurred in seventeen (18 per cent) of these cases. The response in more than half of these cases could be considered good or excellent (table 32). In certain instances wherein wounds and ulcers are complicated by infection of bone underlying the ulcer, the

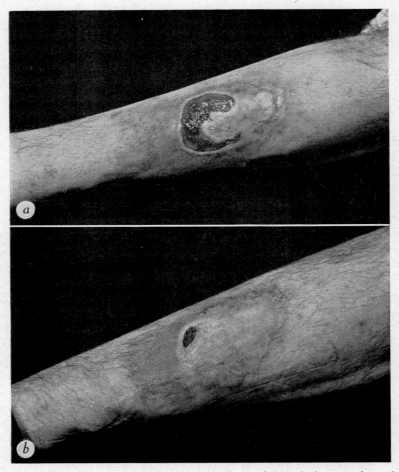

Fig. 45.—Typical ulcer; *a*, before treatment with tyrothricin; *b*, fourteen days after treatment was begun.

results following local use of tyrothricin are not striking. This is to be expected since the method of administration and the low degree of penetration of the antibacterial agent make it impossible to reach these deeper, infected tissues.

Further studies on the local use of tyrothricin in treatment of infected wounds were mentioned by Francis.[47] A sulfonamide resistant infection with Streptococcus pyogenes was said to have been satisfactorily eradicated following local applications of the agent. Likewise, Rankin[48] has reported excellent results from use of tyrothricin in five of six cases of chronic ulcer. According to his report, tyrothricin did not cause toxic symptoms or pain following its local use.

Kvale, Barker and I,[49] in a more extensive study, concluded that tyrothricin was of definite value in treatment of certain types of infected ulcers of both ischemic and stasis origin. Using aqueous suspensions of tyrothricin containing 500 micrograms per cubic centimeter, we were particularly impressed with the low toxic effect of tyrothricin on the extremely delicate tissues concerned. In most instances, the suspension

TABLE 32

RESULTS OF CLINICAL USE OF TYROTHRICIN IN 142 CASES ACCORDING TO TYPE OF LESION

Infection	Cases*	Results					
		Good or excellent		Fairly good		Poor	
		Cases	Per cent	Cases	Per cent	Cases	Per cent
Ulcer and wounds	93	47	51	29	31	17	18
Sinus	21	13	62	2	10	6	28
Bone	19	9	48	5	26	5	26
Bladder and pleura	15	9	60	2	13	4	27

* Multiple types of lesions were present in a few cases.

was applied to the ulcer as a continuous wet dressing. For small ulcers, a sterile cotton pad which barely overlapped the margins of the ulcer was saturated with the solution and applied directly. By means of a medicine dropper, the pad was moistened with the solution every hour. The pads were changed at least every twenty-four hours and oftener if there was much discharge from the lesion. For large ulcers, cotton pads were used and were covered with oiled silk. The pads were moistened before their application and were allowed to overlap the margin of the ulcer only slightly. Occasionally some of the cotton adhered to the base of the ulcer but this was removed before a new pad was applied. It is my opinion that the aqueous suspension is more satisfactory for this type of case than the rather concentrated alcoholic solutions employed by Rammelkamp.

TABLE 33

RESULTS OF TREATMENT WITH TYROTHRICIN IN CASES OF VENOUS STASIS ULCER

Case	Sex	Age, Years	Size and location of ulcer	Type of treatment	Duration of treatment	Comment	Results
1	F.	55	Ulcers anterior surfaces both legs	Tyrothricin	7 days in hospital. 1 month at home	Ulcer almost healed in hospital. Ulcer healed completely at home	Good
2	F.	46	Ulcer 3 by 3 cm. external aspect left leg	Tyrothricin	6 days	50% healing during short period	Good
3	M.	35	Ulcer 4 by 4 cm. above left internal malleolus	Tyrothricin	2½ weeks	Healed	Good
4	M.	32	Multiple small stasis ulcers right ankle	Tyrothricin	10 days	Healed	Good
5	F.	30	Ulcer 5 by 5 cm. lateral surface juncture middle and lower thirds left leg with surrounding cellulitis	Elevation and packs of 1% aluminum subacetate for 7 days until cellulitis had subsided. Tyrothricin thereafter	Tyrothricin for 30 days	Healed	Good
6	F.	37	Ulcer 6 by 6 cm. right leg, 6 years' duration	Sulfanilamide by mouth one week. Tyrothricin	25 days	Healed	Good
7	M.	51	Ulcer 2.5 by 2.5 cm. over right internal malleolus	Tyrothricin	29 days	Healed	Good
8	F.	54	3 ulcers 1 to 2 cm. in diameter left leg	Tyrothricin	14 days	Healed	Good
9	M.	19	2 deep, indolent ulcers lateral surface left leg	Tyrothricin	11 days	Ulcers 25% healed	Fair
10	F.	35	2 large and 1 small ulcer left leg	Tyrothricin	10 days	Skin grafts eventually necessary	Fair
11	F.	70	Ulcer 3 by 1 cm. medial surface left leg	Tyrothricin	1 month together with sulfathiazole ointment and aluminum subacetate packs	Ulcer partially healed on tyrothricin	Fair
12	M.	47	Recurrent stasis ulcer 2 by 2.5 cm. medial surface left ankle	Aluminum subacetate packs for 13 days. Tyrothricin for 25 days	38 days total	No change after 13 days' treatment with aluminum subacetate. 90% healed after 25 days with tyrothricin	Fair
13	F.	48	Large ulcer left leg	Tyrothricin	13 days	50% healed and clean	Fair
14	F.	59	Large deep infected ulcer and one small ulcer left leg	Tyrothricin	14 days	20% healed and clean. Ulcer later healed at home with sulfathiazole ointment and rest in bed	Fair
15	M.	65	3 stasis ulcers 1 to 3 cm. in area of eczema	Tyrothricin	10 days	Ulcers 50% healed	Fair

TABLE 34

RESULTS OF TREATMENT WITH TYROTHRICIN IN CASES OF ISCHEMIC ULCER ASSOCIATED WITH THROMBO-ANGIITIS OBLITERANS

Case	Sex	Age, Years	Size and location of lesion	Type of treatment	Duration of treatment	Comment	Results
1	M.	51	Ulcer L 1 toe. Large necrotic ulcer left calf	One injection typhoid vaccine. Sander's bed. Tyrothricin	30 days	Ulcer L 1 toe healed. Ulcer left calf 50% healed	Good
2	M.	50	Ulcers R 2, 3, 4 fingers	Tyrothricin. Cervicothoracic sympathectomy	28 days	Ulcers healed	Fair
3	M.	37	Large gangrenous ulcer at site of previously amputated R 2 toe and mass gangrene R 3 toe	Injections of typhoid vaccine. Tyrothricin	51 days	Ulcer base R 2 toe 50% healed. R 3 toe then amputated. Tyrothricin continued with entire ulcer healed in 1 month	Good
4	M.	41	Necrotic ulcer L 1 toe. Small ulcer lateral aspect left foot	Injections of typhoid vaccine. Sander's bed. Tyrothricin	10 days with tyrothricin	No results after 10 days' treatment with tyrothricin. Thereafter with sulfathiazole ointment. Ulcer 95% healed in 6 weeks	Failure
5	M.	33	Ulcer nail bed L 1 toe	Injections of typhoid vaccine. Sander's bed. Tyrothricin	30 days	Dismissed with ulcer painless but still unhealed	Fair
6	M.	44	Large ulcer lateral aspect right foot with osteomyelitis base R 5 metatarsal	Ulcer and sinus curetted with drainage persisting for 28 days. Tyrothricin then started	15 days	Ulcer and sinus healed	Good
7	M.	52	Small open lesion site of amputated stump left leg	Tyrothricin	30 days	Nonhealing of lesion. Subsequent excision of ulcerated area	Failure
8	M.	47	Ulcers dorsum both first toes, L 2, and R 3	Tyrothricin	47 days	All lesions practically healed	Good
9	M.	49	Ulcers L 4 and 5 fingers and gangrene R 4 finger	Tyrothricin	21 days	Ulcer L 4 and 5 fingers healed. Amputation R 4 finger	Fair
10	M.	27	Ulcers dorsum base L 1 and 2 toes and over L 5 metatarsal head	Tyrothricin intermittently. Typhoid vaccine. Sander's bed. Lumbar sympathectomy	Total 2 months	Eventual spread of ulcerations to gangrene of left leg and amputation	Failure
11	M	37	Ulcer R 1 toe	Tyrothricin	14 days	Ulcer not healed	Failure
12	M.	55	Large gangrenous ulcer R 1 toe	Tyrothricin intermittently. Sander's bed. Typhoid vaccine. Powdered red blood cells. Sulfathiazole ointment	4 months	Nonhealing of ulcer. Eventual amputation of leg	Failure

TABLE 35

Results of Treatment with Tyrothricin in Cases of Ischemic Ulcer Associated with Arteriosclerosis Obliterans

Case	Sex	Age, Years	Diabetes mellitus	Size and location of ulcer	Type of treatment	Duration of treatment	Comment	Results
1	F.	44	Yes	Ulcer 4 by 4 cm. right anterior tibial region. Stasis as well as ischemic	Tyrothricin	45 days	Ulcer healed	Good
2	M.	60	Yes	Gangrenous ulcer L 1 toe	Tyrothricin	54 days	Ulcer 50% healed	Fair
3	F.	69	Yes	Large gangrenous ulcers lateral and medial surfaces left foot	Tyrothricin	57 days	General opinion that ulcers would not heal. After 57 days treatment, ulcers unquestionably healing	Good
4	F.	80	No	Gangrenous ulcer ball R 1 nail bed. Small ulcer over R 2 midphalangeal joint	Tyrothricin	13 days	Ulcer R 1 toe healed. Nonhealing ulcer R 2 toe.	Fair
5	M.	54	No	Sloughing, infected ulcer stump of amputated R 5 toe with edema and cellulitis dorsum of foot	Elevation scales for 9 days. Tyrothricin thereafter for 41 days	Total 50 days	Ulcer healed	Good
6	M.	59	Yes	Gangrenous ulcer L 1 toe	Tyrothricin	3 weeks	Ulcer healing	Fair
7	M.	71	No	Nonhealing ulcer site of amputated R 2 toe	Tyrothricin	7 days	Ulcer healed	Good
8	M.	67	No	Gangrenous ulcer base mesial side nail R 1 toe	Tyrothricin	15 days	Ulcer healed	Good
9	M.	56	No	Ulcer site of amputated R 5 toe	Tyrothricin	3 weeks	Ulcer 98% healed	Good
10	M.	60	No	Ulcer site of amputated L 1 toe	Sander's bed. Tyrothricin	11 days	Relief of pain, ulcer became cleaner, but base of ulcer was head of metatarsal	Failure
11	M.	76	No	Infected fissure between L 4 and 5 toe	Tyrothricin	14 days	Nonhealing of lesion	Failure
12	M.	58	No	Gangrene dorsum of right foot	Tyrothricin	10 days	Spread of gangrene. Patient died of mesenteric thrombosis	Failure
13	F.	73	No	Infected gangrene R 1 toe	Tyrothricin	11 days	Progression of gangrene. Eventual amputation of leg	Failure
14	F.	56	No	Infected ulcer right leg	Tyrothricin	14 days	Progression in size of ulcer. Eventual amputation of leg	Failure
15	M.	62	Yes	Deep 1 by 1 cm. ulcer base L 5 metatarsal	Tyrothricin. Débridement	1 month	25% healing after 1 month in hospital 90% healed after 1 more month's treatment at home	Good

As part of the study just mentioned,[49] we analyzed the results obtained with tyrothricin when applied to three different types of ulcer: (1) venous stasis ulcer (table 33); (2) ischemic ulcer associated with thrombo-angiitis obliterans (table 34); and (3) ischemic ulcer associated with arteriosclerosis obliterans (table 35). We pointed out that the good results which were obtained in many cases did not necessarily imply that tyrothricin alone was responsible for the result. There seemed little doubt that some of the ulcers might have healed with standard forms of treatment; however, in cases in which tyrothricin was used, the ulcers healed more rapidly than in cases in which it was not used. Furthermore, failures which occurred were not always due entirely to ineffectiveness of tyrothricin. In some instances of infected gangrenous ulcer severe enough to justify consideration of amputation, response to tyrothricin was satisfactory. Of twelve cases of ulcer of ischemic origin, good results were obtained in four, fair results in three, and failure occurred in five. Failure also occurred in five of fifteen cases in which the ulcers were associated with arteriosclerosis obliterans and good or fair results occurred in ten of the fifteen. In general, good results were more frequently obtained in treatment of venous stasis ulcers. Of a total of fifteen such cases, good or excellent results were obtained in eight; fairly good results in seven, and in none could the result be considered to represent failure.

Clinical results in 573 cases have been reported by the Russian investigators, Gause and Brazhnikova,[50] on the use of gramicidin S, which is said to be similar to tyrothricin but somewhat more effective. This series included infected gunshot wounds, empyema and osteomyelitis. According to the investigators, application of gramicidin S led to rapid disappearance of bacteria from the wounds and the substance was effectively used in preparation of these wounds for subsequent surgical treatment.

Tyrothricin has proved useful in preparation for skin grafting of infected ulcers and wounds. It often is possible to eradicate bacterial infections owing to such organisms as Streptococcus pyogenes and Staphylococcus aureus and thereby to hasten the time of successful skin grafting. If grafting is attempted in the presence of infection, the graft is likely to be lost. In addition to ridding surfaces of bacteria, a clinical impression is that application of tyrothricin results in definite stimulation to the formation of granulation tissue. A similar observation also has been reported by Rankin.[48]

Infections of the Nose and Throat.—One of the first reports on the use of tyrothricin in treatment of diseases of the nose and throat was that by Schoenbach, Enders and Mueller.[51] Five persons who carried Streptococcus pyogenes in the rhinopharynx were treated locally with tyrothricin. Two of these persons had been persistent nasal carriers for two months following scarlet fever; three were in the third week of the disease. In one of the five cases there was immediate reduction in the number of streptococci following local administration of tyrothricin. In the remaining four, the number of organisms had become diminished, or the organisms had disappeared, after the fifth day. The authors attributed the abrupt change on the fifth day to increasingly intensive application of tyrothricin. They were inclined to the opinion that tyrothricin was of value in elimination of Streptococcus pyogenes from carriers. In their studies, the alcohol soluble fraction (tyrothricin) was diluted 1:100 in physiologic saline solution containing 2.5 per cent glycerin. This material was copiously sprayed in an attempt to cover the entire nasopharynx. Administration usually was preceded by preliminary cleansing and shrinking of the mucous membranes. The investigators stressed the importance of vigorously shaking the suspensions of tyrothricin immediately before using them.

In a very few selected cases of sinusitis the effectiveness of tyrothricin was investigated at the Mayo Clinic.[8, 45] Again in a few instances, encouraging results were obtained. Unfortunately, reports of the work secured certain unauthorized publicity which created undesirable enthusiasm for the use of tyrothricin in treatment of sinus infections in general. It should be understood that tyrothricin has, if any use at all, a very limited field of usefulness in treatment of sinusitis. Nasal douching with tyrothricin is of little or no value in the treatment of these infections. If the substance is to be employed for sinusitis, its use must be limited to those instances wherein definitely susceptible bacteria can be isolated from cultures of material from the sinuses and wherein the agent can be introduced into sinus cavities by means of the Pretz displacement technic. In other words, adequate openings already must have been established to permit introduction of the material by means of this technic. The tyrothricin suspension (500 micrograms per cubic centimeter) can be instilled into a sinus every day or every other day. Even under the best circumstances, improvement or results which could be considered good were obtained in only thirteen of twenty-one cases in which treatment was administered at the Mayo Clinic by H. L. Williams,[52] of the Section on Otolaryngology. Williams pointed out that evaluation of results based on his limited number of cases is difficult if not impossible. Furthermore, as Williams indicated, tyrothricin is an antibacterial substance only and cannot be expected to rejuvenate damaged tissue or to correct the physical malformations which are so frequently present in cases of chronic sinusitis.

This whole question of the possible value of tyrothricin for acute and chronic infections of the upper part of the respiratory tract, and for elimination of pathogenic bacteria from the nasopharynx and tonsils of carriers, was thoroughly examined by Lindsay and Judd.[53] They used tyrothricin as a suspension in alcohol and water in strengths of 1:5,000 and 1:1,000. In some instances, propylene-glycol was used as a solvent. One gram of tyrothricin was dissolved in 25 c.c. of propylene-glycol and then was diluted with water to obtain solutions of 1:100, 1:500 and 1:1,000. The 1:500 solution was well tolerated by the mucous membranes, whereas the 1:100 solution caused severe irritation in frontal and ethmoid sinuses. For acute infections of the upper part of the respiratory tract, the suspensions of tyrothricin were instilled into the nasal cavity after shrinkage of the mucous membranes had been accomplished. The average period of treatment of these acute infections was seven days. Acute sinusitis also was treated by instillations of tyrothricin. Duration of the infection definitely was not shortened by use of tyrothricin nor could it be said that the substance produced alleviation of symptoms. Likewise, there seemed little evidence that improvement following use of tyrothricin for chronic infection of the sinuses was any more striking than that which follows customarily conservative treatment. In a group of cases of chronic infection of the nasopharynx and tonsils, the investigators used tyrothricin daily by means of liberal applications. From eight carriers of Streptococcus pyogenes treated for an average of six days, negative cultures could not be obtained. These results, as well as those reported by Rammelkamp,[44] are at variance with the encouraging reports by Schoenbach, Enders and Mueller[51] on the use of tyrothricin in treatment of carriers of Streptococcus pyogenes.

On the other hand, Crowe and his associates[54] are responsible for the following statement: "For two years we have used tyrothricin. . . . locally in the treatment of acute otitis media, acute and chronic mastoiditis, and acute and chronic sinusitis with better results in many cases than we have ever had before." According to these investigators, tyrothricin was not only suitable for local application but its use was not associated with toxic reactions, with evidence of damage to tissue or with interference with wound healing. They found that repeated irrigations with tyrothricin greatly reduced the number of bacteria present in chronically infected sinuses; however, results were not permanent and tyrothricin was most valuable when it was used as a supplement to surgical procedures. The investigators were of the opinion, however, that in acute sinus infections, wherein bacteria had not penetrated the deeper layers, a satisfactory result could be obtained.

As the matter stands, it is difficult to evaluate the role of tyrothricin in treatment of infections of the nose and its accessory sinuses. This explains the difference of opinion among investigators. Local sprays and instillations, however, are not likely to accomplish a great deal. If suitable methods can be devised for keeping tyrothricin in contact with susceptible pathogenic organisms, the bacteria will be eliminated. Even then, use of the substance will not replace surgical operation but it may be of some value when administered in combination with surgical drainage. At least some authors[55] still feel that further clinical trials are justifiable.

Mastoiditis.—Rammelkamp[44] reported on the use of tyrothricin combined with surgical drainage in treatment of acute mastoiditis in twenty-seven cases in which the etiologic organism was Streptococcus pyogenes. In the twenty-seven cases, thirty-two mastoidectomies were performed. Twelve of the mastoid cavities were used as controls; each of fifteen received a single application of tyrothricin and five received many applications. Cultures were made of material from the mastoid cavities at the time of operation and at frequent intervals afterwards. From eleven of the twelve mastoid cavities which served as controls, Streptococcus pyogenes was obtained in cultures made at the time of operation. In the fifteen cases, in each of which a single application of 20 to 70 mg. of tyrothricin was made at the time of operation, there was not any material difference in the amount of discharge or in the time required for healing when comparison was made with the controls. Furthermore, both in the controls and in the mastoid cavities treated with tyrothricin, staphylococci frequently were found on culture. These studies, therefore, indicated that a single application of tyrothricin at the time of operation was not sufficient to sterilize the cavity nor to shorten the postoperative course. In the five cases in which tyrothricin was administered repeatedly following operation, the results, according to Rammelkamp, were considerably better. In one case, 25 to 50 mg. of tyrothricin suspended in glycerin was applied daily for several weeks. After this treatment, Streptococcus pyogenes disappeared from the mastoid cavity and the wound healed. Rammelkamp, therefore, concluded that mastoid cavities infected with Streptococcus pyogenes could be sterilized by frequent applications of tyrothricin. Untoward reactions were not observed; however, when tyrothricin in alcohol was applied at the time of operation, hemolysis of the erythrocytes present in the cavity occurred occasionally. These studies, as well as those of Crowe and his associates,[54] seem to be in agreement that local use of tyrothricin is indicated for eradication of infection after mastoidectomy. On the other hand, the results are difficult to evaluate.

Empyema.—Rammelkamp[44] attempted to use tyrothricin intrathoracically in a few cases of empyema. In one group of cases, the tyrothricin was administered before surgical drainage. The tyrothricin injected was suspended in physiologic saline solution or in 10 per cent glucose solution, and the final concentration was 0.1 to 2 mg. per cubic centimeter. As much as 100 mg. of tyrothricin was administered to some patients in this way. There was some evidence of considerable reduction in the number of organisms but sterilization of the cavity could not be effected if the infecting organisms were pneumococci or staphylococci. It was evident, therefore, that although tyrothricin might prove of some value in treatment of empyema, it was better to combine its use with surgical drainage. After open drainage has been established in cases of empyema, suspensions of tyrothricin in physiologic saline solution, or in glucose solution, have proved of value for irrigation and instillation. In one such case reported by Rammelkamp, the pleural cavity was rapidly sterilized. In this particular instance, the organism present was Streptococcus pyogenes.

The effect of tyrothricin is not so satisfactory in cases of the sort just described if the infections are associated with Staphylococcus aureus. However, at times, in the presence of this organism, I have noted satisfactory results following local instillation of 100 or 200 c.c. of a suspension of tyrothricin into the empyema cavity. The suspension used contained between 0.5 and 1 mg. of tyrothricin per cubic centimeter.

Miscellaneous Infections.—In a few instances, suspensions of tyrothricin have been applied locally in treatment of infections involving the eye, including acute conjunctivitis and keratoconjunctivitis. Tyrothricin in suspensions of 0.5 per cent can be used for local application to the conjunctiva and will not, as a rule, prove irritating. Higher concentrations will cause irritation, however, and are to be avoided. Heath[56] reported favorable results following use of tyrothricin (30 mg. per 100 c.c.) in treatment of epidemic keratoconjunctivitis (shipyard fever). The tyrothricin was administered locally four to six times a day. He also found the same preparation, when combined with cauterization, useful in treatment of dendritic keratitis. This same investigator reported, moreover, that tyrothricin was of some value for treatment in certain cases of blepharitis and punctate keratitis associated with chronic conjunctivitis. Furthermore, Heath successfully administered tyrothricin locally, four to six times a day, for conjunctivitis of pneumococcal origin. Conjunctivitis associated with Friedländer's infection, as would be expected, did not respond to use of tyrothricin.

Further studies on the general subject of the value of tyrothricin in treatment of conjunctivitis have been reported by Streicher.[57] The preparation used by him was prepared by adding 0.1 c.c. of a stock solution of 2 per cent tyrothricin to 8 c.c. of sterile distilled water. The material was dispensed in a dropper bottle and was applied locally.

Tyrothricin occasionally has been instilled into the urinary bladder and the patient has been instructed to retain the instilled material as long as possible. For such instillations a suspension of 500 micrograms per cubic centimeter is satisfactory. If the organism of infection is gram-negative, tyrothricin probably will prove of no value. If the infecting organism is one which is susceptible to the action of tyrothricin, daily instillations may prove effective. On the other hand, if the infection is deep-seated or involves the upper part of the urinary tract, reinfection is likely to occur since tyrothricin cannot reach the infection in the deeper layers of the tissue nor can it reach other inaccessible foci following local use.

Tyrothricin has been applied locally in certain cases of dermatitis and eczema. According to Rammelkamp,[44] skin infections owing to Streptococcus pyogenes have responded satisfactorily at times, whereas infections owing to staphylococci are somewhat more resistant to this form of treatment. This is in agreement with my experience.

Tyrothricin has proved of definite value in treatment of certain vaginal infections owing to susceptible organisms. Piper[58] has found it exceedingly effective in treatment of coccal and certain mixed infections of the vagina. There is no evidence that it is effective against Trichomonas. For treatment of vaginal infections, the powdered preparation (500 mg. of tyrothricin per 100 gm. of dry, powdered boric acid—see p. 287) is employed. The material is introduced into the vagina by means of an insufflator and is left there. This procedure is carried out every other day and is continued until improvement occurs.

Bovine Mastitis.—From the reports of Little, Dubos and Hotchkiss,[59] it appeared that tyrothricin possessed considerable activity against Streptococcus agalactiae and for that reason an attempt was made to use tryothricin in aqueous suspensions in treatment of bovine mastitis. It was found, however, that aqueous suspensions of the material at times would cause irritation following injection or instillation into the udder. Further work by this same group of investigators,[60, 61] revealed that mineral oil was a suitable vehicle for administration of tyrothricin in treatment of bovine mastitis. Of thirty-one quarters treated with emulsion in mineral oil, twenty-six responded to treatment; twenty appeared to clear up entirely following a single injection. Subsequently, other investigators[62-65] reported that tyrothricin was effective in treatment of streptococcal bovine mastitis.

The preparation recommended for treatment of the condition here considered consists of a 50 per cent emulsion in mineral oil. The final mixture contains 1.5 to 2 mg. of tyrothricin per cubic centimeter. Treatment is carried out effectively during lactation periods; however, treatment is not recommended during an acute attack. After the infected quarter has been milked, the emulsion is injected into the teat canal, using a sterile syringe with a blunt needle. The usual amount of emulsion injected is 20 c.c. With the orifice of the teat closed, the teat is collapsed between the thumb and finger and, by the process of milking upward, the material is forced high into the cistern. Light massage also assists in spreading the material throughout the quarter. The emulsion of tyrothricin is allowed to remain in the udder until the next regular milking when it is emptied and the secretion discarded. Seven to ten days later, samples should be obtained from the quarter and examined for the presence of the infecting organism. Treatment is repeated as indicated and there should be no interruption in the milking schedule. In some instances, 15 to 30 c.c. of the emulsion have been injected daily for four consecutive days without severe reaction.

Tyrothricin also may be used during the dry period. After the last milking is completed, and before turning the animal off as dry, 20 c.c. of the emulsion may be injected into the quarter as previously described. The material in this instance is not milked out but is left in place. The animal is then allowed to continue through the dry period. Following freshening, samples can be obtained again for examination for the presence of the infecting organism.

REFERENCES

1. Dubos, R. J.: Bactericidal effect of an extract of a soil bacillus on gram-positive cocci. Proc. Soc. Exper. Biol. & Med. *40*:311–312 (Feb.) 1939.
2. Dubos, R. J.: Studies on a bactericidal agent extracted from a soil bacillus. I. Preparation of the agent, its activity in vitro. J. Exper. Med. *70*:1–10 (July) 1939.
3. Dubos, R. J. and Cattaneo, Carlo: Studies on a bactericidal agent extracted from a soil bacillus. III. Preparation and activity of a protein-free fraction. J. Exper. Med. *70*:249–256 (Sept.) 1939.
4. Hotchkiss, R. D. and Dubos, R. J.: Fractionation of the bactericidal agent from cultures of a soil bacillus. J. Biol. Chem. *132*:791–792 (Feb.) 1940.
5. Hotchkiss, R. D. and Dubos, R. J.: Bactericidal fractions from an aerobic sporulating bacillus. J. Biol. Chem. *136*:803–804 (Dec.) 1940.
6. Dubos, R. J. and Hotchkiss, R. D.: Origin, nature and properties of gramicidin and tyrocidine. Tr. & Stud. Coll. Physicians, Philadelphia. *10*:11–19 (Apr.) 1942.
7. Dubos, R. J.: Utilization of selective microbial agents in the study of biological problems (Harvey Lecture). Bull. New York Acad. Med. *17*:405–422 (June) 1941.
8. Herrell, W. E. and Heilman, Dorothy H.: Experimental and clinical studies on gramicidin. J. Clin. Investigation. *20*:583–591 (Sept.) 1941; also Society Report, p. 433 (July) 1941.
9. King, J. T., Henschel, A. F. and Green, B. S.: The bacteriostatic and antitoxic actions of sulfanilamide; tissue culture studies. J. A. M. A. *113*:1704–1709 (Nov. 4) 1939.
10. King, J. T.: Special incubator for tissue cultures. Arch. f. exper. Zellforsch. *20*:208–212, 1937.
11. Rodaniche, E. C. and Palmer, W. L.: The action of tyrothricin on fecal streptococci in vitro and in vivo. J. Infect. Dis. *72*:154–156 (Mar.-Apr.) 1943.
12. Rammelkamp, C. H.: Observations on resistance of *Staphylococcus aureus* to action of tyrothricin. Proc. Soc. Exper. Biol. & Med. *49*:346–350 (Mar.) 1942.
13. Downs, Cornelia M.: The effect of gramicidin and tyrocidine on various bacteria. J. Bact. *44*:392 (Sept.) 1942.
14. Downs, Cornelia M.: The effect of bactericidal agents on gram-negative cocci. J Bact. *45*:137–142 (Feb.) 1943.

15. Stokinger, H. E., Ackerman, Helen and Carpenter, C. M.: The use of tyrothricin in culture medium as an aid in the isolation of Neisseria gonorrhoeae. (Abstr.) J. Bact. *45*:31 (Jan.) 1943.

16. Dubos, R. J., Hotchkiss, R. D. and Coburn, A. F.: The effect of gramicidin and tyrocidine on bacterial metabolism. J. Biol. Chem. *146*:421–426 (Dec.) 1942.

17. Robinson, H. J. and Graessle, O. E.: In vitro and in vivo studies of gramicidin, tyrothricin and tyrocidine. J. Pharmacol. & Exper. Therap. *76*:316–325 (Dec.) 1942.

18. Trussell, P. C. and Sarles, W. B.: Effect of antibiotic substances upon rhizobia. (Abstr.) J. Bact. *45*:29 (Jan.) 1943.

19. Dubos, R. J.: Studies on a bactericidal agent extracted from a soil bacillus. II. Protective effect of the bactericidal agent against experimental pneumococcus infections in mice. J. Exper. Med. *70*:11–17 (July) 1939.

20. Dubos, R. J. and Hotchkiss, R. D.: The production of bactericidal substances by aerobic sporulating bacilli. J. Exper. Med. *73*:629–640 (May) 1941.

21. Weinstein, Louis and Rammelkamp, C. H.: A study of the effect of gramicidin administered by the oral route. Proc. Soc. Exper. Biol. & Med. *48*:147–149 (Oct.) 1941.

22. Rammelkamp, C. H.: Tyrothricin therapy of experimental hemolytic streptococcal empyema. J. Infect. Dis. *71*:40–46 (July-Aug.) 1942.

23. Tillett, W. S., Cambier, Margaret J. and Harris, W. J., Jr.: Sulfonamide-fast pneumococci. A clinical report of two cases of pneumonia together with experimental studies on the effectiveness of penicillin and tyrothricin against sulfonamide-resistant strains. J. Clin. Investigation. *22*:249–255 (Mar.) 1943.

24. Robson, J. M. and Scott, G. I.: The production and treatment of experimental pneumococcal hypopyon ulcers in the rabbit. Brit. J. Exper. Path. *24*:50–56 (Apr.) 1943.

25. Heilman, Dorothy and Herrell, W. E.: Mode of action of gramicidin. Proc. Soc. Exper. Biol. & Med. *47*:480–484 (June) 1941.

26. Lamar, R. V.: Chemo-immunological studies on localized infections. Second paper: Lysis of the pneumococcus and hemolysis by certain fatty acids and their alkali soaps. J. Exper. Med. *13*,380–386 (Mar.) 1911.

27. Avery, O. T.: A selective medium for B. influenzae. J. A. M. A. 71:2050–2051 (Dec. 21) 1918.

28. Walker, J. E.: The germicidal properties of chemically pure soaps. J. Infect. Dis. *35*:557–566, 1924.

29. Eggerth, A. H.: The germicidal action of hydroxy soaps. J. Exper. Med. *50*:299–313 (Sept.) 1929.

30. Bayliss, Milward and Halvorson, H. O.: Germicidal and detoxifying properties of soaps. (Abstr.) J. Bact. *29*:9 (Jan.) 1935.

31. Baker, Zelma, Harrison, R. W. and Miller, B. F.: Action of synthetic detergents on metabolism of bacteria. J. Exper. Med. *72*:249–271 (Feb.) 1941.

32. Herrell, W. E. and Heilman, Dorothy: Tissue culture studies on cytotoxicity of bactericidal agents. III. Cytotoxic and antibacterial activity of gramicidin and penicillin; comparison with other germicides. Am. J. M. Sc. *206*:221–226 (Aug.) 1943.

33. Pittman, Margaret. The action of mixtures of germicides against gram-negative rods. (Abstr.) J. Bact. *47*:427 (May) 1944.

34. Heilman, Dorothy and Herrell, W. E.: Hemolytic effect of gramicidin. Proc. Soc. Exper. Biol. & Med. *46*:182–184 (Jan.) 1941.

35. Mann, F. C., Heilman, Dorothy and Herrell, W. E.: Effect of serum on hemolysis by gramicidin and tyrocidine. Proc. Soc. Exper. Biol. & Med. *52*:31–33 (Jan.) 1943.

36. Herrell, W. E. and Heilman, Dorothy: Further experimental and clinical studies on gramicidin. (Society Proceedings) J. A. M. A. *118*:1401–1402 (Apr. 18) 1942.

37. MacLeod, C. M., Mirick, G. S. and Curnen, E. C.: Toxicity for dogs of a bactericidal substance derived from a soil bacillus. Proc. Soc. Exper. Biol. & Med. *43:*461–463 (Mar.) 1940.

38. Robinson, H. J. and Molitor, Hans: Some toxicological and pharmacological properties of gramicidin, tyrocidine and tyrothricin. J. Pharmacol. & Exper. Therap. *74:*75–82 (Jan.) 1942.

39. Clapp, Mary P.: *In vitro* effect of tyrothricin and tyrocidine hydrochloride on polymorphonuclear leukocytes. Proc. Soc. Exper. Biol. & Med. *51:*279–281 (Nov.) 1942.

40. Rammelkamp, C. H. and Weinstein, L.: Toxic effects of tyrothricin, gramicidin and tyrocidine. J. Infect. Dis. *71:*166–173 (Sept.-Oct.) 1942.

41. Herrell, W. E. and Heilman, Dorothy: Tissue culture studies on cytotoxicity of bactericidal agents. I. Effects of gramicidin, tyrocidine and penicillin in cultures of mammalian lymph node. Am. J. M. Sc. *205:*157–162 (Feb.) 1943.

42. Herrell, W. E., Heilman, Dorothy and Gage, Robert: Tissue culture studies on cytotoxicity of bactericidal agents. II. Effect of tyrothricin, gramicidin and tyrocidine on culture of mammalian spleen. Am. J. M. Sc. *206:*26–31 (July) 1943.

43. Henle, Gertrude and Zittle, C. A.: Effect of gramicidin on metabolism of bovine spermatozoa. Proc. Soc. Exper. Biol. & Med. *47:*193–198 (June) 1941.

44. Rammelkamp, C. H.: Use of tyrothricin in the treatment of infections; clinical studies. War Med. *2:*830–846 (Sept.) 1942.

45. Herrell, W. E.: Gramicidin and penicillin. S. Clin. North America. (Aug.) 1943, pp. 1163–1176.

46. Rammelkamp, C. H. and Keefer, C. S.: Observations on the use of "gramicidin" (Dubos) in the treatment of streptococcal and staphylococcal infections. J. Clin. Investigation. *20:*433–434 (July) 1941.

47. Francis, A. E.: Sulphonamide-resistant Streptococci in a plastic-surgery ward. Lancet. *1:*408–409 (Apr. 4) 1942.

48. Rankin, L. M.: The use of tyrothricin in the treatment of ulcers of the skin. Am. J. Surg. n.s. *65:*391–392 (Sept.) 1944.

49. Kvale, W. F., Barker, N. W. and Herrell, W. E.: The use of tyrothricin in the treatment of ulcers of the extremities due to peripheral vascular disease. M. Clin. North America. (July) 1944, pp. 849–859.

50. Gause, G. F. and Brazhnikova, M. G.: Gramicidin S and its use in the treatment of infected wounds. War. Med. *6:*180–181 (Sept.) 1944.

51. Schoenbach, E. B., Enders, J. F. and Mueller, J. H.: The apparent effect of tyrothricin on Streptococcus hemolyticus in the rhinopharynx of carriers. Science. n.s. *94:*217–218 (Aug. 29) 1941.

52. Williams, H. L.: Discussion. Tr. Am. Acad. Ophth. *47:*440–441 (July-Aug.) 1943.

53. Lindsay, J. R. and Judd, D. K.: Observations on the local use of sulfonamides and tyrothricin in the upper respiratory tract. Tr. Am. Acad. Ophth. *47:*431–439 (July-Aug.) 1943.

54. Crowe, S. J., Fischer, A. M., Ward, A. T., Jr. and Foley, M. K.: Penicillin and tyrothricin in otolaryngology based on a bacteriological and clinical study of 118 patients. Ann. Otol., Rhin. & Laryng. *52:*541–572 (Sept.) 1943.

55. Kolmer, J. A.: Chemotherapy and biotherapy; their relation to the prevention and treatment of diseases of the ear, nose and throat. Arch. Otolaryng. *40:*17–28 (July) 1944.

56. Heath, Parker: Chemotherapy in ophthalmology. J. A. M. A. *124:*152–155 (Jan. 15) 1944.

57. Streicher, C. J.: Treatment of acute conjunctivitis with tyrothricin. Ohio State M. J. *40:*951 (Oct.) 1944.

58. Piper, M. C.: Personal communication to the author.

59. Little, R. B., Dubos, R. J. and Hotchkiss, R. D.: Action of gramicidin on streptococci of bovine mastitis. Proc. Soc. Exper. Biol. & Med. *44:*444–445 (June) 1940.

60. Little, R. B., Dubos, R. J. and Hotchkiss, R. D.: Effect of gramicidin suspended in mineral oil on streptococci of bovine mastitis. Proc. Soc. Exper. Biol. & Med. *45:*462–463 (Oct.) 1940.

61. Little, R. B., Dubos, R. J. and Hotchkiss, R. D.: Gramicidin, Novoxil and acriflavine for the treatment of the chronic form of streptococcic mastitis. J. Am. Vet. M. A. *98:*189 (Mar.) 1941.

62. Little, R. B., Dubos, R. J., Hotchkiss, R. D., Bean, C. W. and Miller, W. T.: The use of gramicidin and other agents for the elimination of chronic form of bovine mastitis. Am. J. Vet. Research. *2:*305 (July) 1941.

63. Schalm, O. W.: Treatment of bovine mastitis. (Abstr.) J. Am. Vet. M. A. *99:*196 (Sept.) 1941.

64. Martin, F. E.: The eradication of streptococcic mastitis by treatment with tyrothricin. J. Am. Vet. M. A. *101:*23–25 (July) 1942.

65. Bryan, C. A., Weldy, M. L. and Greenberg, J.: The results obtained with tyrothricin in the treatment of 157 cows with streptococcic mastitis. Vet. Med. *37:*364 (Sept.) 1942.

CHAPTER XXII

STREPTOTHRICIN

In 1941, Waksman, Woodruff and Horning[1] briefly mentioned a new antibiotic agent which they were in the process of isolating. This agent, "streptothricin," was described in detail by Waksman and Woodruff[2] in 1942. Unlike penicillin or tyrothricin, which already have been discussed, streptothricin, in addition to possessing antibacterial activity against certain gram-positive pathogenic organisms, appears particularly active against certain gram-negative organisms. Introduction of this substance was of especial interest, therefore, since most antibacterial agents of microbial origin which had been isolated previously acted primarily against gram-positive bacteria and possessed rather feeble action against most gram-negative types.

The organism from which streptothricin was isolated by Waksman and Woodruff[2] is a soil organism of the genus Actinomyces, identified as Actinomyces lavendulae. It has been isolated from soil by Kocholaty, who had used the bacteria-enriched agar plate, while working in Waksman's laboratory. The organism was in many respects similar to a species described by Waksman and Curtis[3] in 1916. It would not grow on tryptophane, phenyl alanine or certain simple inorganic salts of nitrogen. Streptothricin was produced when the organism was grown in a tap-water medium containing 1 per cent glucose or starch, 0.5 per cent tryptone, 0.2 per cent potassium phosphate, 0.2 per cent sodium chloride, 0.001 per cent ferrous sulfate and 0.25 per cent agar. It also was produced when the medium was a variety of simple compounds described by Waksman and Woodruff.[2] Actinomyces lavendulae was grown on one of the suitable media for eight to ten days at 28° C. Subsequent to this, streptothricin was isolated from the medium. According to the description of the method by Waksman and Woodruff, streptothricin is readily soluble in water and dilute mineral acids but is destroyed in the presence of concentrated acids. The substance was found by them to be insoluble in ether, petrol ether or chloroform. It was precipitated from the tryptone medium by substances which precipitated protein but, on isolation, it did not have proteinic characteristics. This was explained by the fact that streptothricin was bound in the culture to a protein, which became inactivated on coagulation. In the crude culture filtrate, and in the alcohol precipitated form, streptothricin was found to be thermo-

303

labile, whereas in the purified form it was thermostable as was evidenced by the fact that it would withstand a temperature of 100° C. for fifteen minutes. Proteolytic enzymes did not reduce its activity.

On completion of growth, the medium was adjusted with acid to pH 3.5. A precipitate was thus produced and the filtrate contained virtually

TABLE 36

COMPARATIVE CHEMICAL AND BIOLOGICAL PROPERTIES OF STREPTOTHRICIN AND STREPTOMYCIN

	Streptothricin	Streptomycin
Source of antibiotic substance	Actinomyces lavendulae	Actinomyces griseus
Medium for production of substance	Tryptone-starch broth	Nutrient glucose broth
Need for growth promoting substance	0	+++
Chemical nature	Organic base	Organic base
Solubility	Soluble in water, acid solutions, not in ether or chloroform	Soluble in water, acid solutions, not in ether or chloroform
Heat stability	Thermostable	Thermostable
Sensitivity to acids	Sensitive	Sensitive
Effect of glucose	Inhibitory	Inhibitory
Bacteriostatic spectrum	Certain gram-positive and gram-negative bacteria; relatively inactive against B. mycoides and S. marcescens	More generalized action against bacteria, including B. mycoides and S. marcescens
Activity against Trypanosoma equiperdum	None	None
Antifungal activity	Active against pathogenic and saprophytic fungi	None
Toxicity to animals	Limited toxicity; 1.0–3.5 gm. of purified material per kg. of body weight	Less toxic; about 7.0 gm. of purified material per kg. of body weight
Activity in vivo	Active	Active

From article by Waksman, Bugie and Schatz, Proceedings of the Staff Meetings of the Mayo Clinic, November 15, 1944.

all the active substance. Streptothricin could be adsorbed at neutrality on charcoal and then removed by treatment for eight to twelve hours with dilute mineral acid. The acid extract was then neutralized and concentrated in a vacuum at 50° C. Next, the dry residue was extracted with absolute alcohol, filtered, evaporated and taken up in water. On electrodialysis the active substance was found to move to the cathode at pH 7.0. According to Waksman and Woodruff,[2] it appeared to behave as an organic base.

In a subsequent report by Waksman, Bugie and Schatz,[4] appeared data on the comparative chemical and biological properties of strepto-thricin and streptomycin (table 36). Streptomycin will be discussed in further detail in the following chapter (Chapter XXIII).

Subsequent to the original report by Waksman and Woodruff,[2] it was reported by Woodruff and Foster,[5] and by Waksman, Bugie and Schatz,[4] that streptothricin is formed much more readily and abundantly under conditions of submersion, combined with agitation and aeration, than under ordinary conditions. Further refinements in preparation of strepto-thricin, including the role of various media and the influence of temper-ature as well as of variation in strain, were reported in 1943 by Waksman[6] and also by Woodruff and Foster.[7]

ACTIVITY OF STREPTOTHRICIN IN VITRO AND IN VIVO

The bacteriostatic action of streptothricin, according to Waksman and Woodruff,[2] is unique. They pointed out that the addition of 0.1 mg. of the crude material to 10 c.c. of nutrient agar inhibited the growth of Escherichia coli as well as that of various other gram-negative bacteria. There was also evidence that certain gram-positive bacteria were sensi-tive (table 37). According to the investigators named, streptothricin possessed bactericidal properties especially against certain gram-negative bacteria. Among the first organisms to be studied both in vitro and in vivo, with reference to the effect of streptothricin thereon, was Brucella abortus. The studies were reported by Metzger, Waksman and Pugh.[8] The results indicated that streptothricin offered some promise as an antibiotic agent against brucellosis of animals. From the tests made in vitro, it appeared that 0.1 mg. or more of crude streptothricin per 10 c.c. of broth was sufficient to prevent growth of the organism. Further studies were carried out in which incubating eggs were employed as the medium. Ten milligrams of the crude material, administered twenty-four hours after inoculation of the eggs with Brucella abortus, resulted in complete destruction of the organism in the living chick embryo. Using the guinea pig as the test animal, the investigators established Brucella abortus infection and each animal in the treated group received a total of 600 mg. of crude streptothricin; the doses were administered at intervals of five days for four weeks. At the conclusion of the experiment, Brucella abortus was recovered from the heart blood of all the untreated controls but from none of the treated guinea pigs. That the infection was not completely eradicated from the body was evident in another experiment, however, wherein Brucella abortus could be recovered from the spleens

TABLE 37

INHIBITORY EFFECT OF STREPTOTHRICIN ON GROWTH OF VARIOUS BACTERIA

Organism	Crude streptothricin added per 10 c.c. agar, mg.					
	3	1	0.3	0.1	0.03	0.01
Bac. subtilis	0‖	0	0	0	0	1
Bac. mycoides	2	2	2	2	2	2
Bac. macerans	2	2	2	2	2	2
Bac. megatherium	0	0	0	0	1	2
Bac. polymyxa	0	0	2	2	2	2
Bac. cereus	2	2	2	2	2	2
Micrococcus lysodeikticus	0	0	0	1	2	2
Staphylococcus muscae	0	0	0	1	2	2
Sarcina lutea	0	0	0	0	1	2
Aërobacter aërogenes*	0	0	1	2	2	2
Aërobacter aërogenes	0	0	0	Tr	2	2
Escherichia coli†	0	0	0	0	2	2
Escherichia coli 4348	0	0	Tr	1	2	2
Serratia marcescens	0	1	2	2	2	2
Serratia marcescens	1	1	2	2	2	2
Pseudomonas fluorescens‡	2	2	2	2	2	2
Shigella gallinarum	0	0	0	0	1	2
Pasteurella pseudotuberculosis	0	0	0	Tr	2	2
Salmonella choleraesuis	0	0	0	Tr	2	2
Salmonella schottmülleri	0	0	0	1	2	2
Salmonella abortivo-equina	0	0	0	Tr	2	2
Salmonella typhimurium	0	0	0	2	2	2
Hemophilus suis	0	0	0	2	2	2
Hemophilus influenzae	0	0	0	0	0	1
Brucella abortus	0	0	0	0	2	2
Azotobacter agile	0	0	0	0	0	2
Azotobacter vinelandii	0	0	0	0	0	2
Azotobacter chroococcum	0	0	0	Tr	2	2
Azotobacter indicum	0	0	0	2	2	2
Mycobacterium phlei	0	0	0	1	2	2
Clostridium butylicum§	2	2	2	2	2	2
Lactobacillus casei§	0	0	0	2	2	2
Actinomyces albus	0	0	0	1	2	2
Actinomyces violaceus-ruber	0	0	—	—	—	—
Actinomyces lavendulae	0	1	2	2	2	2

* Representing 3 distinct strains.
† Representing 5 strains of E. coli obtained from different sources.
‡ Representing 4 strains.
§ Cultured anaerobically.
‖ 0 = no growth, 1 = limited growth, 2 = good growth, Tr = trace of growth.
From article by Waksman and Woodruff, Proceedings of the Society for Experimental Biology and Medicine, February, 1942.

of both the treated and the control guinea pigs. On the other hand, it appeared that there was a greater concentration of organisms in the spleens of the control than of the treated animals.

Additional studies on the activity in vitro of purified streptothricin were reported in 1943 by Waksman.[6] He found Bacillus subtilis, which is

TABLE 38

ANTIBACTERIAL SPECTRUM OF PURIFIED STREPTOTHRICIN

Organism	Units of activity	Organism	Units of activity
Escherichia coli	100,000	Bacillus subtilis	750,000
Aerobacter aerogenes	30,000	Bacillus mycoides	<10,000
Pseudomonas fluorescens	<10,000	Bacillus cereus	<10,000
Shigella gallinarum	300,000	Staphylococcus aureus	200,000
Shigella dysenteriae, 8712	100,000	Sarcina lutea	100,000
Shigella dysenteriae, 8708	100,000		
Shigella dysenteriae, 7424	30,000		
Shigella paradysenteriae	50,000		

From article by Waksman, Journal of Bacteriology, September, 1943.

gram-positive, the most sensitive organism of those studied, whereas a variety of gram-negative organisms, including Escherichia coli, also were sensitive (table 38). A more extensive study of the antibacterial properties of streptothricin subsequently appeared in the report of Foster and Woodruff.[9] These investigators studied not only the effectiveness of streptothricin against a variety of bacteria but also its effect on certain yeasts and fungi. It was again evident that the susceptibility of gram-negative bacteria to streptothricin was in sharp contrast to their susceptibility to the action of another antibiotic agent, penicillin, the effect of which is primarily on gram-positive organisms. Other gram-negative organisms found to be sensitive to the action of streptothricin include Salmonella paratyphi A and B and Eberthella typhi. It was of considerable interest that certain yeasts and pathogenic fungi were found to be sensitive to the action of streptothricin. Examples of sensitive pathogenic fungi include Blastomyces dermatitidis and Achorion schoenleinii. These fungi were inhibited in ranges which compared favorably with the ranges of sensitivity of Escherichia coli. Other studies carried out by Foster and Woodruff indicated that bacteria subjected to inhibition by streptothricin became greatly enlarged and evidenced a tendency towards incomplete fission. These morphologic changes have been noted also when other antibiotic agents, such as penicillin, have been allowed to act on bacteria.

Further significant studies on the activity of streptothricin in vitro and in vivo have been reported by Robinson,[10] by Robinson, Graessle and Smith[11] and by Robinson and Smith.[12] From these reports it was further evident that streptothricin was active against not only a variety of gram-positive pathogens but also against a group of gram-negative organisms, including those of the colon-typhoid-dysentery group. Of especial significance was the fact that as little as 4 units of streptothricin per cubic centimeter of agar (for definition of the unit, see p. 311) was sufficient to inhibit completely the growth of Eberthella typhi (table 39). Among the more resistant organisms were found various members of the genus Clostridium (tetani, welchii, septique and sordellii). Certain other organisms, such as Bacillus pyocyaneus, Bacillus proteus, Streptococcus

TABLE 39

BACTERIOSTATIC ACTION OF STREPTOTHRICIN AGAR PLATE METHOD

Organism	Concentration required to produce complete inhibition
	Streptothricin, units per c.c. of agar
Strep. hemolyticus 1685	32
Strep. hemolyticus MIT	256
Strep. hemolyticus M	256
Strep. viridans	1024
Strep. lactis	1024
Staph. aureus SM	16
Staph. aureus FDA	128
Staph. aureus SD	128
Staph. aureus 155	128
Diplo. pneumoniae Type I	32
B. mycoides	1024
B. subtilis	32
E. typhi	4
S. aertrycke	16
S. enteritidis	64
S. schottmülleri	16
B. flexneri	32
B. sonne	128
P. lepiseptica	32
B. proteus	512
B. pyocyaneus	256
N. meningitidis	256
E. coli	16
S. lutea	256
A. aerogenes	256
	Kolmer's method
Cl. welchii	>855
Cl. tetani	>1080
Cl. sordellii	>1080
Cl. septique	540
Cl. novyi	270

From article by Robinson and Smith, Journal of Pharmacology and Experimental Therapy, August, 1944.

viridans and Streptococcus lactis, were rather resistant to the action of streptothricin.

Robinson, Graessle and Smith[11] and Robinson and Smith[12] further studied in mice the activity of streptothricin against a number of gram-negative and gram-positive organisms. The infections were produced by intraperitoneal injection of 10,000 lethal doses of the test organism.

TABLE 40

EFFICACY OF STREPTOTHRICIN IN MICE INFECTED WITH S. SCHOTTMÜLLERI
(SUBCUTANEOUS THERAPY)

Organism: Salmonella schottmülleri
Age of culture: 6 hours
Infection: 0.5 c.c. of a 10^{-5} culture dilution in 4 per cent mucin
Therapy: Streptothricin given subcutaneously immediately after bacterial inoculation

No. of mice	Drug	Units/dose	No. of doses/day	Culture dilution	1	2	3	4	5	6	7	8	Per cent survival
				(Therapy: A single dose)									
30	Streptothricin	12.5	1	10^{-5}	3	0	0	0	0	0	0	0	0
65	"	25.0	1	"	25	23	18	16	15	15	15	14	21.5
65	"	50.0	1	"	49	44	43	41	37	37	34	34	52.4
65	"	100.0	1	"	65	62	62	60	59	59	59	59	90.8
35	"	200.0	1	"	35	35	35	35	35	35	35	35	100.0
				(Therapy: Single daily doses over a 5-day period)									
20	Streptothricin	12.5	1	10^{-5}	9	2	0	0	0	0	0	0	0
20	"	25.0	1	"	2	5	4	3	1	1	1	1	5
20	"	50.0	1	"	18	13	12	12	12	11	11	11	55
				(Therapy: Every 6 hours over a 5-day period)									
20	Streptothricin	12.5	4	10^{-5}	20	4	3	3	3	3	3	3	15
20	"	25.0	4	"	20	6	3	3	1	1	1	1	5
20	"	50.0	4	"	20	20	20	20	20	20	20	19	95
20	"	100.0	4	"	20	20	20	20	20	20	20	20	100
				(Therapy: None)									
65	Controls	—	—	10^{-5}	6	0	0	0	0	0	0	0	0
30	"	—	—	10^{-6}	3	1	0	0	0	0	0	0	0
30	"	—	—	10^{-7}	16	10	7	5	3	3	3	3	10
30	"	—	—	10^{-8}	16	9	8	7	6	6	6	6	20

From article by Robinson, Graessle and Smith, Science, June 30, 1944.

Treatment consisted of a single dose, or repeated doses, of streptothricin given subcutaneously, intravenously or intraperitoneally. The intervals between the repeated doses varied from once every six hours to once daily over a period of five days. Animals could be protected against lethal infections due to Salmonella schottmülleri, Escherichia coli and Bacillus shigalis. The results of one such experiment are represented in table 40. Streptothricin was found by Robinson, Graessle and Smith to be of little value in protecting animals against infections owing to Bacillus pyocyaneus, Bacillus proteus, Staphylococcus aureus and Diplococcus pneumoniae. Streptothricin had no significant influence on infections due to the virus of epidemic influenza nor to Trypanosoma equiperdum. According to the investigators last named, subcutaneous or oral administration of streptothricin was followed by no significant untoward effects. On the other hand, ten to twelve times the effective dose was followed by some deaths when the material was given intravenously. It was also evident, from the report by Robinson,[10] that streptothricin produced no damaging effect when applied to the conjunctiva of rabbits in concentrations of 0.5 to 1 per cent in physiologic saline solution. He concluded, therefore, that streptothricin should be suitable for local application to infected wounds and mucous membranes.

While Robinson and others[11, 12] were able to protect animals against certain experimental infections by using streptothricin and, at the same time to avoid serious toxic effects, this has not been the experience of all investigators. At the Mayo Foundation,[13] delayed deaths of animals occurred too frequently to justify serious consideration of streptothricin for systemic treatment of infections of human beings. Whether or not the streptothricin differed in some way from that used by Robinson, Graessle and Smith[11] cannot be definitely stated at the moment. At all events, mice, guinea pigs or hamsters were found not to tolerate streptothricin when it was administered systemically in amounts which were considered to be therapeutically effective against a variety of infections. On the other hand, there is little evidence that streptothricin produces any important toxic effects when administered locally and, for that reason, I am inclined to agree with Robinson and Smith[12] that, since streptothricin is so effective against certain gram-negative and gram-positive organisms, the drug should prove of value in local treatment of infected wounds and burns. Furthermore, since the substance, unlike many antibiotic agents, can be given orally and since, as was pointed out by Robinson, Graessle and Smith,[11] lactose-fermenting bacteria in the intestinal tract are greatly reduced in number following administration of the preparation by mouth, there is some hope that it may be of value in treatment of certain types of dysentery and other infections owing to susceptible bacteria (paratyphoid organisms and so forth).

On the basis of present information, however, intravenous or subcutaneous administration of streptothricin in treatment of systemic infections of man is to be avoided.

THE ESTIMATION OF POTENCY OF STREPTOTHRICIN (THE UNIT)

Using the principle of the cup method for estimation of penicillin which was described by Abraham and others,[14] Foster and Woodruff[15] described a method for estimation of the potency of streptothricin. Since different batches of streptothricin vary somewhat in potency, it is essential, as in the case of penicillin and other antibiotic agents, to determine the potency of the material in terms of units. As in the case of the penicillin unit (Oxford unit), the streptothricin unit is simply that amount by weight of streptothricin which will completely inhibit growth of the test organism. However, the unit has no relation to the Oxford unit. The test organism recommended by Foster and Woodruff is Bacillus subtilis. Others, including Robinson, Graessle and Smith,[11] as well as Waksman, Bugie and Schatz,[4] use for the test organism a given strain of Escherichia coli. Their unit of streptothricin is the minimal quantity of the drug which, when added to 1 c.c. of nutrient broth, will inhibit growth of the inoculum of Escherichia coli.

Some idea of the quantity of streptothricin in units, which is used in the treatment of experimental animals, can be obtained from the following data. For example, in a typical experiment, such as the one reported by Robinson, Graessle and Smith,[11] 100 units of streptothricin were administered subcutaneously four times a day, or every six hours, over a period of five days. This amount of streptothricin was sufficient to protect 100 per cent of animals infected with lethal doses of certain gram-negative pathogens (Salmonella schottmülleri). When given orally, doses of as much as 3,000 units per mouse have been employed.

POSSIBLE CLINICAL USE OF STREPTOTHRICIN

Streptothricin, when administered subcutaneously or intravenously to experimental animals, at times will result in either early or delayed death. Accordingly, as was said earlier in this chapter, it does not seem wise, at the time of preparation of this monograph, to recommend its systemic use in treatment of infections of man that are due to susceptible organisms. Streptothricin, however, can be used successfully in local treatment of certain infections.

Preparations Suitable for Local Treatment.—Streptothricin is usually supplied in ampules containing 100,000 units. It is a fairly stable, dry powder. The material is readily soluble in physiologic saline solution or in distilled water. Solutions can be prepared which contain from 500 to 1,000 units per cubic centimeter. Such a solution can be applied locally to infected wounds, ulcers or burns. It also can be introduced into certain infected body cavities, such as the pleural space. Following its use, such lesions may at times become sterile.

A preparation of 0.5 to 1 per cent streptothricin in physiologic saline solution can be used for irrigation of the conjunctiva.

REFERENCES

1. Waksman, S. A., Woodruff, H. B. and Horning, Elizabeth S.: The distribution of antagonistic properties among actinomycetes. J. Bact. 42:816 (Dec.) 1941.

2. Waksman, S. A. and Woodruff, H. B.: Streptothricin, a new selective bacteriostatic and bactericidal agent, particularly active against gram-negative bacteria. Proc. Soc. Exper. Biol. & Med. 49:207–210 (Feb.) 1942.

3. Waksman, S. A. and Curtis, R. E.: Quoted by Waksman, S A. and Woodruff, H. B.[2]

4. Waksman, S. A., Bugie, Elizabeth and Schatz, Albert: Isolation of antibiotic substances from soil micro-organisms, with special reference to streptothricin and streptomycin. Proc. Staff Meet., Mayo Clin. 19:537–548 (Nov. 15) 1944.

5. Woodruff, H. B. and Foster, J. W.: Cultivation of actinomycetes under submerged conditions, with special reference to the formation of streptothricin. J. Bact. 45:30 (Jan.) 1943.

6. Waksman, S. A.: Production and activity of streptothricin. J. Bact. 46:299–310 (Sept.) 1943.

7. Woodruff, H. B. and Foster, J. W.: Microbiological aspects of streptothricin. I. Metabolism and streptothricin formation in stationary and submerged cultures of Actinomyces lavendulae. Arch. Biochem. 2:301–315 (Aug.) 1943.

8. Metzger, H. J., Waksman, S. A. and Pugh, Leonora H.: In vivo activity of streptothricin against Brucella abortus. Proc. Soc. Exper. Biol. & Med. 51:251–252 (Nov.) 1942.

9. Foster, J. A. and Woodruff, H. B.: Microbiological aspects of streptothricin. II. Antibiotic activity of streptothricin. Arch. Biochem. 3:241–255 (Dec.) 1943.

10. Robinson, H. J.: Some toxicological, bacteriological and pharmacological properties of antimicrobial agents produced by soil micro-organisms. Thesis, Rutgers University, 1943.

11. Robinson, H. J., Graessle, O. E. and Smith, Dorothy G.: Studies on the toxicity and activity of streptothricin. Science. n.s. 99:540–542 (June 30) 1944.

12. Robinson, H. J. and Smith, Dorothy G.: Streptothricin as a chemotherapeutic agent. J. Pharmacol. & Exper. Therap. 81:390–401 (Aug.) 1944.

13. Heilman, F. R. and Herrell, W. E.: Unpublished data.

14. Abraham, E. P., Chain, E., Fletcher, C. M., Gardner, A. D., Heatley, N. G., Jennings, M. A. and Florey, H. W.: Further observations on penicillin. Lancet. 2:177–188; 189 (Aug. 16) 1941.

15. Foster, J. W. and Woodruff, H. B.: Quantitative estimation of streptothricin. J. Bact. 45:408–409 (Apr.) 1943.

CHAPTER XXIII

STREPTOMYCIN

In the preceding chapter it was pointed out that streptothricin possesses activity against gram-negative organisms. Most other antibiotic substances, including penicillin and other mold products, as well as tyrothricin, are primarily effective against gram-positive organisms. With the exception of their effect on organisms of the genus Neisseria, they possess little if any activity against gram-negative organisms. Subsequent to isolation of streptothricin by the group of investigators[1, 2] at the Agricultural Experimental Station at Rutgers University, the search for other antibiotic substances which might possess activity against gram-negative bacteria was continued. Since streptothricin had been obtained from Actinomyces lavendulae, other actinomycetes were intensively studied by these same investigators. After detailed examination of a number of cultures either isolated at random from different natural and enriched soils or selected from a culture collection, another organism was found by Schatz, Bugie and Waksman[3] which produced a promising antibiotic substance. This substance was named "streptomycin" and was described by them in January, 1944.

The organism of the genus Actinomyces which produced this substance apparently was a strain of Actinomyces griseus, which had been described some twenty-five years before by Waksman. The name "streptomycin" was given to the substance because it was produced by one of the actinomycetes which sporulates and produces aerial mycelia and to which the generic name "Streptomyces" had been given by Waksman and Henrici[4] in 1943. While, in some respects, streptomycin resembled streptothricin, it differed from streptothricin in that it possessed greater activity against various gram-negative bacteria.[3, 5] In fact, it was effective against certain organisms which were resistant to the action of streptothricin.

Whereas streptothricin was produced most abundantly when Actinomyces lavendulae was grown in tryptone starch medium, streptomycin was produced when Actinomyces griseus was grown in ordinary nutrient broth (peptone-meat extract). Schatz, Bugie and Waksman[3] further pointed out that production of streptomycin required the presence of a specific growth-promoting substance supplied by meat extract and that corn steep liquor could be substituted for the meat extract. The yield of streptomycin increased following addition of glucose to the medium.

313

Growth was much more rapid in shaken cultures than when cultures remained stationary, although fairly good growth could be obtained when the organism was grown under stationary conditions. Growth of Actinomyces griseus (suitable strains) was allowed to proceed for five to twelve days, at which time streptomycin was isolated from the culture filtrates by a method similar to that described previously by Waksman and Woodruff[2] for isolation of streptothricin (p. 304).

Streptomycin chemically behaves as an organic base. It is soluble in water and dilute acid solutions. It is insoluble in ether or chloroform. It is thermostable. It is considerably less toxic than the related substance, streptothricin. For comparison of the chemical and biological properties of streptomycin with those of streptothricin, see table 36 (Chapter XXII).

ACTIVITY OF STREPTOMYCIN IN VITRO AND IN VIVO

Schatz, Bugie and Waksman[3] compared the antibacterial behavior of streptomycin with that of the related substance, streptothricin. Examination of the bacteriostatic spectra of the two substances brought out some rather interesting differences in their activity in vitro (table 41). It was evident from these data that, taking the gram-negative organism Escherichia coli as a standard, streptomycin was found to have about the same activity as streptothricin against such organisms as Bacillus subtilis, Aerobacter aerogenes and Proteus vulgaris. While streptomycin was less active than streptothricin against Staphylococcus aureus and against one species of Salmonella, it was more active than streptothricin against a variety of other organisms. That Mycobacterium tuberculosis was considerably more sensitive to the action of streptomycin than to the action of streptothricin was evident from the reports by Waksman, Bugie and Schatz[5] (table 42) and by Schatz and Waksman.[6] Students of chemotherapy were, therefore, considerably stimulated by these reports. If, for example, streptomycin was found to possess antibacterial activity against Mycobacterium tuberculosis, its discovery might inaugurate an entirely new approach to the problem of chemotherapy of tuberculosis.

The investigators at Rutgers University[7] subsequently extended their studies on streptomycin to include experiments on the activity of the agent in vivo against a variety of susceptible organisms. The preparation of streptomycin used in these early studies contained 30 units per milligram. *The unit of streptomycin is that quantity of the dry material which will inhibit the growth of a given strain of Escherichia coli in 1 c.c. of nutrient broth or agar.* Mice were inoculated with fatal doses of Salmonella schottmülleri. The treated animals received 190 units (6.4 mg.) of streptomycin. The total amount was divided into four doses and one dose was administered every six hours. All control animals died within the first twenty-four hours, whereas the majority of the treated animals were alive and well at termination of the experiment (table 43). Equally striking results were obtained with streptomycin in treatment of animals infected with fatal doses of Pseudomonas aeruginosa. Fully as good, also, were results obtained in study, on chick embryos, of the effectiveness

TABLE 41

COMPARATIVE BACTERIOSTATIC SPECTRA OF STREPTOMYCIN AND STREPTOTHRICIN ON BASIS OF CRUDE, ASH-FREE DRY MATERIAL

Organism	Gram stain	Units of activity per gram ash-free dry material	
		Streptomycin × 1000	Streptothricin* × 1000
B. subtilis 0	+	125	500
B. mycoides 0	+	250	<3
B. mycoides 317–911	+	20	<3
B. cereus	+	30	<3
B. mesentericus	+	15	—
B. megatherium	+	100	150
S. aureus	+	15	200
S. lutea	+	100	150
M. phlei	+	100	50
M. tuberculosis	+	30	—
Phytomonas pruni	−	100	400
Listerella monocytogenes	−	10	—
Shigella gallinarum	−	—	150
E. coli	−	25	100
S. marcescens	−	25	5
A. aerogenes	−	10	50
P. vulgaris	−	10	50
S. aertrycke	−	2.5	—
S. schottmülleri	−	—	50
Ps. fluorescens	−	2	<3
Ps. aeruginosa	−	1	<3
Cl. butylicum	−	3	<3

* These results are partly based on data reported previously; data obtained more recently with purified preparations give the same type of spectrum. Since streptothricin represented a more purified and, therefore, more concentrated preparation than streptomycin, a better comparison would be with the activity against E. coli as a unit; the units for the other test organisms would, therefore, have to be multiplied by 4.

From article by Schatz, Bugie and Waksman, Proceedings of the Society for Experimental Biology and Medicine, January, 1944.

of streptomycin against fowl typhoid. The results, according to the investigators, proved that streptomycin, if used in sufficient amounts, offered full protection against fowl typhoid. Even the dead embryos were completely free of the infecting organisms. Another interesting observation was the effectiveness of streptomycin against Brucella abortus infection of chick embryos. According to the observers, the protection following use of streptomycin against experimental infections owing to Brucella abortus was excellent. Likewise, following use of the agent, experimental animals were protected against experimental infections owing to Proteus vulgaris.

TABLE 42

BACTERIOSTATIC SPECTRA OF CRUDE PREPARATIONS OF STREPTOMYCIN AND STREPTOTHRICIN: COMPARATIVE ACTIVITY IN DILUTION UNITS, AS DETERMINED BY PLATE METHOD

Test organism	Streptomycin	Streptothricin
Bacillus subtilis	25,000	30,000
Bacillus mycoides	7,500	<100
Staphylococcus aureus	1,500	2,000
Mycobacterium phlei	10,000	5,000
Mycobacterium tuberculosis (Human, H37)	3,000	100
Escherichia coli	2,000	2,000
Shigella gallinarum	2,000	5,000
Salmonella pullorum	3,000	5,000
Serratia marcescens	2,500	200
Pseudomonas aeruginosa	300	50

From article by Waksman, Bugie and Schatz, Proceedings of the Staff Meetings of the Mayo Clinic, November 15, 1944.

TABLE 43

ACTIVITY OF STREPTOMYCIN IN MICE INFECTED WITH S. SCHOTTMÜLLERI

No. of mice	Treatment	Dilution of bacterial culture used for infection	Survival of mice, in hours					
			18	24	30	42	48	72
5	Control*	10^{-5}	2	0	0	0	0	0
3	Control	10^{-6}	1	0	0	0	0	0
3	Control	10^{-7}	1	0	0	0	0	0
3	Control	10^{-8}	2	0	0	0	0	0
5	Streptomycin, 6.4 mg.†	10^{-5}	5	5	5	5	5	5
5	Streptomycin, 12.8 mg.†	10^{-5}	5	5	5	5	4	4

* No streptomycin.
† Divided in 4 doses, every 6 hours.
From article by Jones, Metzger, Schatz and Waksman, Science, August 4, 1944.

From these preliminary reports, therefore, it became evident that a new antibiotic substance had been introduced, which appeared to possess therapeutic possibilities against such diseases as tuberculosis, dysentery, fowl typhoid, possibly undulant fever, as well as, possibly, infections owing to organisms of the genus Pseudomonas and the genus Proteus. For the most part, this group of infections had resisted treatment with antibiotic substances previously available. It is not surprising, therefore, that intensive investigation of streptomycin immediately was begun by many investigators.

Feldman and Hinshaw[8] were the first to study the possible effectiveness of streptomycin on experimental tuberculosis. They established rather severe tuberculous infections by inoculating guinea pigs subcutaneously with virulent cultures of Mycobacterium tuberculosis.

TABLE 44

SUMMARY OF RESULTS OBTAINED WITH STREPTOMYCIN
AGAINST EXPERIMENTAL TUBERCULOSIS

Experiment	Ani- mals	Duration of infection, days		Duration of treatment, days	Organs showing macroscopic tuberculosis			Index of infection determined micro- scopically*
		Died	Killed		Spleen	Liver	Lungs	
1 Controls (8 animals)	1	43		0	0	1	1	81.9
	1	53		0	1	1	1	
	2		54	0	2	2	2	
	4		60	0	4	3	2	
1 Treated (4 animals)	2		54	39	1	0	0	2.8
	2		54	54	0	0	0	
2 Controls (9 animals†)	9		61	0	8	7	7	67
2 Treated (9 animals†)	4		61	47	1	0	0	5.8
	5		61	61	0	0	0	

* Tissues examined included spleen, liver, lungs, tracheobronchial lymph nodes, sub-cutis at the site of injection and the axillary lymph nodes (100 units represents theoretical maximal amount of tuberculosis possible).
† Of the ten animals in the group originally, one died prematurely.
From article by Feldman and Hinshaw, Proceedings of the Staff Meetings of the Mayo Clinic, December 27, 1944.

Treatment with streptomycin was begun at varying intervals following inoculation and, in some instances, was continued for as long as sixty-one days. A rather striking suppressive effect on the course of tuberculosis of guinea pigs was obtained (table 44). Based on the arbitrary selection of the numeral 100 as representing the theoretical maximal amount of tuberculosis possible (index of infection), it appeared that 81.9 represented the index of infection in one series of controls and 67 the index

11

of infection in another series of control animals. On the other hand, the index of infection was reported as 2.8 and 5.8 in two separate series of animals who had been treated for varying periods of time with streptomycin. The investigators concluded that, in addition to the suppressive effect of streptomycin on infections in guinea pigs owing to a human variety of Mycobacterium tuberculosis, streptomycin was well tolerated by the experimental animals.

Another contribution in connection with the possible use of streptomycin as a chemotherapeutic agent was the report by F. R. Heilman[9] on the effect of streptomycin on Pasteurella tularensis in vitro and on the use of the substance in treatment of experimental tularemia. Chemotherapeutic agents in general, including sulfonamides and penicillin, have little effect on the course of this important disease. On the basis of studies in vitro, however, it appeared that growth of a virulent strain of Pasteurella tularensis was inhibited completely by concentrations of 0.15 unit of streptomycin per cubic centimeter. Furthermore, when lethal infections owing to Pasteurella tularensis were established in mice, of thirty untreated animals, all died of tularemia within ninety-six hours after inoculation. This is a mortality rate of 100 per cent. Thirty mice received 1,000 units each of streptomycin subcutaneously per day for ten days. All thirty survived. In treatment of these animals, 150 units of streptomycin dissolved in physiologic solution of sodium chloride was administered at 8 a.m., 12 noon, 3 p.m. and 6 p.m.; 400 units suspended in 0.05 ml. of 1 per cent beeswax and sesame oil was administered at 9 p.m. In view of the fact that the disease is so highly virulent for mice, and because all of the treated animals survived, Heilman suggested that streptomycin might prove useful in treatment of tularemia of man.

Further studies on the chemotherapeutic properties of streptomycin have been reported by Robinson, Smith and Graessle.[10] These investigators found that streptomycin was considerably less toxic for experimental animals than was the related substance, streptothricin. For example, in one of their experiments it was found that 5,000 units of streptothricin administered subcutaneously to mice weighing 20 gm. resulted in death of 100 per cent of the animals. On the other hand, 10,000 units of streptomycin of high potency, administered subcutaneously to mice weighing 20 gm., resulted in no significant evidence of toxicity. The investigators further reported that streptomycin possessed greater activity in vivo than streptothricin possessed, not only against gram-negative bacteria but also against gram-positive bacteria.

Another significant observation has been reported by F. R. Heilman which concerns the possible chemotherapeutic value of streptomycin.[11] He found that streptomycin was exceedingly effective against the microorganisms of the Friedländer group (Klebsiella). Heilman reported that five strains of Klebsiella were inhibited completely in vitro in the presence of concentrations varying from 0.15 to 0.37 unit of streptomycin per milliliter of culture medium. He also established lethal infections in mice with five different strains of these organisms. In one experiment, the mice received 10,000 lethal doses of the infecting organism. Half of the infected group received streptomycin for forty-eight to seventy-two hours; all survived. The other half of the animals, which received no streptomycin, all died.

In the past, treatment of the severe type of pneumonia caused by the micro-organisms of the Friedländer group has not been entirely satisfactory. These experimental results reported by Heilman give reason to hope that streptomycin may prove of value in treatment of this disease in man. In his report, Heilman further pointed out that these organisms are not infrequently present as secondary invaders in various types of respiratory infections due to other causes. He further emphasized the fact that the organisms are commonly present in the nasal mucous membranes of patients suffering with ozena and in the affected tissues of patients who have rhinoscleroma.

CLINICAL USE OF STREPTOMYCIN

Dosage and Method of Administration.—Streptomycin is dispensed in ampules which contain one million units each. The material is a stable powder and is readily soluble in physiologic saline solution or in distilled water. It can be administered satisfactorily by the intramuscular route in a manner similar to that commonly used for administration of penicillin. I[12] have administered, intramuscularly, to human beings, as much as 100,000 units of streptomycin every three hours day and night without evidence of toxicity. Single intramuscular injections of as much as 250,000 units of streptomycin also have been administered without evidence of local or systemic untoward effects. Pyrogen-free streptomycin can be administered intravenously, either in single injections or by the intravenous drip method, in a manner similar to that commonly used for administration of penicillin (see Chapter IX).

Absorption, Distribution and Excretion.—Following intramuscular administration, streptomycin appears to be readily absorbed and reaches the general circulation. Using an adaptation of the Fleming slide-cell technic (p. 94) Dorothy Heilman and I[13] have found that the concentration of streptomycin in the serum of patients who are receiving the substance falls rather sharply and that little or none of it remains in the serum three hours following its intramuscular administration. Not unlike penicillin, streptomycin is readily excreted by the kidneys and, on occasions, 60 to 70 per cent of the total amount administered is excreted in the urine. Just as is true of penicillin, so streptomycin also appears not to diffuse readily into the cerebrospinal fluid even when the blood serum contains fairly large amounts of the substance.

Clinical Results.—At the time of this writing, enough clinical data have not been accumulated to justify final statements concerning the use of streptomycin in treatment of infections of man owing to susceptible organisms. Included among the conditions which I have treated with streptomycin are brucellosis, typhoid fever and infections owing to the micro-organisms of the Friedländer group (Klebsiella) and bacteriemia owing to Escherichia coli. Final evaluation of results must await further clinical trials. At least it can be stated that patients will tolerate therapeutic doses of the material without evidence of serious toxic effects. In order to maintain therapeutic levels of the material in the blood, it must be administered by the intravenous drip method or at least every three hours by the intramuscular method. For recent developments in streptomycin see page 336 and following.

REFERENCES

1. Waksman, S. A., Woodruff, H. B. and Horning, E. S.: The distribution of antagonistic properties among actinomycetes. J. Bact. *42*:816 (Dec.) 1941.

2. Waksman, S. A. and Woodruff, H. B.: Streptothricin, a new selective bacteriostatic and bactericidal agent, particularly active against gram-negative bacteria. Proc. Soc. Exper. Biol. & Med. *49*:207–210 (Feb.) 1942.

3. Schatz, Albert, Bugie, Elizabeth and Waksman, S. A.: Streptomycin, a substance exhibiting antibiotic activity against gram-positive and gram-negative bacteria. Proc. Soc. Exper. Biol. & Med. *55*:66–69 (Jan.) 1944.

4. Waksman, S. W. and Henrici, A. T.: The nomenclature and classification of the actinomycetes. J. Bact. *46*:337–341 (Oct.) 1943.

5. Waksman, S. A., Bugie, Elizabeth and Schatz, Albert: Isolation of antibiotic substances from soil micro-organisms, with special reference to streptothricin and streptomycin. Proc. Staff Meet., Mayo Clin. *19*:537–548 (Nov. 15) 1944.

6. Schatz, Albert and Waksman, S. A.: Effect of streptomycin and other antibiotic substances upon Mycobacterium tuberculosis and related organisms. Proc. Soc. Exper. Biol. & Med. *57*:244–248 (Nov.) 1944.

7. Jones, Doris, Metzger, H. J., Schatz, Albert and Waksman, S. A.: Control of gram-negative bacteria in experimental animals by streptomycin. Science. n.s. *100*:103–105 (Aug. 4) 1944.

8. Feldman, W. H. and Hinshaw, H. C.: Effects of streptomycin on experimental tuberculosis in guinea pigs; a preliminary report. Proc. Staff Meet., Mayo Clin. *19*:593–599 (Dec. 27) 1944.

9. Heilman, F. R.: Streptomycin in the treatment of experimental tularemia. Proc. Staff Meet., Mayo Clin. *19*:553–559 (Nov. 29) 1944.

10. Robinson, H. J., Smith, Dorothy G. and Graessle, O. E.: Chemotherapeutic properties of streptomycin. Proc. Soc. Exper. Biol. & Med. *57*:226–231 (Nov.) 1944.

11. Heilman, F. R.: Streptomycin in the treatment of experimental infections with micro-organisms of the Friedländer group (Klebsiella). Proc. Staff Meet., Mayo Clinic, *20*:32–39 (Feb. 7) 1945.

12. Herrell, W. E.: Unpublished data.

13. Heilman, Dorothy and Herrell, W. E.: Unpublished data.

CHAPTER XXIV

MISCELLANEOUS ANTIBIOTIC AGENTS

In the introduction to this section (Chapter XX) it was said that antibiotic agents which, at the time of this writing, do not appear to possess great clinical value would be dealt with in the present chapter.

PYOCYANASE AND PYOCYANINE

According to Schoental,[1] Pseudomonas pyocyanea is one of the oldest examples known of a micro-organism producing substances antagonistic to other bacteria. It appears that Bouchard[2] had observed that this organism produced an antagonistic substance. The substance, however, was named "pyocyanase" by Emmerich and Loew[3] (1899), who considered it to be an enzyme.

It was subsequently found by Wrede and Strack[4] (1924), that the organism produced not only the enzyme pyocyanase but also pyocyanine. Pyocyanase is a thermostable substance and is lipoid in nature. According to Waksman,[5] its activity is largely due to the presence of unsaturated fatty acids. Pyocyanine is a blue pigment, soluble in chloroform, which is also thermostable. Although these antibiotic agents were somewhat active in vitro against a variety of gram-positive and gram-negative pathogens, they were found to be considerably toxic for experimental animals. For example, Schoental found that intraperitoneal injection of as little as 2 mg. of pyocyanine resulted in death of animals. Neither pyocyanase nor pyocyanine has proved of any significant clinical value although each has been used at times in the treatment of infections of human beings.

ACTINOMYCIN A AND B

Actinomycin A and B, both elaborated from Actinomyces antibioticus (Waksman and Woodruff[6]), possess considerable activity against a variety of gram-positive pathogenic organisms. Actinomycin A is soluble in ether and alcohol. It is orange colored and highly toxic. It appears to be a thermostable, nitrogen bearing, ring compound. Actinomycin B is soluble in ether but is relatively insoluble in alcohol. The two substances, therefore, are not identical but are closely related. From an experimental standpoint these antibiotic agents are interesting. Both, however, have proved exceedingly toxic for experimental animals and, to date, efforts to remove the toxic properties and, at the same time, to preserve antibacterial activity, have been unsuccessful. At present, neither substance appears to have any place in treatment of diseases of man.

PENICILLIC ACID

Penicillic acid, which is derived from both Penicillium puberulum and Penicillium cyclopium, is a colorless substance which is rather readily soluble in water. Something is known of its chemical nature. According to reports by Oxford, Raistrick and Smith,[7] by Oxford,[8] and by Page and Robinson,[9] its chemical formula is as follows: $CH_3C(:CH_2) COC(OCH_3)$:CHCOOH. It appears to possess considerable activity not only against gram-positive bacteria but also against members of the colon-typhoid-Salmonella group of gram-negative organisms. Little information has been obtained as to its possible therapeutic value.

CITRININ

The source of citrinin is a strain of Penicillium citrinum. It is a yellow substance which has been obtained in crystalline form. The chemical formula suggested for it by Hetherington, Raistrick and their associates[10,11] is $C_{13}H_{14}O_5$. The material is predominantly active against gram-positive organisms. It is practically insoluble in cold water. Unfortunately, it has been found to be toxic for experimental animals when administered either orally or intraperitoneally. The toxic signs in animals, described by Robinson,[12] include ataxia, irregular respiration, tonic convulsions and a fall in body temperature which occurs shortly after administration. Obviously, therefore, the toxicity of this substance precludes its consideration as a therapeutic agent.

GLIOTOXIN

Gliotoxin, which was obtained from Trichoderma lignorum,[13] appears also to be obtainable from filtrates of Aspergillus fumigatus.[14] This antibiotic substance appears to be a sulfur bearing, ring compound which in crystalline form appears as elongated plates. The empirical formula for gliotoxin, suggested by Johnson, Bruce and Dutcher,[15] is $C_{13}H_{14}N_2O_4S_2$.

The substance appears to be active against certain gram-positive organisms, as well as against certain gram-negative pathogens. As is true of many other antibiotic agents, so this one is exceedingly toxic. As was pointed out by Robinson,[12] its toxicity approaches that of actinomycin which, as I have said, is exceedingly toxic. Gliotoxin, therefore, holds little promise as a chemotherapeutic agent.

FUMIGATIN

Fumigatin was obtained in crystalline form from the organism Aspergillus fumigatus by Anslow and Raistrick.[16] The empirical formula which they suggested for it was $C_8H_8O_4$. It was found to be fairly soluble and to be active especially against certain gram-positive organisms. In its present form, this substance is too toxic to consider for therapeutic use.

CLAVIFORMIN, CLAVACIN AND PATULIN

Claviformin obtained from cultures of Penicillium claviforme, clavacin obtained from Aspergillus clavatus, and patulin obtained from Penicillium patulum were described by three different groups of investigators.[17-19] It is now generally agreed[20-22] that all three of these antibiotic agents, although they are derived from different organisms, are identical. They appear to have the same empirical formula: $C_7H_6O_4$. Patulin received some clinical investigation. Since it was effective against both gram-positive and gram-negative organisms that commonly are present in the nasopharynx, Raistrick and his colleagues[19] used the substance locally for treatment of patients suffering with common colds. Solutions of patulin, 1:10,000, were sprayed into the nose or snuffed up from the hand. The investigators reported that 57 per cent of the treated patients recovered completely within forty-eight hours, as compared with only 9.4 per cent of the control group. Unfortunately, these results have not been confirmed, as was evidenced by the reports of Stansfeld, Francis and Stuart-Harris[23] and of the Patulin Clinical Trials Committee of the British Medical Research Council.[24]

Neither claviformin, clavacin nor patulin is suitable for subcutaneous or intravenous administration. Experimental animals may die shortly after intraperitoneal administration of these substances. According to Robinson,[12] one of these agents, clavacin, is surpassed in toxicity only by actinomycin and gliotoxin. A high degree of toxicity for mice also was evident from the report by Katzman and his associates.[25] Whether any of these substances will prove of value as local agents for treatment of bacterial infections remains to be seen.

FUMIGACIN AND HELVOLIC ACID

The antibiotic substance fumigacin, obtained from Aspergillus fumigatus by Waksman, Horning and Spencer,[18] and helvolic acid, subsequently obtained from the same organism by Chain and others,[26] appear now, from reports by Waksman and Geiger,[27] and by Waksman,[22] to be identical substances. In pure form, fumigacin appears as very fine white needles and the empirical formula suggested for the substance by Waksman and Geiger[27] (1944) is $C_{32}H_{44}O_8$. This same formula had been suggested by Chain and his associates[26] for helvolic acid (1943).

It was suggested by Chain and Florey[28] that helvolic acid merited attention as a chemotherapeutic agent because it appeared to be stable and possessed low toxicity for tissue as measured by tissue culture methods. It was also found to possess relatively low toxicity for animals following single intravenous injections. On the other hand, prolonged administration resulted in severe damage to the liver. Furthermore, Robinson[12] examined the identical substance, fumigacin, and found that doses of 4 to 8 mg., administered intraperitoneally, produced depression and ataxia although the experimental animals eventually recovered. When 12 mg. of the substance was administered intraperitoneally to experimental animals, death resulted within one to two hours. It seems unlikely, therefore, in view of these studies, that the identical substances, fumigacin and helvolic acid, deserve at this time serious consideration as chemotherapeutic agents.

ASPERGILLIC ACID

Aspergillic acid was isolated by White and Hill[29] from a strain of Aspergillus flavus. The substance was obtained in crystalline form and the empirical composition appeared to be $C_{12}H_{20}N_2O_2$. It was found to be effective against both gram-positive and gram-negative bacteria, as well as against the organisms associated with gas gangrene. Unfortunately, the substance is too toxic to be administered systemically. White and Hill quoted certain studies to suggest that aspergillic acid might be of value in local treatment of gas gangrene.

FLAVICIN

Flavicin was isolated by Bush and Goth[30] from broth filtrates of Aspergillus flavus. The crude extracts were toxic, as was partially purified flavicin; however, the latter was considerably less toxic than the former. Although the chemical nature of this substance is not well known, it appears to resemble rather closely penicillin. It is soluble in water and in ether. Just as is true of penicillin, it is highly active against most gram-positive organisms. As is true of penicillin also, it is unstable in acid media and appears to be unstable on shaking with air. From the studies reported by Bush and Goth, however, it seemed that flavicin was a little more active than penicillin against certain organisms. If purified preparations of this antibiotic agent prove to have low toxicity and high antibacterial activity, another therapeutic agent may be available which is comparable to penicillin.

GIGANTIC ACID

Gigantic acid was obtained from Aspergillus giganteus by Philpot.[31] This substance was reported to possess properties rather closely similar to penicillin. Whether or not it will prove of value as a therapeutic agent cannot be stated at the moment. Its isolation, however, would tend to indicate further that substances which resemble penicillin can be produced by certain species of Aspergillus.

FLAVACIDIN

Further evidence to suggest that substances which resemble penicillin can be obtained from organisms of the genus Aspergillus was brought out in the report of McKee, Rake and Houck.[32] A strain of Aspergillus flavus was grown in submerged culture in a modified Czapek-Dox medium. The antibiotic substance elaborated by this organism, and isolated by the investigators just mentioned, has been named "flavacidin." Although the chemical nature of flavacidin was not known when McKee, Rake and Houck made their report, there was considerable evidence of biologic similarity between flavacidin and penicillin. Both are highly active against gram-positive organisms and both possess only feeble action against gram-negative pathogens. Flavacidin and penicillin protect mice to an equal degree against pneumococcal infections. Flavacidin, as is true also of penicillin, is highly soluble, readily absorbed by the tissues of the body and quickly excreted by the kidneys. Of further interest is the fact that organisms rendered resistant to penicillin were found to be resistant to flavacidin, whereas other antibiotic substances still would produce inhibition of growth of these organisms. Moreover, an enzyme which is antagonistic to penicillin was also antagonistic to flavacidin but not to other antibiotic substances. Whether or not this new agent is to be considered chemically the same as penicillin will depend on further investigations.

REFERENCES

1. Schoental, R.: The nature of the antibacterial agents present in *Pseudomonas pyocyanea* cultures. Brit. J. Exper. Path. *22*:137–147 (June) 1941.

2. Bouchard, L.: Quoted by Schoental, R.[1]

3. Emmerich, R. and Loew, C.: Quoted by Schoental, R.[1]

4. Wrede, F. and Strack, E.: Quoted by Waksman, S. A.: Antagonistic relations of microörganisms. Bact. Rev. *5*:231–291 (Sept.) 1941.

5. Waksman, S. A.: Antibiotic substances, production by micro-organisms—nature and mode of action. Am. J. Pub. Health. *34*:358–364 (Apr.) 1944.

6. Waksman, S. A. and Woodruff, H. B.: Bacteriostatic and bactericidal substances produced by a soil Actinomyces. Proc. Soc. Exper. Biol. & Med. *45*:609–614 (Nov.) 1940.

7. Oxford, A. E., Raistrick, H. and Smith, G.: Antibacterial substances from moulds. II. Penicillic acid, a metabolic product of Penicillium puberulum Bainier and Penicillium cyclopium Westling. Chem. & Ind. *61*:22 (Jan. 10) 1942.

8. Oxford, A. E.: Antibacterial substances from moulds. III. Some observations on the bacteriostatic powers of the mould products citrinin and penicillic acid. Chem. & Ind. *61*:48 (Jan. 24) 1942.

9. Page, J. E. and Robinson, F. A.: An examination of the relationship between the bacteriostatic activity and the normal reduction potentials of substituted quinones. Brit. J. Exper. Path. *24*:89–95 (June) 1943.

10. Hetherington, A. C. and Raistrick, H.: Studies in the biochemistry of micro-organisms. Part XIV. On the production and chemical constitution of a new yellow colouring matter, citrinin, produced from glucose by Penicillium citrinum, Thom. Tr. Roy. Soc. London, s.B., *220*:269–295, 1931. (Abstr.) Chem. Abstr. *26*:2486 (May 10) 1932.

11. Coyne, F. P., Raistrick, Harold and Robinson, Robert: Studies in the biochemistry of micro-organisms. Part XV. The molecular structure of citrinin. Tr. Roy. Soc. London, s. B., *220*:297–300, 1931. (Abstr.) Chem. Abstr. *26*:2486 (May 10) 1932.

12. Robinson, H. J.: Some toxicological, bacteriological and pharmacological properties of antimicrobial agents produced by soil micro-organisms. Thesis, Rutgers University, 1943.

13. Weindling, R. and Emerson, O.: Quoted by Waksman, S. A.: Antagonistic relations of micro-organisms. Bact. Rev. *5*:231–291 (Sept.) 1941.

14. Menzel, A. E. O., Wintersteiner, O. and Hoogerheide, J. C.: The isolation of gliotoxin and fumigacin from culture filtrates of Aspergillus fumigatus. J. Biol. Chem. *152*:419–429 (Feb.) 1944.

15. Johnson, J. R., Bruce, W. F. and Dutcher, J. D.: Gliotoxin, the antibiotic principle of *Gliocladium fimbriatum*. I. Production, physical and biological properties. J. Am. Chem. Soc. *65*:2005–2009 (Oct.) 1943.

16. Anslow, W. K. and Raistrick, Harold: Studies in the biochemistry of micro-organisms. LVII. Biochem. J. *32*:687–696, 1938.

17. Chain, E., Florey, H. W. and Jennings, M. A.: An antibacterial substance produced by *Penicillium claviforme*. Brit. J. Exper. Path. *23*:202–205 (Aug.) 1942.

18. Waksman, S. A., Horning, E. S. and Spencer, E. L.: The production of two antibacterial substances, fumigacin and clavacin. Science. n.s. *96*:202–203 (Aug. 28) 1942.

19. Raistrick, Harold and others. Patulin in the common cold. Collaborative research on a derivative of *Penicillium patulum* Bainier. Lancet. *2*:625–635 (Nov. 20) 1943.

20. Chain, E., Florey, H. W. and Jennings, M. A.: Identity of patulin and claviformin. Lancet. *1*:112–114 (Jan. 22) 1944.

21. Hooper, I. R., Anderson, H. W., Skell, P. and Carter, H. E.: The identity of clavacin with patulin. Science. n.s. *99*:16 (Jan. 7) 1944.

22. Waksman, S. A.: Purification and antibacterial activity of fumigacin and clavacin. Science. n.s. *99*:220–221 (Mar. 17) 1944.

23. Stansfeld, J. M., Francis, A. E. and Stuart-Harris, C. H.: Laboratory and clinical trials of patulin. Lancet. *2*:370–372 (Sept. 16) 1944.

24. Report of the Patulin Clinical Trials Committee, Medical Research Council: Clinical trial of patulin in the common cold. Lancet. *2*:373–375 (Sept. 16) 1944.

25. Katzman, P. A., Hays, E. E., Cain, C. K., Van Wyk, J. J., Reithel, F. J., Thayer, S. A. and Doisy, E. A.: Clavacin, an antibiotic substance from Aspergillus clavatus. J. Biol. Chem. *154*:475–486 (July) 1944.

26. Chain, E., Florey, H. W., Jennings, M. A. and Williams, T. I.: Helvolic acid, an antibiotic produced by Aspergillus fumigatus, mut. helvola Yuill. Brit. J. Exper. Path. *24*:108–119 (June) 1943.

27. Waksman, S. A. and Geiger, W. B.: The nature of the antibiotic substances produced by Aspergillus fumigatus. J. Bact. *47*:391–397 (Apr.) 1944.

28. Chain, E. and Florey, H. W.: Penicillin. Endeavour. vol. 3, no. 9, (Jan.) 1944.

29. White, E. C. and Hill, Justina H.: Studies on antibacterial products formed by molds. I. Aspergillic acid, a product of a strain of Aspergillus flavus. J. Bact. *45*:433–442 (May) 1943.

30. Bush, M. T. and Goth, Andres: Flavicin; an antibacterial substance produced by an Aspergillus flavus. J. Pharmacol. & Exper. Therap. *78*:164–169 (June) 1943.

31. Philpot, Flora J.: A penicillin-like substance from *Aspergillus giganteus* Wehm. Nature. *152*:725 (Dec. 18) 1943.

32. McKee, Clara M., Rake, Geoffrey and Houck, Carol L.: Studies on Aspergillus. flavus. II. Production and properties of a penicillin-like substance—flavacidin. J. Bact. *47*:187–197 (Feb.) 1944.

CHAPTER XXV

ANTIBIOTIC SUBSTANCES ORIGINATING FROM SOURCES OTHER THAN MICROBES

The antibiotic substances which have been considered in the foregoing chapters are of microbial origin. Other antibiotic agents have been derived from other natural sources. Examples are lysozyme, chlorellin, canavalin and allicin. These substances will be discussed briefly in the present chapter.

LYSOZYME

According to Waksman[1] and to Waksman and his colleagues,[2,3] certain Russian investigators had claimed that actinomycetes produced a substance resembling lysozyme and it was believed also that various bacteria were capable of producing lysozyme. On the other hand, it appears from the studies of Welsch[4] that there was no evidence for production of true lysozyme by actinomycetes.

Lysozyme then can be considered to have been discovered by Fleming[5] in 1922. He named the substance "lysozyme" since it possessed properties akin to those of ferments. The observation on lysozyme was first made in connection with a case of acute coryza. The nasal secretion of the patient was cultured on blood-agar plates daily for the first three days of the infection. With the exception of an occasional colony of staphylococci Fleming noted that there was no other growth. Cultures made on the fourth day of the infection revealed large numbers of small colonies which proved to be composed of gram-positive cocci which tended to group in twos and fours. This organism was identified as Micrococcus lysodeikticus. Fleming extended his observations and reported that the nasal mucus possessed powerful inhibitory and lytic action on different organisms. He further was able to demonstrate that this inhibitory action was possessed by tissues and various secretions of the human body, by tissues of other animals, by vegetable tissues and, to a marked degree, by egg white. Lysozyme was not found in normal urine, cerebrospinal fluid or sweat (table 45). According to Fleming and Allison,[6] lysozyme appeared to be stable and to maintain its activity in fluids for many weeks. Neither did the dry material appear to deteriorate. These authors pointed out, for example, that the material was found in large quantities in commercial dried egg albumin which had been prepared months, or even years, before. It was found, also, that lysozyme was soluble in water but that it was insoluble in alcohol, ether, chloroform, toluol, xylol or acetone.

Further studies on the nature and distribution of this substance were reported by Goldsworthy and Florey[7] and by Florey[8] in 1930. Seven years later, lysozyme was purified by Roberts.[9] According to his report, the substance appeared to be a protein of rather low molecular weight. In the meantime, studies of Meyer and his associates[10] indicated that the substance was a carbohydrate-splitting enzyme. That lysozyme was an enzyme belonging to the class of carbohydrases was further evident from the report of Epstein and Chain[11] in 1940. It seemed fairly clearly established, therefore, that lysozyme was a powerful antibacterial agent.

TABLE 45

THE PRESENCE OR ABSENCE OF LYSOZYME WITH REFERENCE TO VARIOUS FLUIDS

Fluids containing lysozyme	Fluids not containing lysozyme
Tears	Normal urine
Sputum	Cerebrospinal fluid
Nasal mucus	Sweat (one sample only tested)
Saliva	
Blood serum	
Blood plasma	
Peritoneal fluid	
Pleural effusion	
Hydrocele fluid	
Ovarian cyst fluid	
Sebum	
Pus from acne pustule	
Sero pus from a "cold" abscess in the popliteal space	
Urine containing much albumin and pus	
Semen (very weak)	

From article by Fleming, Proceedings of the Royal Society, London, May, 1922.

On the other hand, an enzyme is not particularly suitable for treatment of bacterial infections in vivo. Therefore, lysozyme has not proved of significant value as a chemotherapeutic agent. It is interesting, however, that the Oxford investigators turned from lysozyme to investigate a variety of antibacterial agents and, happily, next investigated penicillin. It is further interesting that other investigators (Meyer and his associates at Columbia University) who had examined lysozyme also turned next to penicillin.

CHLORELLIN

This product was described by Pratt and his colleagues.[12] It was obtained from unicellular algae, Chlorella vulgaris and Chlorella pyrenoidosa. These cells were cultured in solutions of the mineral nutrients usually used for algal cultures. After a suitable period of growth, the cells and the solution were separated and the substance was extracted from the solution. Biologic tests carried out by the investigators indicated that the material would inhibit growth of staphylococci and of Streptococcus pyogenes as well as growth of the gram-negative Escherichia coli. It was further evident that the presence of rabbit serum did not interfere with antibacterial activity of the substance. Reports have not yet appeared on the exact nature of the product nor on its chemical or possible toxic properties. Knowledge of whether or not the material is of practical clinical value must await further studies.

CANAVALIN

This substance is obtained from flour made from soy beans or jack beans. It was described and named "canavalin" by Farley.[13] The substance is extracted from the flour in a mixture of water and an organic solvent, such as alcohol. The clear supernatant fluid is separated from the rest of the material by centrifugation. Next, acetone is added to this supernatant fluid and a precipitate forms. The resulting second supernatant fluid is recovered, again by centrifugation. From this second supernatant fluid, Farley obtained the enzyme by adding a solution of a heavy metal salt which, according to him, hypothetically results in formation of a compound composed of the heavy metal and the enzyme. The heavy metal is removed, leaving the enzyme in solution. To this solution is added a co-enzyme, called "vitatropin." To obtain vitatropin, a mixture of cellular tissue and thiamin chloride is allowed to stand for a week, but with frequent shaking and daily heating for one hour at 70° C. The vitatropin is then "absorbed on" insoluble barium sulfate and is removed from the barium sulfate by means of a weak solution of ammonia, from which it is crystallized. Canavalin is prepared, therefore, by mixing the solutions of the enzyme and the co-enzyme.

From preliminary studies, it appeared that canavalin was effective against Staphylococcus aureus and it was further claimed that canavalin, in vitro, rendered both gram-positive and gram-negative organisms incapable of growth. Large doses of canavalin were said to be tolerated by both animals and human beings without evidence of ill effects. Included in Farley's report is a summary of thirteen cases, most of which were examples of pneumococcal pneumonia, complicated, in some instances, by empyema and bacteriemia. Beneficial effects or cures were claimed in nearly all of these cases. Data are lacking concerning the quantity of canavalin solution administered, although in one instance it was stated that a very large amount (300 c.c.) was used over a period of eleven days and that the material was administered by the continuous, slow, intravenous method. The average dose per day, then, was nearly 30 c.c. Whether or not this substance, which appears to be a mixture of an enzyme and a co-enzyme, will prove of permanent value in treatment of infections owing to susceptible organisms must await further studies.

ALLICIN

The antibacterial principle of Allium sativum (the common garlic) has been isolated and given the name "allicin" by Cavallito and Bailey[14] and by Cavallito, Buck and Suter.[15] According to these investigators, the substance was isolated in the pure state as a colorless liquid The compound was said to contain approximately 40 per cent sulfur, no nitrogen and no halogens. The empirical formula suggested by them was $C_6H_{10}OS_2$ and the molecular weight of the substance was given as 162.

According to these preliminary reports, allicin is considerably more bacteriostatic than bactericidal. It was further claimed that the substance was equally effective against gram-positive and gram-negative organisms. According to the method used in study of its antibacterial effectiveness against Staphylococcus aureus, the activity of allicin was equivalent to approximately 15 Oxford units of penicillin per milligram. Its activity was unaffected by the presence of para-aminobenzoic acid. On the basis of certain studies made in vitro, in dilutions of 1:125,000 this substance inhibited growth of a large number of gram-positive and gram-negative organisms. Included in this group of organisms were Staphylococcus aureus, Streptococcus viridans, Bacillus subtilis, Eberthella typhi and other members of the colon-typhoid-dysentery group.

Cavallito and Bailey[14] reported certain studies on the toxicity of allicin. The LD_{50} for allicin in aqueous solutions was found to be of the order of 60 mg. per kilogram intravenously and 120 mg. per kilogram subcutaneously. Whether or not this substance will prove of clinical value will not be known until further investigations have been made.

COMMENT

Many other antibacterial agents or antibiotic substances occur in nature. Certain flowering plants and weeds have been found to contain them. The hope of investigators is that antibiotic agents will be obtained which are inhibitory for all forms of pathogenic bacteria. In the meantime, much investigative work remains to be done.

REFERENCES

1. Waksman, S. A.: Antagonistic relations of microörganisms. Bact. Rev. 5:231–291 (Sept.) 1941.

2. Waksman, S. A. and Woodruff, H. B.: Selective antibiotic action of various substances of microbial origin. J. Bact. 44:373–384 (Sept.) 1942

3. Waksman, S. A., Woodruff, H. B. and Horning, Elizabeth S.: The distribution of antagonistic properties among actinomycetes. J. Bact. 42:816 (Dec.) 1941.

4. Welsch, Maurice: Bacteriostatic and bacteriolytic properties of actinomycetes. J. Bact. 44:571–588 (Nov.) 1942.

5. Fleming, Alexander: On a remarkable bacteriolytic element found in tissues and secretions. Proc. Roy. Soc. London. s.B., *93:*306–317 (May) 1922.

6. Fleming, Alexander and Allison, V. D.: Observations on a bacteriolytic substance ("Lysozyme") found in secretions and tissues. Brit. J. Exper. Path. *3:*252–260 (Oct.) 1922.

7. Goldsworthy, N. E. and Florey, Howard: Some properties of mucus, with special reference to its antibacterial functions. Brit. J. Exper. Path. *11:*192–208 (June) 1930.

8. Florey, Howard: The relative amounts of lysozyme present in the tissues of some mammals. Brit. J. Exper. Path. *11:*251–261 (Aug.) 1930.

9. Roberts, E. A. H.: Preparation and properties of purified egg-white lysozyme. Quart. J. Exper. Physiol. *27:*89–98 (July) 1937.

10. Meyer, Karl, Palmer, J. W., Thompson, Richard and Khorazo, Devorah: On the mechanism of lysozyme action. J. Biol. Chem. *113:*479–486 (Mar.) 1936.

11. Epstein, L. A. and Chain, E.: Some observations on the preparation and properties of the substrate of lysozyme. Brit. J. Exper. Path. *21:*339–355 (Dec.) 1940.

12. Pratt, Robertson, Daniels, T. C., Eiler, J. J., Gunnison, J. B., Kumler, W. D., Oneto, J. F., Strait, L. A., Spoehr, H. A., Hardin, G. J., Milner, H. W., Smith, J. H. C., and Strain, H. H.: Chlorellin, an antibacterial substance from Chlorella. Science. n.s. *99:*351–352 (Apr. 28) 1944.

13. Farley, D. L.: Canavalin, a new enzymatic bactericidal agent; preliminary report. Surg., Gynec. & Obst. *79:*83–88 (July) 1944.

14. Cavallito, C. J. and Bailey, J. H.: Allicin, the antibacterial principle of *Allium sativum*. I. Isolation, physical properties and antibacterial action. J. Am. Chem. Soc. *66:*1950–1951 (Nov.) 1944.

15. Cavallito, C. J., Buck, J. S. and Suter, C. M.: Allicin, the antibacterial principle of *Allium sativum*. II. Determination of the chemical structure. J. Am. Chem. Soc. *66:*1952–1954 (Nov.) 1944.

CHAPTER XXVI

RECENT DEVELOPMENTS WITH REGARD TO PENICILLIN AND OTHER ANTIBIOTIC AGENTS

Since this book was first issued in April, 1945, the two most significant developments with regard to penicillin and other antibiotic agents include (1) studies concerning the possibility of oral administration of penicillin and (2) continued studies on the experimental and therapeutic possibilities of streptomycin. The present chapter, therefore, deals with these two subjects.

ORAL ADMINISTRATION OF PENICILLIN

The desirability of administering penicillin orally was early recognized by the Oxford investigators.[1] They, therefore, carried out certain studies on the subject which were discussed on pages 72 and 73 of this monograph. It was evident from their work that the failure of penicillin to be absorbed from the gastro-intestinal tract is due to its inactivation by gastric acids. It was further evident from their studies that penicillin could be absorbed from the gastro-intestinal tract once it was introduced beyond the stomach. These investigators reported that concentrations sufficiently great to inhibit growth of susceptible micro-organisms could be obtained in the blood following administration of penicillin through a tube, the tip of which was placed in the duodenum. It was still further evident, from the studies of Rammelkamp and Helm,[2] that when penicillin was given by mouth therapeutic concentrations of the substance were obtainable in the blood serum of patients suffering with pernicious anemia because their gastric juice contained no free hydrochloric acid. Patients with achlorhydria owing to any cause, therefore, would absorb penicillin when it was administered orally. However, since most of the penicillin given orally to normal subjects was likely to be inactivated by the gastric acids, as has been said, this method of administration was impractical during the early period of investigation of penicillin, when supplies were exceedingly small. That some penicillin reached the general circulation following oral administration of large doses (100,000 Oxford units) was evident from the report of Free and his colleagues.[3]

When supplies of penicillin increased, further attempts were made to assess its possible effectiveness if administered orally. Efforts directed toward increased absorption of penicillin from the gastro-intestinal tract entailed the use of methods to protect the substance from inactivation by gastric acids. Sodium bicarbonate was one of the vehicles first employed. Libby,[4] applying the general principle that little fat-splitting occurs in the presence of acidity such as exists in the stomach, combined penicillin with various oils and administered the mixture orally. These studies showed that relatively large amounts of penicillin would be required to obtain satisfactory therapeutic levels following oral administration. Furthermore, the time between ingestion of food and administration of the substance materially affected its absorption.

Simultaneously with the report of Libby there appeared a report by the British investigators, Little and Lumb,[5] on the use of penicillin by mouth. The method of administration was essentially as follows: 1 dram (4 c.c.) of sodium bicarbonate or of magnesium trisilicate was given with $\frac{1}{4}$ pint (about 125 c.c.) of milk. Ten minutes later a solution of penicillin mixed with raw egg was administered. The investigators reported that effective bacteriostatic levels of penicillin were maintained in the blood for several hours. In fact, this method of administration resulted in maintenance of higher concentrations of penicillin in the blood serum for a longer period than resulted following the standard parenteral or intramuscular methods of administration. However, these results could not be confirmed by Heatley,[6] who pointed out that the difference in the results obtained by Little and Lumb on the one hand, and by himself on the other hand, might be explainable on the basis of the assay technic employed. Heatley's report disclosed that if penicillin were to be administered orally, several times the intramuscular dose must be given.

Furthermore, McDermott and his colleagues[7] reported that after oral administration of penicillin it is possible to attain, in the blood serum, concentrations of the substance that are comparable to those attained after intramuscular injection; the amount given by mouth, however, must be at least five times as much as that given intramuscularly. McDermott and his associates administered penicillin orally in various vehicles, including peanut oil and beeswax, corn oil, antacids and water. Likewise, Perlstein and his associates[8] have prepared penicillin for oral administration by suspending it in equal parts of corn oil and lanolin. That the use of antacids in combination with penicillin would result in some absorption of the substance following oral administration was clear from the report of Charney, Alburn and Bernhart.[9] Moreover, they found that fasting (which in turn resulted in decreased gastric acidity) was important in connection with absorption of the substance. It was further evident from their studies that individual differences in absorption of orally administered penicillin are significant. I am inclined to believe that these differences are dependent entirely on variation in gastric acidity.

That relatively mild infections, such as localized gonorrhea, could be treated successfully by oral administration of penicillin together with antacids was reported by György and his colleagues.[10] They used 1 gm. of trisodium citrate per 10,000 Oxford units oi penicillin. The dose varied from 10,000 units for children to 15,000 to 40,000 units for adults and was given every three to four hours until the desired effect was obtained.

Further studies on oral administration of penicillin have been reported by Burke, Ross and Strauss.[11] They used aluminum hydroxide as an antacid. Two tablets of aluminum hydroxide were administered thirty minutes before the administration of gelatin capsules which contained 100,000 Oxford units of penicillin. By this method, therapeutic concentrations of penicillin could be maintained for three to four hours. In other words, 100,000 Oxford units of penicillin administered every three hours would be expected to result in therapeutic concentrations in the blood serum. This represents a total daily dose of penicillin that is at least four to eight times that ordinarily used for systemic treatment. That the presence in, or absence from, the stomach of recently ingested food influenced the rate of absorption of penicillin following its oral administration also was evident from this report by Burke, Ross and Strauss.

Further studies on the concentrations attainable in the blood following oral administration of penicillin combined with antacids have been made by Welch, Price and Chandler.[12] They administered various amounts of penicillin combined with aluminum hydroxide or magnesium hydroxide. At the end of the second hour following administration of 100,000 Oxford units of penicillin dissolved in 20 c.c. of water, to which had been added dropwise with constant agitation 30 c.c. of U. S. P. aluminum hydroxide, the concentrations of penicillin in the blood, according to the report, were approximately 0.03 to 0.06 unit per cubic centimeter. Furthermore, when 100,000 Oxford units were administered orally in four doses of 25,000 units each, over a period of six hours, a rather surprising result was obtained; namely, the concentrations of penicillin in the serum were said not to have fallen below what could be considered an effective therapeutic level until sometime after the twenty-fourth hour from the time when the first dose had been administered; this in spite of the fact that penicillin and the antacid had not been given after the sixth hour of the experiment. In some cases, therapeutic concentrations were found thirty hours after the beginning of administration of the substance in the manner just described. While it is true that penicillin activity of 0.03 to 0.06 unit per cubic centimeter can be considered therapeutically effective, it is difficult to understand how detectable concentrations of penicillin in the blood could be found twenty-four hours after oral administration when little or no penicillin activity can be detected three hours following a single intramuscular or intravenous injection of the material. If these results are misleading, the difficulty, as so frequently is the case, may stem from the method of assay used. For determining penicillin activity in this study, a serial dilution technic was employed and Bacillus subtilis was used as the test organism. That the blood of man contains a substance which has a marked inhibitory effect on the test organism, Bacillus subtilis, was evident from the studies reported by Stebbins and Robinson.[13] Their observations were recorded in their report on the determination of another antibiotic substance, streptomycin, in the blood of patients who had received this substance. It seems possible, therefore, that what was interpreted as penicillin activity in the blood of these subjects was the antisubtilis factor rather than penicillin activity. Until the results of Welch, Price and Chandler have become established, the physician would do well to guard against acquiring a false sense of security concerning the method used by these investigators. Otherwise, if my conjecture is correct, infections might progress and patients who were severely ill might be seriously jeopardized by being deprived of systemic treatment.

Dosage and Vehicles for Oral Administration of Penicillin.—Either the sodium or the calcium salt of penicillin is satisfactory for oral use. The dose to be administered is usually dissolved in 10 to 20 c.c. of physiologic saline solution. This quantity of solution can be administered in cold water alone or with various antacids or oils. Penicillin is best absorbed from the fasting stomach or from the stomach which is low in content of acid. The dose selected should be administered every two or three hours until improvement occurs. On the basis of present knowledge, I am inclined to recommend at least 25,000 Oxford units per dose for children and 50,000 to 100,000 Oxford units per dose for adults if the oral method of administration is employed.

Comment.—What I have written concerning oral administration of penicillin is not to be construed as condemnation of this procedure. Penicillin, as it exists at the time of this writing (August, 1945), can be given satisfactorily by the oral route in treatment of mild infections which do not endanger life. Examples of such infections include localized gonorrhea, mild pneumonia without bacteriemia, perhaps impetigo, as well as many other conditions which usually are of limited seriousness.

Patients who have moderately severe or severe infections, including bacteriemia, should, at least for the first period of their illness, receive systemic therapy not by the oral method but by one of the standard methods of administration (Chapter IX).

Penicillin Pastilles for Oral Infection.—MacGregor and Long[14] have reported on the use of pastilles containing 500 units of penicillin. To determine how much antibacterial effect would be communicated to the saliva, single pastilles were allowed to melt in the mouth, each for fifteen minutes. After each such experiment, the saliva contained antibacterial amounts of penicillin for a short time. For therapeutics, the patient received the medication in the following manner: A pastille was placed in the buccal sulcus and was left there to dissolve without chewing or sucking. When it was dissolved, the next pastille was inserted. The time required for a pastille to dissolve varied with the individual; however, the average was about forty-five minutes. Included among the conditions so treated were acute ulcerative gingivostomatitis (Vincent's infection) and acute streptococcal tonsillitis. Also, persons who chronically carried streptococci in the throat were treated in this manner. These preparations were used, moreover, following certain operations on the mouth and throat, such as tonsillectomy, for various ulcerative conditions in these regions and for fractures about the mouth. The results given in the preliminary report were encouraging. Greey and Macdonald[15] also have reported satisfactory clinical results from use of similar preparations of penicillin.

While this form of treatment may prove of value in certain types of mild infection of the mouth or throat, systemic therapy unquestionably will be required for the more severe infections. I agree with others that to rely on this form of treatment for such a severe and life-endangering infection as diphtheria would be, indeed, hazardous.[16]

STREPTOMYCIN: RECENT DEVELOPMENTS

As was pointed out earlier in this chapter, certain studies on the experimental and therapeutic possibilities of the antibiotic agent streptomycin (Chapter XXIII) have occurred since this book was first issued in April, 1945. The recent developments of importance are, therefore, summarized in this section.

In Vitro and in Vivo.—As was mentioned in Chapter XXIII, streptomycin was described by Schatz, Bugie and Waksman,[17] of Rutgers University, in January, 1944. The source of this antibiotic agent was a strain of Actinomyces griseus. The investigators named have emphasized that even a strain of Actinomyces griseus capable of producing streptomycin has varied in certain characteristics.[15] For example, a freshly isolated strain of Actinomyces griseus which has the capacity of producing streptomycin forms typical aerial mycelia and is resistant to the antibiotic action of streptomycin. On the other hand, the non-sporulating variant of the strain produces no aerial mycelia, forms no streptomycin and is sensitive to the antibiotic action of the substance. The variant which produces no mycelia is classified with the genus

Nocardia. This variant of the streptomycin-producing strain is, therefore, of considerable importance in connection with preparation of the substance. Further studies by Waksman and his colleagues[19] brought out other interesting facts concerning the activity of streptomycin. For example, it was shown that different strains of the same bacterial species varied greatly in their sensitivity to streptomycin. The ratio of sensitivity of Escherichia coli varied from 100 to 10 units; of Proteus vulgaris, from 75 to 10 units; of Staphylococcus aureus, from 20 to 75 units; and of Bacillus subtilis, from 30 to 250 units. The practical significance of these observations lies in the fact that it becomes increasingly important to know the relative sensitivity not only of different bacterial species but also of different strains of the same species.

Studies have been reported which indicate that streptomycin, as is true of other antibiotic agents, can be inactivated by certain organic compounds. For example, Denkelwater, Cook and Tishler[20] have reported that streptomycin is inactivated by cysteine. On the other hand, a related substance, streptothricin, is not inactivated by cysteine. Furthermore, streptomycin is inactivated by 2-aminoethanethiol but not to any significant extent by thioglycollic acid. It appears, therefore, that cysteine can be used not only to distinguish between the two substances but also to estimate the relative amounts of each in a mixture of the two. It may be possible, then, to use cysteine to eliminate streptomycin from certain body fluids and, therefore, to make it possible to avoid false negative cultures.

The isolation of a salt of streptomycin (reineckate) in crystalline form was first reported by Fried and Wintersteiner.[21] The compound was obtained from submerged culture filtrates. The substance crystallizes from water in thin plates. Following the analysis made by Fried and Wintersteiner, certain inconsistencies rendered it difficult for them to report a definite empirical formula for the substance. However, the formulae suggested were $(C_{14}H_{26}O_7N_9S_4Cr)_n$ or $(C_{14}H_{26}O_8N_9S_4Cr)_n$ corresponding to $(C_{10}H_{19}O_{7-8}N_3)_n$ for the basic component. Since the two preparations which were analyzed assayed 370 and 410 units per milligram, the investigators suggested that the potency of pure streptomycin base should lie between 800 and 910 units per milligram. For definition of the streptomycin unit, see page 314.

A further report on the isolation of crystalline salts of streptomycin has been made by Kuehl and his colleagues.[22] However, their analytic data were not considered sufficient to establish firmly the true empirical formula of streptomycin hydrochloride or of streptomycin helianphate, the two salts examined by these investigators. They did point out, however, that the molecular weight of streptomycin hydrochloride was approximately 700.

Certain experimental studies on the activity of streptomycin in vivo have recently appeared. F. R. Heilman[23] has reported experimental studies which indicate that streptomycin possesses some antispirochetal activity. Experimental infections were established with Borrelia novyi and Leptospira icterohaemorrhagiae. Streptomycin was found to exert considerable protective effect against these spirochetal infections; however, it appeared that streptomycin was relatively less effective than penicillin. F. R. Heilman suggested, therefore, that streptomycin may be useful as an adjunct to penicillin in treatment of spirochetal infections of man.

Previously I have mentioned (p. 317) that Feldman and Hinshaw[24] were the first to report on in vivo studies of the possible effectiveness of streptomycin in experimental tuberculosis. Their results were encouraging. Feldman, Hinshaw and Mann[25] recently have extended these studies with equally encouraging results. In a crucial experiment carried out by these investigators, guinea pigs were inoculated with virulent strains of Mycobacterium tuberculosis of the human variety. Treatment was not begun until forty-eight days thereafter. After the disease obviously had become well established, biopsy of the livers of all the animals was carried out. By this means it was possible to record accurately the extent of the infection before and after treatment. The treated group consisted of twenty-five guinea pigs and the untreated control group consisted of twenty-four guinea pigs. Each of the treated series received 1,500 units of streptomycin every six hours daily for 166 days. When the experiment was terminated, seventeen (70 per cent) of the control, untreated animals had died; only two (8 per cent) of the group that had received streptomycin died. Practically all of the untreated animals which survived had widely disseminated tuberculosis. Only minimal evidence of tuberculosis was found in examination of the animals that had received treatment. In addition to the suppressive effect of streptomycin on the course of experimental tuberculosis, these studies further emphasized the low toxicity of streptomycin, since animals which received the material over this long period of time gave no recognizable evidence of toxic effects. The investigators further emphasized that the effect was suppressive rather than sterilizing. They also observed that in some instances successful treatment by streptomycin resulted in the reversal of a positive to a negative tuberculin test. They expressed the opinion that it was unwise to conjecture as to the clinical potentialities of streptomycin at the time their report was made, although they did feel that streptomycin, because of its low toxicity, was worthy of limited clinical trial.

Standardization of Streptomycin.—The original unit of streptomycin, as described by the investigators at Rutgers University, was that quantity of the dry material which would inhibit the growth of a given strain of Escherichia coli in 1 c.c. of nutrient broth or agar (p. 314). Waksman[26] has pointed out that a situation now has arisen with regard to streptomycin which is similar to that which existed with respect to penicillin. For example, when crystalline penicillin was finally obtained, the value of the Oxford unit was adjusted to the weight of the product. Waksman has pointed out further that while the original designation of the unit was satisfactory for early studies in production and isolation, as well as for certain pharmacologic and animal experiments, clinical studies require too many units, thus giving the impression that extremely large doses of the material are needed for effective therapeutic purposes. Because of these reasons, Waksman has proposed to establish the following three units for designating streptomycin:

(1) An S unit, or that amount of material which will inhibit the growth of a standard strain of E. coli in 1 ml. of nutrient broth or other suitable medium. This unit will thus correspond to the original E. coli unit.

(2) An L unit, or that amount of material which will inhibit the growth of a standard strain of E. coli in 1 liter of medium. An L unit is thus equivalent to 1,000 S units.

(3) When crystalline material becomes available, a weight unit will become possible. One can even now prepare for it by recognizing a G unit, comparable to one gram of the crystalline material. Should this material show an activity of 1,000 E. coli units per 1 mg., it will be equivalent to 1,000,000 S units, to 1,000 L units and to 1 G unit, per gram of material.

Waksman has suggested, therefore, that for the purpose of measuring concentrations of streptomycin in the blood, urine and other body fluids, the new S unit, or the old E. coli unit, may still be used. For clinical studies, however, he suggests that the new L unit, or even the G unit, would be preferable.

Methods Suitable for Determining Streptomycin in Body Fluids.— *Slide-cell Method.*—Dorothy Heilman[27] has reported on a method which has been found satisfactory for determining the concentration of streptomycin in body fluids. It is an adaptation of the Fleming slide method which has been used for determination of penicillin in studies reported from the Mayo Clinic.[28] The Fleming slide-cell method has been described in detail earlier in this book (p. 94). The principal change in the method described by Dorothy Heilman for determination of streptomycin in body fluids has been to use a culture of Bacillus megatherium instead of Streptococcus pyogenes as the test organism. Strains of many bacterial species were examined and a strain of Bacillus megatherium was selected because it would grow in whole blood, would cause definite hemolysis and, in addition, was fairly sensitive to the action of streptomycin. Additional details of the modification of the slide-cell method used for determining the presence of streptomycin, as reported by Dorothy Heilman, are as follows:

The bacteriologic medium used in the test is sterile human blood, defibrinated by shaking with glass beads. The blood is heated in a water bath at 50° C. for thirty minutes to kill the leukocytes. When unheated, freshly drawn blood is inoculated with Bacillus megatherium and incubated in slide cell preparations, bacterial growth occurs in some of the cells but growth of the test organism is completely prevented in about half of the preparations. Blood that is insufficiently heated will also prevent the growth of the test organism in a certain number of slide cells even when streptomycin is not present, with the result that such blood is unsuitable for use in the test. Blood that has been stored in the refrigerator for three days or longer may be used without being heated. Just before the blood is used, it is inoculated with the test organism. For each cubic centimeter of blood is added 0.005 c.c. of a twenty-four hour broth culture of Bacillus megatherium. It is convenient to store suitable preparations of the test organism in solid carbon dioxide. For this purpose an equal volume of nutrient broth is added to a twenty-four hour culture of Bacillus megatherium before freezing. Small amounts (approximately 1 c.c.) of the diluted culture are placed in small sterile glass tubes which are corked and put in a vacuum jar with solid carbon dioxide. By this means a uniform bacterial suspension is available at all times. It is necessary to use 0.01 c.c. of the diluted culture for each cubic centimeter of blood.

Suitable dilutions of standard streptomycin hydrochloride are included in each day's work. If more than one lot of whole blood is used as medium, tests with standard streptomycin are repeated with each lot used. A stock solution is made containing 25 units of streptomycin hydrochloride per cubic centimeter of 0.84 per cent solution of sodium chloride. Serial one-to-one dilutions of the stock solution are made with 0.84 per cent solution of sodium chloride so that solutions are prepared which contain 25, 12.5, 6.25, 3.12, 1.56 and 0.78 units per cubic centimeter respectively. For each test employing the standard, 0.2 c.c. of each dilution is placed in a separate tube. To each tube containing 0.2 c.c. of different dilutions of the standard is added 0.2 c.c. of whole blood inoculated with the test organism. The tubes are shaken and part of the contents of each tube is run into slide cells with a capillary pipet in a manner previously described. When all of the compartments of a slide have been filled, it is sealed to a glass plate with a heated mixture of paraffin and petrolatum.

Specimens of blood serum, spinal fluid and so forth to be tested are centrifuged to remove leukocytes, erythrocytes and other particulate material. The presence of living leukocytes causes erroneous results. Specimens that are known to be contaminated with bacteria may be heated in a water bath to 70° C. for thirty minutes to kill vegetative forms of bacteria without causing a loss of streptomycin activity. Serial one-to-one dilutions of each specimen are made with 0.84 per cent solution of sodium chloride in 0.2 c.c. or 1 c.c. amounts, depending on the accuracy desired. To tubes containing 0.2 c.c. of each dilution of the test material and 0.2 c.c. of the undiluted specimen is added 0.2 c.c. of blood inoculated with the test organism. The tubes are well shaken and part of the contents of each tube is run into individual slide cells, which in turn are sealed on a glass plate. Several slide cell preparations may be placed close together on the same glass plate and the spaces between them filled with the heated mixture of paraffin and petrolatum. Photographs of slide cell preparations appear in articles by Fleming and by Heilman and Herrell in the American Journal of Clinical Pathology, January, 1945.

Slide cell preparations are incubated in the horizontal position at 37° C. for eighteen hours. In reading the test, one examines the slide cells containing standard streptomycin for the presence of hemolysis resulting from the growth of Bacillus megatherium. The smallest concentration of streptomycin that completely prevents hemolysis is chosen as an end point. The end point is usually 3.125 units per cubic centimeter but, when whole blood that is more than one week old is used, an end point of 1.56 units per cubic centimeter is frequently obtained. After an end point is established for the standard, a determination is made of the highest dilution of each test substance that has prevented hemolysis. The dilution factor is multiplied by the number of units of the standard causing inhibition in the same test. For instance, if a 1/16 dilution of serum prevents hemolysis, and the end point with the standard is 3.125 units per cubic centimeter, the undiluted serum contains approximately 50 units per cubic centimeter of streptomycin.

Dorothy Heilman has pointed out that this method is fairly satisfactory for determination of the streptomycin content of blood, spinal fluid, bile and other body fluids. Although it can be used for determination of streptomycin in the urine, the cup method of assay is a little more reliable for this purpose.

Cup Method.—Stebbins and Robinson[13] have described a modification of the cup method for the determination of streptomycin in body fluids. Their method is an adaptation of the one described by Foster and Woodruff[29] for the determination of streptothricin in aqueous solutions. As I have mentioned earlier in this chapter, it was evident that the test organism, Bacillus subtilis, was not satisfactory for determination of the amount of streptomycin in the blood, owing to the antisubtilis factor (p. 335). Stebbins and Robinson, therefore, recommended the use of a sensitive strain of Staphylococcus aureus in performing the test. The method recommended by them is as follows:

Materials.—A strain of *Staphylococcus aureus SM* is used as the test organism. The culture is maintained in a uniform condition by daily transfer in F. D. A. nutrient broth at 37° C. The assay medium is a modified F. D. A. nutrient agar. Including the beveled glass cylinders known as penicylinders, the glassware required is ordinary standard bacteriological equipment.

Procedure.—Using a 6-hour culture of the test organism grown in F. D. A. broth, a serial 10-fold dilution is made through 10^{-4} in broth. A final dilution to 10^{-5} is then made directly into the melted nutrient agar which has previously been cooled to 45° C. With the aid of a calibrated wide mouth pipette, 10 c.c. of this melted seeded agar is added to each of a series of petri dishes and these are set aside until the agar solidifies. Next, the beveled glass cylinders are warmed slightly by passage through a Bunsen flame and immediately placed upon the surface of the agar plate. In this manner a seal between the glass cylinder and the agar is effected. Four such cylinders are placed in each agar plate. The glass cylinders are then filled with the properly diluted samples for assay and the plates incubated at 30° C. for 16–18 hours. At the end of this period the diameters of the zones of inhibition are measured in millimeters.

Assay of Blood, Urine and Tissue Extracts.—In determining the concentration of streptomycin in blood, it is necessary to construct a standard curve of reference for each assay using an aliquot of the drug solution which is being administered to the patient. This is done by making dilutions of streptomycin containing 1, 2, 4, 8 and 16 units per c.c. in serum obtained from each individual prior to treatment or from any normal donor. The diameters of the resulting zones of inhibition are plotted as ordinates (arithmetic scale) against the concentrations of streptomycin as abscissa (logarithmic scale).

Absorption, Distribution and Excretion.—As was pointed out earlier in this book (p. 319), it appeared that following systemic administration of streptomycin the substance was readily absorbed and reached the general circulation. It also was pointed out that streptomycin was excreted fairly readily by the kidneys. Further studies on the general subject have been reported by Elias and Durso.[30] It was evident from their studies that following intramuscular and intravenous injections of streptomycin, demonstrable concentrations in the blood could be obtained and that a fairly large amount of the material was excreted in the urine. Following systemic administration little could be found in the feces. After oral administration little or none of the material became diffused into the blood stream and only a very small amount appeared to be excreted in the urine. Following this method of administration, the concentration of streptomycin in the feces was said to be very high.

It appears from the report of Reimann, Elias and Price[31] that small amounts of streptomycin became diffused into the cerebrospinal fluid following administration of the substance by repeated intramuscular injection over a period of several days. From another report,[32] it appears that little or no streptomycin can be demonstrated in the spinal fluid two to three hours following a single intramuscular injection of 200,000 units. Subsequent to continued administration of relatively large amounts of streptomycin, however, antibacterial amounts have been demonstrated in the spinal fluid of patients suffering with meningitis.

In connection with studies on the diffusion of streptomycin, Dorothy Heilman and her colleagues[32] have found that the streptomycin passes fairly readily through the placenta and reaches the fetal circulation following administration of the agent to pregnant women. Judging from these same studies, it also seems likely that streptomycin is concentrated and excreted to some extent in the bile.

Methods of Administration and Dosage.—As was mentioned earlier (p. 319), human subjects tolerate without serious toxic effects repeated intramuscular injections of streptomycin. This also was evident from the report by Reimann and his colleagues.[31] Certain studies also have been carried out at the Mayo Clinic[32] to examine the possible methods of administration of streptomycin and, as a result of these studies, certain facts became established.

Intravenous Administration.—The preparation may be administered intravenously, either by continuous drip or by intermittent injection. Patients were given as much as 4,000,000 units of streptomycin per day by the intravenous drip method. Local irritation at the site of injection occurred at times but was not serious. Likewise, single intravenous injections of as much as 200,000 units of streptomycin, dissolved in 10 c.c. of physiologic saline solution, were administered every three hours.

Intramuscular Administration.—Streptomycin likewise may be administered by the intermittent intramuscular or continuous intramuscular method. For intermittent intramuscular injections, the amount used for each injection was, as a rule, 100,000 units per cubic centimeter. For continuous intramuscular administration, the contemplated daily dose may be dissolved in 1 liter (or less) of physiologic saline solution and the rate of flow regulated to deliver the entire amount in twenty-four hours.

Subcutaneous Administration.—Furthermore, it appears that streptomycin may be administered satisfactorily by the subcutaneous route.

When preparations of high potency are available, 100,000 units of streptomycin may be administered subcutaneously every three hours. The amount is administered in 1 c.c. of physiologic saline solution or distilled water.

Intrathecal Administration.—When necessary, streptomycin also may be administered satisfactorily by the intrathecal route. For this purpose, 100,000 units of streptomycin dissolved in 5 or 10 c.c. of physiologic saline solution may be administered every twenty-four to forty-eight hours.

Administration by Means of Nebulization.—It was further evident in the report from the Mayo Clinic that streptomycin could be administered satisfactorily by means of nebulization in a manner similar to that used for the administration of penicillin (p. 116). For this method of administration, 50,000 units of streptomycin per cubic centimeter may be introduced into the nebulizer and inhaled. Patients have received as much as 500,000 units per day by this method, without interruption, for periods as long as four weeks in the treatment of such conditions as tuberculous involvement of the larynx and tracheobronchial tree.[33]

Oral Administration.—While streptomycin may be administered satisfactorily by mouth, as was mentioned above, little or no streptomycin reaches the general circulation following this method of administration. The substance is not destroyed in the intestinal tract and, therefore, its oral administration may at times be indicated under conditions wherein reduction of the number of susceptible organisms present in the bowel is desirable. Amounts of streptomycin varying from 500,000 to several million units per day may be given in divided doses by this method.

Consideration of Toxicity.—At the time of this writing (August, 1945) no serious, irreversible toxic reactions have been reported following administration of fairly large amounts of streptomycin by means of single or repeated injection. In the beginning of studies on streptomycin, material of low potency was used. Whether or not certain toxic reactions will become less frequent as material of high potency, and consequently greater purity, becomes available cannot as yet be stated. Local irritation at the site of intravenous, intramuscular or subcutaneous injection may occur occasionally. This is especially true when streptomycin of low potency is used. It is important that the size of the inoculum be kept small (no more than 2 or 3 c.c.) if this reaction is to be kept at a minimum. On occasions, chill and fever may follow administration of certain batches of streptomycin. This reaction may result from the presence of pyrogens or possibly may occur for other reasons. Toxic erythema and cutaneous eruptions of urticarial type have occurred at times following administration of streptomycin. This may represent individual sensitivity to the substance on the part of the patient. On occasion, patients have complained of joint and muscle pains following administration of certain batches of the substance. Likewise, headache with nausea and vomiting has occurred on occasion. At the time of this writing (August, 1945), it appears that administration of streptomycin in therapeutic amounts has not been followed by any evidence of serious impairment of renal function. Likewise, no evidence of serious impairment of hepatic function has followed its administration in therapeutically effective doses. Furthermore, no serious damage to the hemopoietic system has been encountered following administration of streptomycin to human beings.

Clinical Results.—As was pointed out earlier in this book (p. 320), enough clinical data have not been accumulated to allow final statements to be made concerning the use of streptomycin in treatment of those infections in which it unquestionably should be tried.

Based on experimental studies which have been discussed in a previous chapter (XXIII) and in the present chapter, it would appear that streptomycin is worthy of clinical trial against certain infections owing to organisms susceptible to its action. Included among those conditions in which experimental evidence seems ample to justify clinical trials are tuberculosis, tularemia, typhoid fever, paratyphoid fever, infections owing to Escherichia coli, as well as infections owing to those organisms included in the dysentery group. There is some evidence to suggest that use of streptomycin should be thoroughly studied in treatment of brucellosis, of infections owing to micro-organisms of the Friedländer group (Klebsiella) and of infections owing to Hemophilus influenzae (influenzal meningitis). Likewise, it would appear that use of streptomycin might be justified in treatment of certain spirochetal infections, including leptospirosis icterohaemorrhagica, relapsing fever and perhaps syphilis. In view of the sensitivity of certain organisms such as Proteus vulgaris and Aerobacter aerogenes, it should prove of value in treatment of infections of the urinary tract owing to sensitive strains of these gram-negative pathogens or to other sensitive gram-negative organisms commonly associated with urinary infection.

One of the first reports on the clinical use of streptomycin was that by Reimann, Elias and Price.[31] They used streptomycin in treatment of five patients suffering with typhoid fever. These patients received from 1,000,000 to 4,000,000 units of streptomycin daily by the intravenous or intramuscular route. The authors were inclined to feel that streptomycin offers promise as a substance capable of sterilizing the blood stream and urinary tract of the patient suffering with this disease. It was further evident from their report that when given orally the substance would eliminate typhoid bacilli from the feces. Of the five cases reported, recovery occurred in three during treatment with streptomycin.

The investigators were inclined to advise that the substance be given orally as well as systemically in treatment of this disease. As was mentioned earlier (p. 320), I have administered streptomycin to two patients suffering with typhoid fever. The dosage employed was small; however, it was possible to sterilize the urine of these patients. While the two patients recovered, it is impossible at the time of this writing to say that streptomycin was entirely responsible for their recovery.

Hinshaw and Feldman[34] for some time have had under way clinical studies to assess the possible value of streptomycin in treatment of twenty-two patients with clinical tuberculosis.

In view of the apparent sensitivity of certain spirochetes, as suggested by the studies of F. R. Heilman,[23] O'Leary and I[35] have treated four patients who had early syphilis and one patient who had gummatous syphilis of the skin with streptomycin. These patients received only small amounts of streptomycin for short periods (between 320,000 and 1,000,000 units per day for ten days). In the cases of primary syphilis, darkfield positive lesions became darkfield negative within a period of twenty to eighty hours. These studies would suggest that streptomycin has some antispirochetal activity; however, these patients all underwent relapse during the follow-up period of two to three months and resort was had to other standard methods of treatment. If streptomycin is to be studied further in relation to this infection, it is recommended that larger doses (2,000,000 to 4,000,000 units per day) be given over a period of perhaps three to four weeks.

REFERENCES

1. Abraham, E. P., Chain, E., Fletcher, C. M., Gardner, A. D., Heatley, N. G., Jennings, M. A. and Florey, H. W.: Further observations on penicillin. Lancet. 2:177–188; 189 (Aug. 16) 1941.

2. Rammelkamp, C. H. and Helm, J. D., Jr.: Studies on the absorption of penicillin from the stomach. Proc. Soc. Exper. Biol. & Med. 54:324–327 (Dec.) 1943.

3. Free, A. H., Leonards, J. R., McCullagh, D. R. and Biro, Barbara E.: The urinary excretion of penicillin after oral administration to normal human subjects. Science. n. s. 100:431–432 (Nov. 10) 1944.

4. Libby, R. L.: Oral administration of penicillin in oil. Science. n. s. 101:178–180 (Feb. 16) 1945.

5. Little, C. J. H. and Lumb, George: Penicillin by mouth. Lancet. 1:203–206 (Feb. 17) 1945.

6. Heatley, N. G.: Administration of penicillin by mouth. Lancet. 1:590–591 (May 12) 1945.

7. McDermott, Walsh, Bunn, P. A., Benoit, Maria, DuBois, Rebeckah and Haynes, Willetta: Oral penicillin. Science. n. s. 101:228–229 (Mar. 2) 1945.

8. Perlstein, D., Kluener, R. G., Liebmann, A. J. and Dorrell, I.: Oral administration of penicillin in corn oil and lanolin. Science. n. s. 102:66–67 (July 20) 1945.

9. Charney, Jesse, Alburn, H. E. and Bernhart, F. W.: Urinary excretion of penicillin in man after oral administration with gastric antacids. Science. n. s. 101:251–253 (Mar. 9) 1945.

10. György, Paul, Vandegrift, H. N., Elias, Williams, Colio, L. G., Barry, F. M. and Pilcher, J. D.: Administration of penicillin by mouth. J. A. M. A. 127:639–642 (Mar. 17) 1945.

11. Burke, F. G., Ross, Sidney and Strauss, Clifton: Oral administration of penicillin. J. A. M. A. *128*:83–87 (May 12) 1945.

12. Welch, Henry, Price, C. W. and Chandler, Velma L.: Prolonged blood concentrations after oral administration of modified penicillin. J. A. M. A. *128*:845–847 (July 21) 1945.

13. Stebbins, R. B. and Robinson, H. J.: A method for determination of streptomycin in body fluids. Proc. Soc. Exper. Biol. & Med. *59*:255–257 (June) 1945.

14. MacGregor, A. B. and Long, D. A.: The use of penicillin pastilles in oral infections; a preliminary report. Brit. M. J. *2*:686–689 (Nov. 25) 1944.

15. Greey, Philip and Macdonald, I. B.: Penicillin agar pastilles. Canad. M. A. J. *52*:327–330 (Apr.) 1945.

16. Symposium: Oral administration of penicillin. Internat. M. Digest. *46*:369–372 (June) 1945.

17. Schatz, Albert, Bugie, Elizabeth and Waksman, S. A.: Streptomycin, a substance exhibiting antibiotic activity against gram-positive and gram-negative bacteria. Proc. Soc. Exper. Biol. & Med. *55*:66–69 (Jan.) 1944.

18. Schatz, Albert and Waksman, S. A.: Strain specificity and production of antibiotic substances. IV. Variations among actinomycetes, with special reference to Actinomyces griseus. Proc. Nat. Acad. Sc. *31*:129–137 (May) 1945.

19. Waksman, S. A., Reilly, H. C. and Schatz, Albert: Strain specificity and production of antibiotic substances. V. Strain resistance of bacteria to antibiotic substances, especially to streptomycin. Proc. Nat. Acad. Sc. *31*:157–164 (June) 1945.

20. Denkelwater, R., Cook, M. A. and Tishler, M.: The effect of cysteine on streptomycin and streptothricin. Science. n. s. *102*:12 (July 6) 1945.

21. Fried, J. and Wintersteiner, O.: Crystalline reineckates of streptothricin and streptomycin. Science. n. s. *101*:613–615 (June 15) 1945.

22. Kuehl, F. A., Jr., Peck, R. L., Walti, Alphonse and Folkers, Karl: Streptomyces antibiotics. I. Crystalline salts of streptomycin and streptothricin. Science. n. s. *102*:34–35 (July 13) 1945.

23. Heilman, F. R.: Streptomycin in the treatment of experimental relapsing fever and leptospirosis icterohaemorrhagica (Weil's disease). Proc. Staff Meet., Mayo Clin. *20*:169–176 (May 30) 1945.

24. Feldman, W. H. and Hinshaw, H. C.: Effects of streptomycin on experimental tuberculosis in guinea pigs: a preliminary report. Proc. Staff Meet., Mayo Clin. *19*:593–599 (Dec. 27) 1944.

25. Feldman, W. H., Hinshaw, H. C. and Mann, F. C.: Personal communication to the author.

26. Waksman, S. A.: Standardization of streptomycin. Science, n. s. *102*:40–41 (July 13) 1945.

27. Heilman, Dorothy H.: A method for estimating the concentration of streptomycin in body fluids. Proc. Staff Meet., Mayo Clin. *20*:145–150 (May 16) 1945.

28. Heilman, Dorothy H. and Herrell, W. E.: The use of Fleming's modification of the Wright slide cell technic for determining penicillin in body fluids. Am. J. Clin. Path. *15*:7–9 (Jan.) 1945.

29. Foster, J. W. and Woodruff, H. B.: Quantitative estimation of streptothricin. J. Bact. *45*:408–409 (Apr.) 1943.

30. Elias, W. F. and Durso, Jane: Blood, urine and fecal levels of streptomycin in the treatment of human infections of E. typhosa. Science. n. s. *101*:589–591 (June 8) 1945.

31. Reimann, H. A., Elias, W. F. and Price, Alison H.: Streptomycin for typhoid; a pharmacologic study. J. A. M. A. *128*:175–180 (May 19) 1945.

32. Heilman, Dorothy H., Heilman, F. R., Hinshaw, H. C., Nichols, D. R. and Herrell, W. E.: Streptomycin: absorption, diffusion, excretion and toxicity. Scheduled for publication in Am. J. M. Sc. for Oct., 1945.

33. Hinshaw, H. C.: Personal communication to the author.

34. Hinshaw, H. C. and Feldman, W. H.: Observations on chemotherapy of clinical and experimental tuberculosis. M. Clin. North America. (July) 1945, pp. 918–922.

35. O'Leary, P. A. and Herrell, W. E.: Unpublished data.

INDEX